T0201538

HANDBOOK OF APPLIED DOG BEHAVIOR AND TRAINING

Volume Two

Etiology and Assessment of Behavior Problems

HANDBOOK OF APPLIED DOG BEHAVIOR AND TRAINING

Volume Two

Etiology and Assessment of Behavior Problems

Steven R. Lindsay

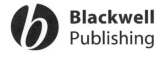

STEVEN R. LINDSAY, MA, is a dog behavior consultant and trainer who lives in Philadelphia, Pennsylvania, where he provides a variety of behavioral training and counseling services. In addition to his long career in working with companion dogs, he previously evaluated and trained highly skilled military working dogs as a member of the U.S. Army Biosensor Research Team (Superdog Program). Mr. Lindsay also conducts workshops and seminars and is the author of numerous publications on dog behavior and training.

© 2001 Iowa State University Press
A Blackwell Publishing company
All rights reserved

Blackwell Publishing Professional
2121 State Avenue, Ames, Iowa 50014

Orders: 1-800-862-6657
Office: 1-515-292-0140
Fax: 1-515-292-3348
Web site: www.blackwellprofessional.com

Cover image: "Puppy Carrying a Pheasant Feather," 16th century by Yi Om (Korean). Courtesy of the Philadelphia Museum of Art.

Authorization to photocopy items for internal or personal use, or the internal or personal use of specific clients, is granted by Blackwell Publishing, provided that the base fee is paid directly to the Copyright Clearance Center, 222 Rosewood Drive, Danvers, MA 01923. For those organizations that have been granted a photocopy license by CCC, a separate system of payments has been arranged. The fee code for users of the Transactional Reporting Service is 978-0-8138-2868-8/2001.

First edition, 2001
    Volume Two: Etiology and Assessment of Behavior Problems

The Library of Congress has catalogued Volume One as follows:

Lindsay, Steven R.
Handbook of applied dog behavior and training/Steven R. Lindsay;
    foreword by Victoria Lea Voith.—1st ed.
      p. cm
    Contents: v. 1. Adaptation and learning.
    ISBN 978-0-8138-0754-6

    1. Dogs—Behavior. 2. Dogs—Training. I. Title.

  SF433.L56 1999
  636.7¢0887—dc21

                                              99-052013

Printed in United States of America
SKY10054062_090123

Contents

8   *Social Competition and Aggression*   229

9   *Appetitive and Elimination Problems*   273

IN VOLUME 1, *Adaptation and Learning,* it was argued that the functional epigenesis of behavior takes place under the influence of various environmental and biological constraints, including species-typical tendencies, genetic predispositions, and the alteration of various behavioral thresholds brought about by domestication and selective breeding. Clearly, although extraordinarily flexible and adaptive, dog behavior expresses itself in relatively uniform and consistent ways. The causes of this behavioral regularity are found in both phylogenic and ontogenic influences that continuously act on dogs from their conception to their senescence and death. As the result of selection pressures exerted upon the canine genotype during its evolution or phylogenesis, the dog's behavior has been biologically shaped and prepared to express itself in a limited set of ways. During the dog's development or ontogeny, the environment continues to exert selection pressures on the behavioral phenotype through learning. The dog's behavioral phenotype is the composite of evolutionary mutation and selection (organized in the canine genotype) together with selected refinements and modifications as the result of interaction with the environment and learning. In other words, the dog's behavior is conjointly influenced by both phylogenic and environmental determinants via experience and learning. In addition, the behavioral phenotype at each stage of ontogeny affects subsequent development (prepared and regulated by genes operating on a physiological level) and undergoes further modification by maturational demands and environmental pressures. Finally, it was shown in Volume 1 that successful adaptation and learning depend on the presence of an orderly environment composed of highly predictable and controllable events. Without the presence of a stable and orderly environment, neither natural selection nor selection by learning is possible. Learning is primarily concerned with obtaining predictive information about the environment and refining phenotypic routines and strategies for controlling and exploiting significant events. In the present volume, *Etiology and Assessment of Behavior Problems,* these general theoretical assumptions and principles are applied toward better understanding how adjustment problems develop in dogs. Certainly, whether adaptive or maladaptive, a dog's behavioral adjustment is ever under the dynamic influence of experience and learning operating within the context of biological and environmental constraints. Both learning and biology contribute to a dog's adaptive success or failure.

Borrowing from Tinbergen's terminology, the canine *Merkwelt* or perceptual world significantly differs from the human Merkwelt. As species, we inhabit very different sensory, cognitive, emotional, motivational, and social worlds but still succeed generation upon generation to reach across millions of years of evolutionary divergence to form a profoundly enriching and affectionate bond with one another and to share the same living space cooperatively. Although domestication has helped to bridge the gap, much phylogenic room remains for mutual misunderstanding and interactive tension. Further, as people and dogs live together in closer social arrangements and progressively artificial environments, the likelihood of behavioral tensions and problems is simply bound to increase. In fact, it is nothing short of a biological wonder that we get along together as well as we do. However, not only are we apt to misunderstand one another, dogs are also often exposed to neglect, abuse, detrimental rearing practices, and various other adversarial and environmental pressures, many of which appear capable of disrupting or disorganizing a dog's ability to learn and adjust effectively. Naturally, problems are bound to occur and do. Every year, thousands of distraught dog owners haul their wayward dogs off to obedience classes or to private animal behavior consultants, seeking advice or training for some puppy or dog behavior problem. Estimates vary, but the vast majority of dogs appear to exhibit at least one undesirable habit that its owner would like to change. Most of these behavior problems are an outcome of inadequate training or socialization and are usually responsive to remedial training and brief counseling. Besides social sources of causation, behavior problems may also develop as the result of chronic mismanagement or neglect of the dog's basic biological needs and requirements for stimulation. Some problems, however, are the result of a more complex etiology, involving cognitive deficiencies, distressing emotional activity, and pervasive behavioral disorganization. Volume 2 is especially concerned with exploring the collective epigenetic causes underlying the development of these more disruptive adjustment problems.

Many behavior problems appear to be strongly influenced by classical and instrumental learning, especially learning strained or disturbed under the adverse influences of stressful anxiety and frustration. Disruptive anxiety and frustration result when a dog's social and physical environment lacks sufficient order and stability in terms of overall predictability and controllability. Social interaction consisting of unpredictable and uncontrollable aversive or attractive exchanges between the owner and the dog is prone to disrupt effective lines of communication, promote stress and distrust, and result in behavioral maladjustment. Other problems appear to stem from trauma and deprivation occurring early in life, resulting in phenotypic disturbances that persist and disrupt the subsequent course of the dog's behavioral development. Finally, some severe behavior problems are under the exacerbating influence of species-typical tendencies and appetites, genetically altered behavioral thresholds, and various physiological and neurobiological sources of causation that may require adjunctive veterinary differential diagnosis and treatment.

A goal of Volume 2 is to examine these and other causes underlying the development of behavior problems. Without accurately identifying and properly assessing the various contributory causes underlying a behavioral adjustment problem, it is not possible to intervene with a truly rational plan of behavior modification and therapy. Despite significant advances in our understanding and treatment of dog behavior problems over the past 20 years, much yet remains to be accomplished in this and related fields of professional activity. Unfortunately, many theories and assumptions in wide public circulation are either dated or unproven. For example, perusing any random selection of dog-care and dog-training books that address dog behavior problems reveals a perplexing and sometimes irritating array of opinions, beliefs, and methods about how such problems ought to be modified or managed. These various texts often espouse conflicting or contradictory information, some encouraging very intrusive or forceful techniques as the necessary prerequisites for controlling undesirable dog behavior, while others admonish the reader to never raise an impatient voice to the errant dog. Much of the contemporary popular literature is confounded by moralistic and ideological agendas that deflect from an honest and rational search for an objective understanding of dog behavior and its effective control and management. Unfortunately, the acceptance of a training system is often based more on an author's personal charisma and fame than on its actual efficacy or scientific merit. The overall result of these influences has been the accumulation of widely divergent and sometimes baffling opinions, theories, and practices performed in the name of companion-dog training and counseling.

An important focus of Volume 2 is to collect and evaluate the relevant applied and scientific literature, with the goal of clarifying what is known about the etiology of dog behavior problems and to highlight what yet remains to be done by way of additional analysis and behavioral research. Although the applied literature is somewhat more consistent and uniform, it also suffers from many of the same maladies found in the popular literature. In spite of an ostensible dedication to the scientific method, many common diagnostic assumptions and treatment protocols are based largely on anecdotal evidence, isolated impressions, and personal opinions. This state of affairs is compounded by a dearth of confirming evidence that the methods used to treat behavior problems actually function in the ways suggested by the rationales given for their use. Furthermore, notwithstanding the optimistic success rates claimed by some practitioners, no one knows within a reasonable degree of scientific certainty whether the methods work as claimed. The lack of scientific validation is a significant practical and legal concern with respect to the treatment of some potentially dangerous behavior problems such as *dominance* aggression, especially since homologous interspecific models of such aggression remain to be developed and studied under laboratory conditions. Although a few provisional clinical studies have been recently performed to evaluate the efficacy of some behavioral protocols (especially those involving the adjunctive use of drugs), much remains to be done in this important area to place the field of applied dog behavior on a more respectable scientific foundation. In lieu of the needed clinical and laboratory research, it is incumbent upon behavioral practitioners to apply scientifically demonstrated learning and ethological principles for the control and management of dog behavior problems. Most significant progress in the field of applied dog behavior has occurred in the areas of description, classification, and incidence, but even here much confusion remains to be worked out. In addition to challenging conventional wisdom and questioning some widely held (but unproven) assumptions and beliefs, Volume 2 introduces and discusses other ways of understanding dog behavior and adjustment problems in the light of the scientific concepts and principles of ethology and learning covered in Volume 1.

In addition to the various causes discussed above, behavior adjustment problems often reflect an underlying failure of the owner and the dog to connect and bond with each other harmoniously. Such problems may require diligent cynopraxic counseling to resolve. Ultimately, a dog's domestic success depends on the formation of a harmonious and satisfying relationship with human companions and other animals sharing the same home and life experience. Consequently, intervention should always include efforts that simultaneously address social, environmental, and quality of life concerns. At the minimum, a healthy and successful human-dog relationship depends on the establishment of clear lines of communication, interspecies appreciation and understanding, leader-follower cooperation, playfulness, and the lifelong nurturance of mutual affection and trust.

Volume 2 begins with a brief history of applied dog behavior and training. Selecting the content for this chapter was difficult and, admittedly, much of importance has been regretfully omitted for sake of brevity and focus. In general, areas of historical significance for applied dog behavior are emphasized that have been neglected in the past. In Chapter 2, various methods for collecting and assessing behavioral information are introduced, together with a general discussion of etiological factors believed to underlie the development of many behavior problems. The remainder of the text includes reviews, analyses, and criticism of the scientific and applied literature insofar as it is relevant to the etiology, assessment, and treatment of fear, separation anxiety, aggression, behavioral excesses (compulsions and hyperactivity), and appetitive and elimination problems. The volume concludes with a chapter devoted to the cynopraxic counseling process and the role of interactive dynamics and social bonding on the etiology of behavior problems. Although treatment strategies are occasionally discussed, behavior modification and therapy protocols are the subject of a forthcoming text: *Dog Behavior Modification and Therapy: Procedures and Protocols* (Ames: Iowa State University Press, 2001).

Acknowledgments

OVER THE years, I have had the good fortune to benefit from the knowledge of many of the world's most prominent and respected authorities working in the field of applied dog behavior and training. However, special appreciation and recognition are due Drs. Peter Borchelt, Mary Burch, Jaak Panksepp, Barbara Simpson, Victoria Voith, and John Wright for critically reading and commenting on various chapters or portions of the book. Their advice and guidance have been invaluable. Much appreciation is due to Christina Cole for her help in collecting research materials and sundry other forms of assistance that helped keep the loose ends together. The expert editorial guidance of John Flukas has been consistently constructive and sincerely appreciated. I also wish to thank the wonderful staff at Iowa State University Press. I am very grateful for their patience and confidence in the project and deeply appreciative for their care and professionalism.

Volume Two

Etiology and Assessment of Behavior Problems

History of Applied Dog Behavior and Training

To his master he flies with alacrity, and submissively lays at his feet all his courage, strength, and talent. A glance of the eye is sufficient; for he understands the smallest indications of the will. He has all the ardour of friendship, and fidelity and constancy in his affections, which man can have. Neither interest nor desire of revenge can corrupt him, and he has no fear but that of displeasing. He is all zeal and obedience. He speedily forgets ill-usage, or only recollects it to make returning attachment the stronger. He licks the hand which causes pain, and subdues his anger by submission. The training of the dog seems to have been the first art invented by man, and the fruit of that art was the conquest and peaceable possession of the earth.

G. L. L. COMTE DE BUFFON, *quoted in* JACKSON (1997)

OUR SPECIES is the only one that keeps and purposefully modifies the behavior of another species to make it a more compatible and cooperative companion and helper. The process of domestication involves at least three interdependent elements: (1) selective breeding for conducive traits, (2) controlled socialization with their keepers, and (3) systematic training to obtain desirable habits. In addition to the effects of selective breeding, socialization, and training, a dog's basic needs are largely provided by a human caregiver. The overall effect of domestication is to perpetuate paedomorphic characteristics into adulthood and to enhance a dog's dependency on its keeper for the satisfaction of its biological and psychological needs, including affection and a sense of belonging to a group. The origins of this process began far back into prehistoric times.

SOCIAL PARALLELISM, DOMESTICATION, AND TRAINING

Close social interaction between early humans and dogs was probably facilitated by the evolution of parallel social structures, especially the tendency to form cooperative hunting groups and extended families. Both wolves and early humans shared sufficient similarity of social custom to communicate well enough to lay a foundation and bridge for the development of a lasting relationship. One possible scenario is that early humans coming out of Africa approximately 140,000 years ago encountered wolves dispersed throughout the Eurasian land mass. These early humans, perhaps numbering only a few hundred individuals, are believed to have beeen the direct ancestors of contemporary humans. Over a relatively short period, these migrant humans were able to supplant indigenous humans already living in Eurasia. In *Evolving Brains,* John Allman (1999) speculates that the primary advantage needed to achieve this biological precedence and hegemony may have been the domestication of wolves. According to this view, the two species were preadapted to fit each other's ecology and family structure, thus making the transition to domestication relatively easy and natural. By cooperating, the two species may have attained an enormous competitive advantage over other species competing for the same resources. Interestingly, the migration out of Africa by this small group of humans roughly coincides with the first evidence of domestication as indicated by the analysis of mitochondrial DNA sequences. These studies indicate that the domestication of dogs was probably initiated approximately 135,000 years ago (Wayne and Ostrander, 1999). To fully exploit the advantages presented by domestication, early humans must have developed relatively sophisticated means of behavioral control and training. Undoubtedly, our ancestors engaged in activities aimed at limiting some sorts of dog behavior while encouraging other forms as opportunities and needs may have presented themselves. The obvious necessity of training as an integral part of the domestication process prompted Comte de Buffon to conclude that dog training was *the* first art invented by humans (see the introductory epigraph). Whether dog training was the first art will remain the subject of debate; however, one can safely assume that dog training, in one form or another, emerged long before the advent of recorded history.

Cave Art and the Control of Nature

Clearly, early humans were acute observers and sensitive social organizers, living in close-knit and cooperative hunting-gatherer groups. That they were interested in animal habits and their control is attested to by the masterful cave paintings found at Altamira (Spain) and Lascaux (France). These artworks were produced at about the same time that dogs began to appear in the archeological record, between 12,000 to 17,000 years ago (Jansen, 1974). The paintings depict with extraordinary sensitivity and realism a procession of various prey animals (e.g., bison, and deer) captured in line and color and transfixed in time to await rediscovery after many millennia shrouded in darkness. The animals are beautifully rendered in moments of flight or after falling from mortal wounds inflicted on them by the artist-hunter. The purpose of this early art was presumably to exert magical control over the prey animal by capturing its image and "killing" it, thereby giving the hunter success during the chase. One can hardly imagine that the Magdalenian people responsible for cave painting had not also discovered other means of control besides sympathetic magic, just as they had certainly learned how to use many natural forces long before they had names or adequate means to describe them.

Evolution of Altruism and Empathy

The ancient emergence of dog keeping appears to coincide with the evolutionary appearance of altruism and empathy among humans. According to Eccles (1989), the likely foundation of human altruism is the emergence of food sharing, followed closely by the development of the nuclear family and extended family groups. As humans evolved into food-sharing communities composed of individuals cooperating with one another, the emerging tendency toward altruism may have been extended to semidomesticated canids living at the outermost perimeter of their encampments. These early canids also appear to have evolved significant altruistic tendencies and social structures, perhaps sufficient to attract empathic interest by early humans, if not to mediate symmetrical altruistic reciprocation and exchange. Eccles characterizes *altruistic actions* as purposeful efforts intended to benefit others without regard to how they might benefit oneself. He rejects Dawkins's (1976) more severe definition in which *altruism* denotes actions that benefit another at some expense or sacrifice to the altruistic actor. Eccles appears to assume that the advent of human altruism entailed an awareness of self and empathy for others. As a result of such evolutionary elaborations and social developments, altruistic humans may have been prompted to feel sympathy and pity for dogs living and suffering in their midst, thereby facilitating a growing sense of commonality and responsibility toward dogs.

Early training activities probably included the contingent sharing of food based on dogs behaving in some particular way (e.g., begging). The power of empathy would have offered early humans the ability to consider how their actions might influence dogs. In fact, the development of human empathy and its extension to dogs provides a viable means for understanding how the evolutionary gap between our two species was narrowed sufficiently to enable close interspecies cohabitation and domestication. Human altruism, coupled with empathy for others (especially those belonging to a common group that are acted toward altruistically), may have provided the foundation for the dog's domestication and behavioral incorporation. Human altruism and empathy seem to be especially strong toward the young, perhaps explaining the evolutionary trend toward paedomorphosis in dogs (see *Paedomorphosis* in Volume 1, Chapter 1). Paedomorphic dog types may have enjoyed a significant survival advantage by evoking altruistic caregiving and protective behavior in human captors.

DOGS AND THE ANCIENT WORLD

The earliest historical records of dogs come mainly from the art of Egypt and Assyria (Merlin, 1971). Archeological findings suggest that at least a dozen different breeds existed in ancient Egypt, ranging from the greyhound-

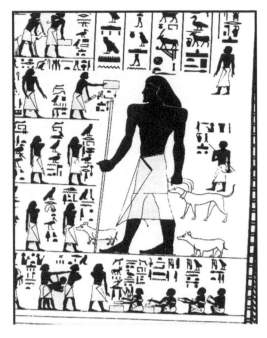

FIG. 1.1 Egyptian hunters developed a variety of breeds for different tasks, ranging from the sleek coursing hounds to short-legged dogs that may have been used for chasing prey to earth. (Detail from an Egyptian tomb painting, Beni Hasan, 1900 B.C.)

like coursing hound and mastifflike hunting dogs to dogs resembling the modern dachshund. Egyptian hunters primarily used coursing hounds that were slipped to chase down fleeing game. Egyptian breeders selected for traits and structural attributes conducive to this sort of hunting activity, as well as short-legged dogs, perhaps, used for digging into burrows after fleeing animals (Figure 1.1). As such, all breeding is a form of antecedent control over behavior that is subsequently refined and brought into practical expression by the agency of training. As remains common today, the breeding and training of dogs were probably overseen by the same person.

By the time Herodotus visited Egypt in the mid-5th century B.C., the dog was found living in homes as companions. When house dogs and cats died, the household experienced a period of mourning. The dead animals were mummified and given ritual burials. Other evidence of highly developed breeding and

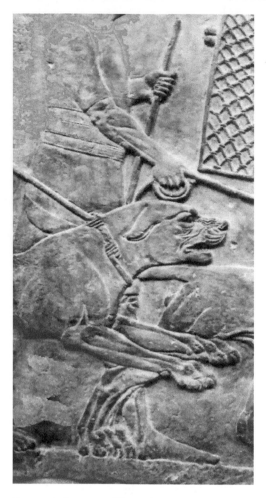

FIG. 1.2 Large mastiff-type dogs were used by Assyrian hunters to hunt large prey. Note the early use of slip collars. Assyrian dogs also wore bronze collars shaped in the form of a spiralling ring (Assyrian bas-relief, 7th-century BC).

training practices comes from Assyrian bas-relief depictions of powerful mastiffs used for various hunting purposes (Figure 1.2). Unfortunately, details from this period are lacking with respect to the methods of training used, but there can be little doubt that training played an important role in the way such dogs were prepared for the hunt and to live in close contact and harmony with humans.

As suggested by Homer's verses describing the sorrow felt by Odysseus for his dying dog Argos ("Swift"), Greek dogs were held as

objects of sincere affection and symbols of devotion and faithfulness (see *Dog Devotion and Faithfulness* in Volume 1, Chapter 10). However, the Greek attitude toward dogs was complex, with many common expressions of contempt and personal insult involving reference to dogs. By the 5th century B.C., various dog breeds had been developed for specific hunting tasks and other purposes, such as guarding and shepherding flocks. In addition to working dogs, the Greeks also kept household or "table" dogs and small Melitean lapdogs as pets (Halliday, 1922). The breeding and training of hunting dogs appear to have been significant pastimes for ancient Greeks. Xenophon (circa 380 B.C.), a student of Socrates, wrote a valuable tract on dog husbandry and training entitled *Cynegeticus* (Hull, 1964; Merchant, 1984; see Xenophon, 1925/1984a), which gives the reader a rare glimpse into the breeding and management of Greek hunting dogs. For hunting hare, Xenophon recommends the Castorian and vulpine breeds, the latter of which was believed to be the result of an admixture of dog and fox lineage—a false belief that was widely accepted at the time. Aristotle perpetuated the vulpine-cross belief in his *History of Animals* and further suggested that the Indian hound (a particularly aggressive variety) was the result of crossing a male tiger with a female dog. These Indian hounds (mastiff-type dogs) were used for deer hunting and other pursuits that required bigger and stronger breeds. For wild boar, a variety of dogs were employed in a mixed pack, including the Indian, Cretan, Locrian, and Laconian breeds. Apparently, great care was taken to keep these breeds unadulterated. Control over undesirable matings was discouraged by the use of a spiked *surcingle,* or girth strap, that was wrapped around the female dog's body (Hull, 1964). However, Merlin (1971) has suggested that another possible function of this piece of equipment was to protect the dog from injury when hunting dangerous game like wild boar.

Xenophon recognized the value of early training and recommended that a dog's education be started while it was still young and most eager to learn. During the early stages of training, hare-hunting dogs were trained to drive fleeing prey into snag nets by feeding the dogs near the location of the nets, at least until they developed a sufficient appetite for the hunt itself to perform the task of coming to the nets without such aid. Young trailing dogs were placed on long leashes and paired up with more experienced dogs to hunt hare. As their training progressed, novice dogs were restrained until the hare was out of sight and then released to ensure that they relied on scent rather than sight to follow and locate the fleeing prey. If a puppy failed to trail an animal in the correct direction, the puppy was recalled and the procedure repeated until the behavior was mastered (Hull, 1964).

Xenophon (1925/1984b) also anticipates with surprising accuracy a number of modern training theories and techniques. Although Thorndike has been credited with the discovery of the *law of effect,* stating that behavior is strengthened (stamped in) by reward and weakened (stamped out) by punishment (see *Basic Mechanisms of Behavioral Change: Stamping In and Stamping Out* in Volume 1, Chapter 7), Xenophon enunciated this basic rule of animal training well over 2000 years ago in his essay *On the Art of Horsemanship:*

> Now, whereas the gods have given to men the power of instructing one another in their duty by word of mouth, it is obvious that you can teach a horse nothing by word of mouth. If, however, you reward him when he behaves as you wish, and punish him when he is disobedient, he will best learn to do his duty. This rule can be stated in few words, but it applies to the whole art of horsemanship. (341)

It is easy to recognize how closely this dictum anticipates Thorndike's formulation. In addition to possessing a clear understanding of the value of behavioral consequences for the control of behavior, Xenophon also appreciated the usefulness of presenting rewards and punishers in a timely manner, stressing the importance of a close temporal connection between the action to be influenced and the consequences used to achieve that effect:

> He [the horse] will receive the bit, for example, more willingly if something good happens to him as soon as he takes it. (341)

He then continues:

> He will also leap over and jump out of anything, and perform all his actions duly if he can expect a rest as soon as he has done what is required of him. (341)

This latter passage describes a practice anticipating the *Premack Principle,* which states "for any pair of responses, the independently more probable one will reinforce the less probable one" (Premack, 1962:255). In addition to appreciating the usefulness of reward training, Xenophon was also fully aware of the methods for establishing escape, avoidance behavior, successive approximation, fading, and stimulus control:

> When a man has a raw horse quite ignorant of leaping, he must get over the ditch himself first, holding him loosely by the leading-rein, and then give him a pull with the rein to make him leap over. If he refuses, let someone strike him as hard as he can with a whip or a stick: whereupon he will leap, and not only the necessary distance, but much further than was required. In future there will be no need to beat him, for if he merely sees a man approaching behind him, he will leap. As soon as he has grown accustomed to leap in this way, let him be mounted and tried first at narrow, and then at wider ditches. Just as he is on the point of springing touch him with the spur. (337)

This list of parallels between ancient training methods and modern learning theory could go on to include many other examples demonstrating the existence of a sophisticated understanding of training methodology already current during Xenophon's time and probably in existence long before. In addition, Xenophon was aware of the value of such modern techniques as direct exposure (habituation), counterconditioning, and modeling for modifying fears. All of these methods are implied in the following passages:

> One should also handle those parts in which the horse likes most to be cherished, that is to say the hairiest parts and those where the horse has least power of helping himself, if anything worries him. Let the groom be under orders also to lead him through crowds, and accustom him to all sorts of sights and all sorts of noises. If the colt shies at any of them, he must teach

him, by quieting him and without impatience, that there is nothing to be afraid of. (307, 309)

A few pages later, he continues on the subject of fear and its management:

The one best rule and practice in dealing with a horse is never to approach him in anger; for anger is a reckless thing, so that it often makes a man do what he must regret. Moreover, when the horse is shy of anything and will not come near it, you should teach him that there is nothing to be afraid of, either with the help of a plucky horse—which is the surest way—or else by touching the object that looks alarming yourself, and gently leading the horse up to it. To force him with blows only increases his terror; for when horses feel pain in such a predicament; they think that this too is caused by the thing at which they shy. (325, 327)

Animal training has been operating at a fairly sophisticated level over the ensuing centuries since the appearance of Xenophon's *Cynegeticus* in the 4th century B.C. Like the Greeks, the Romans also appear to have been well versed in the art of dog training. In addition to companionship, several practical uses were made of dogs, such as hunting, pulling carts and chariots, guarding, and military work (Figure 1.3). Dogs were trained to perform in Roman circuses and on the stage. During one of these performances, a dog reportedly walked on two feet, danced, and feigned death after eating a bit of "poisoned" food (Griffith, 1952; Riddle, 1987). Immediately upon taking the food, the dissimulating dog appeared to become sick, thereupon staggering about the stage, until at last it fell down and remained perfectly still on the floor, as though dead. Actors then proceeded to grab and abuse the "corpse," dragging the dog around the stage, thereby making the illusion even more convincing. Throughout the performance, the dog remained motionless. At last, the trainer signaled the dog to break the trance, and it suddenly jumped up and rushed affectionately toward the trainer as the crowd looked on with amazed delight at the training feat.

Although Romans often lived in close association with dogs as domestic protectors and companions, affectionate care and treatment of pet animals were looked upon with some degree of official contempt by Roman leaders.

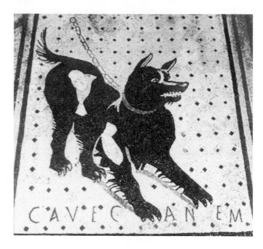

FIG. 1.3 The Romans used guard dogs to watch over their homes. This ancient warning inscribed is *Cave Canem,* "Beware of the Dog" (Pompeii mosaic).

Plutarch, for example, recorded an anecdote revealing Caesar's apparent disdain for the public display of such affection for pet animals, suggesting that such behavior was neither accepted nor considered natural by the Roman elite:

On seeing certain wealthy foreigners in Rome carrying puppies and young monkeys about in their bosoms and fondling them, Caesar asked, we are told, if the women in their country did not bear children, thus in right princely fashion rebuking those who squander on animals that proneness to love and loving affection which is ours by nature, and which is due only to our fellow-men. (Plutarch, 1914: Pericles 1.1)

In China, merchants made use of messenger dogs to communicate over long distances (Humprey and Warner, 1934). These canine messengers carried valuable advance information about cargo and progress from camel caravans approaching remote population centers. In addition to shepherds and guards, the presence of such messenger dogs 1000 years ago in China makes it certain that a fairly sophisticated level of understanding about dog behavior and training was widely dispersed throughout the ancient world. Over the centuries, animal training has provided the means to conform the dog's behavior to utilitarian purposes and the amusement of crowds (Figure 1.4).

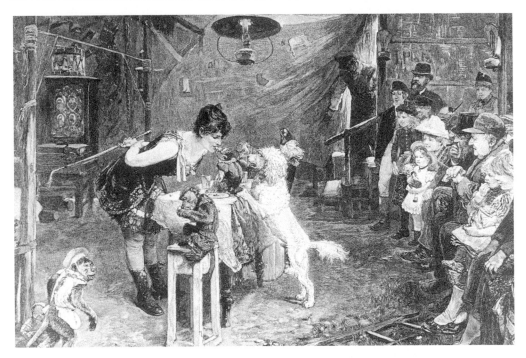

FIG. 1.4 A 19th-century German animal trainer performing with monkeys and a poodle. (Detail from *Ein Bravourstück,* an etching by Paul Meyerheim.)

ROOTS OF MODERN TRAINING

From the earliest times onward, countless conflicts between the dog's behavior and our expectations of it have tested and tempered our relationship. Even today—as any dog owner will testify—a dog's adjustment to family life rarely occurs without some tension and conflict. Little is known about how problem dogs were handled in the ancient past, but the methods employed were probably not much different from those used at the time to educate and discipline children. Corporal punishment certainly played an important role, with whipping being a very popular form of punishment until very recent times (Blaine, 1858; Hammond, 1894).

Although whipping was widely accepted and used to control unwanted dog behavior, it would be unfair to paint the picture of historical dog training with an overly broad brush. For example, H. W. Horlock (1852), a leading authority on the subject, wrote at length in his *Letters on the Management of Hounds* praising the virtues of reward and

gentle training methods. Horlock clearly recognized the incendiary effect of corporal punishment on aggression, describing several cases in which whipping resulted in attacks against the "whipper-in." In one of his letters, he described a telling incident involving a highly aggressive hound that he attempted to punish for fighting:

> There was one [hound] particularly cross and savage with the other hounds, and, catching him one day fighting and quarrelling, I called the other hounds out of the kennel, and resolved to make him know better. I laid the whip upon him sharply; but, at every cut I gave him, he jumped at me, with his bristles up, as savage as a lion. Seeing I might kill but could not subdue him, I threw the whip down on the floor, and, holding out my hand, called him to me by name. He immediately approached, with his bristles and stern well up still, and licked the hand held out to him. The lesson was never forgotten by me. (211)

Following this insight, Horlock goes on to describe a rather contemporary-sounding management strategy for controlling disruptive and injurious fighting that was occurring in his kennels nightly:

> I adopted afterwards the plan of separating at night the most quarrelsome, but in the summer it was difficult to keep them from fighting without constant and long exercise. More, however, was done by the voice than the whip, which I found only made them more irritable. With kind words they would do anything, and, as I always made pets of them, their tractability was shown in various ways. (211–212)

Horlock also emphasized the use of rewards for establishing control, describing the following steps for training the dog to come to its name:

> First give them names, and make them understand them. If you can find time to feed them yourself, do so, calling them by name to their food; if not take them out walking with you every day for an hour or two; put some hard biscuits in your pocket, give the dog a few bits at starting [establishing operation], call him by name occasionally when running forward, and every time he returns to you when called, give him a piece of biscuit; pat him and caress him the while. Follow this lesson for a week or ten days, and the dog will soon begin not only to know but to love his master. (223)

His emphasis on kindness and *connecting* with the dog for promoting cooperative behavior is further underscored by the following insightful passage:

> There are some persons to whom dogs become more readily attached than to others. The eye and the voice are a terror to some, as they are also an attraction to other animals. A soft eye, beaming with gentleness and good temper, is a point to which the instinct of the canine race naturally directs them, nor are they often deceived in its expression. Kind and benevolent looks have as great an influence over the animal as they have over the human species. They are, moreover, a sure criterion of temper. (223)

European Influences

Konrad Most is considered by many authorities to be the "father of modern dog training." As a captain in the German army, he was responsible for the formation of the German military-dog service during World War I, and from 1919 to 1937 he served as the director of the Canine Research Department of the Army High Command. Originally published in 1910, his book *Training Dogs* (1955, English) anticipates the articulation of many behavioral concepts and principles (e.g., shaping, primary and secondary reinforcement, stimulus control, punishment, and extinction) subsequently developed and refined by experimental analysis (Burch and Pickel, 1990). Although Most's work had its greatest influence in Europe, many American trainers have also benefited from his insights. Despite being dated and containing some problematic content, *Training Dogs* remains a "must read" for professional trainers and a useful resource for those interested in the history of dog training.

The reports of heroic dogs used during World War I led to heightened public interest in dog training, with high demand for dogs capable of performing specialized tasks such as police work and guiding the blind. The first official police dogs were reportedly trained and deployed in 1886 by Captain Schoenherr to control criminal activity in Hildesheim, Germany (Humphrey and Warner, 1934), although some evidence suggests that police-type dogs had been trained for police work long beforehand. Systematic efforts to train "police" dogs appears to have been already under way by the 15th century and probably much earlier. A description of such training appears in the writings of Heinrich Mynsinger published in 1473 (Von Stephanitz, 1925). These early police dogs were trained to stand ground against a human agitator (protected by a cloak of heavy hides) and to "track out the thief and the knave" (Figure 1.5). The brutal deployment of dogs by the Spaniards during the conquest of the Caribbean reveals that the Spanish already had a fairly advanced understanding of such matters by the 15th century (Varner and Varner, 1983).

By 1903 in Germany, various tests and efficiency trials were developed for evaluating police service dogs (Von Stephanitz, 1925) and, by 1914, as many as 6000 dogs were ready for military use (Griffith, 1952), with approximately 28,000 being requisitioned during World War I by the German

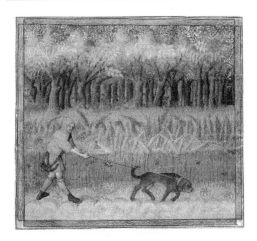

FIG. 1.5 A 15th-century tracker using a hound to trail a thief. (From *Treatise on Hunting* by Gaston Phébus. Bibliothèque Nationale, Paris.)

army (Von Stephanitz, 1925). Such police dogs gradually became a prominent feature of law enforcement in Europe. In England, Col. E. H. Richardson (1910) promoted the use of military rescue and ambulance dogs at around this date, and in 1916 established the War Dog Training School. Guide dogs appeared in Germany in 1917, primarily trained to assist soldiers blinded during the war, but strong evidence suggests that guide dogs were trained and used by the blind long before this date (Coon, 1959). In 1927, Dorothy Harrison Eustis, a Philadelphian living in Switzerland, enthusiastically described the training of guide dogs taking place at the Potsdam School for the Blind. The article, printed in the October 1927 issue of the *Saturday Evening Post,* caught the attention of a blind man, Morris Frank, who wrote a letter to Eustis expressing his appreciation and desire to come to Fortunate Fields (see below) to receive a guide dog of his own. Eustis agreed and, by 1928, Frank was back in America with a female German Shepherd guide dog named Buddy. Frank and Buddy rapidly became a media sensation and, in 1929, together with the financial support of Eustis, The Seeing Eye was founded in Morristown, New Jersey, where it has operated continuously up to the present. Canine guides for the blind were such a success that by the early 1930s several thousand

guide dogs were already in use throughout Europe and the United States (Humphrey and Warner, 1934).

At about this time, several trainers schooled in German training techniques came to the United States to establish various dog-training schools. Especially prominent in this regard was Carl Spitz (1938), Hans Tossutti (1942), and Joseph Weber (1939). Spitz, who had been trained as a military-police dog handler in Germany, immigrated to Chicago in 1926. After 2 years in Chicago, he relocated to Southern California, where he established a training kennel. Although most famous for his work with dog actors (e.g., Buck, in *The Call of the Wild* with Clark Gable), Spitz strongly emphasized the importance of training for family pets, specifically, for the improvement of a dog's character and adaptation to life with humans: "Only a well-behaved dog can possibly be 'man's best friend'" (101). On the East Coast, Weber, an experienced German trainer who had been schooled at the Berlin Police School and Potsdam School for the Blind, established a dog-training school in Princeton and made significant contributions to the development of competitive obedience training (see below). Like Weber, Tossutti was associated with the Potsdam School for the Blind and the Berlin Police School, where he was an instructor. Tossutti established a successful dog-training school in Boston.

Famous Dogs

Enthusiastic public interest in dog training was propelled by the sensational appearance of highly trained, intelligent, and well-behaved canine actors like Fellow, Rin-Tin-Tin, and Strongheart. The appearance of these dogs in motion pictures set the stage for a growing awareness of dogs' capabilities to learn. For example, Fellow, a German shepherd dog, was reputed to respond to 400 vocal commands and perform a variety of complex sequences of behavior (see *Nora, Roger, and Fellow: Extraordinary Dogs* in Volume 1, Chapter 4). His fame caught the attention of two prominent psychologists at Columbia University, who subsequently verified many of the dog's unusual abilities by testing them under stringent laboratory conditions (Warden and

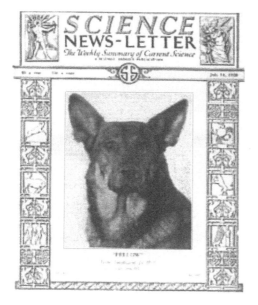

FIG. 1.6 The *Science-Newsletter* (now *Science News*) of July 14, 1928, featured a photo of Fellow on its cover, reporting that C. J. Warden, together with J. B. Watson, had set up a "Fellow Fund" in hopes of raising $100,000 in public donations to support continued dog behavior research at Columbia Univeresity.

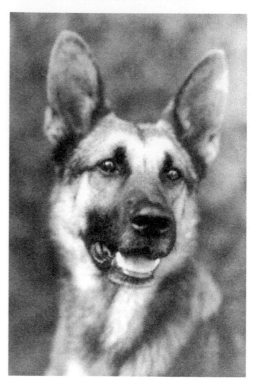

FIG. 1.7 Strongheart exerted a tremendous fascination on the public, both as the result of his film work and the inspired literary efforts of J. Allen Boone. (Trimble-Murphin Productions, 1924.)

Warden, 1928) (Figure 1.6). The trainer-owner (J. Herbert) attributed his success with Fellow to a habit of talking to the dog "constantly almost from birth." The trainer also stressed the importance of avoiding corporal punishment.

The original Rin-Tin-Tin (named after a good-luck doll given to soldiers by French girls) was one of five puppies found by Lee Duncan that had been abandoned with their mother in a shelled German bunker in 1918 at Metz, France (Duncan, 1958). Rinty made his first film debut in *The Man from Hell's River* in 1922. Until his death in 1932, the canine film star made a total of 24 movies for Warner Brothers, followed by numerous other movie and television appearances by a long line of Rin-Tin-Tin descendants. Rinty's sensational success on the screen was certainly influenced by a craze sparked earlier by another famous German shepherd dog actor named Strongheart, whose film debut occurred 7 months earlier in *The Silent Call*. Strongheart was a highly trained police dog

obtained when he was 3 years old from an impoverished German breeder at the end of World War I (Trimble, 1926). Strongheart (aka Etzel von Oeringen) made a dramatic impression on silent-film enthusiasts, rapidly acquiring international fame for his sagacity and physical prowess on the silver screen (Figure 1.7). Strongheart's lasting fame, however, comes primarily from the profound effect he had on J. Allen Boone, a Hollywood publicity writer, whose life was indelibly changed by the dog's companionship (see *Mysticism* in Volume 1, Chapter 10). Boone carefully recorded how this unique relationship transformed his life in *Letters to Strongheart* and *Kinship with All Life*. Together, Fellow, Rin-Tin-Tin, and Strongheart raised the public image of dogs to a new level of respect and appreciation, while underscoring the value of training for actualizing a dog's potential.

American Field Training

Until the 1930s, dog training in the United States had its largest following of enthusiasts among hunters. Among trainers of field dogs, Hammond (1894), Lytle (1927), and Whitford (1928) stand out as prominent and well-respected authorities. Although writing primarily for hunters, they provided their readership with many tips and methods for general obedience training and problem solving. Carlton (1915), writing at this time on the subject of hunting dogs, made an early effort to bridge the gap between science and the practice of dog training:

> Few breakers are aware that the dog's mind, in common with that of other animals, has been scientifically studied and that many patient observations and careful experiments are recorded in an extensive literature on the subject of "Animal Psychology." It is remarkable that the accepted principles of dog-breaking—which in most cases have been arrived at empirically and handed down by tradition—are to a great extent in accord with the scientist. This chapter is a first attempt to interest breakers in the subject. . .. Although the scientist abhors mere anecdote, he is at the same time conscious of the great disadvantages accompanying test conditions, and recognizes the value of observations and suggestions of the breaker when founded on a careful record of fact. (173–175)

Carlton goes on to interpret and summarize Thorndike's various laws and rules of learning in terms relevant to efficient dog training (see *Thorndike's Basic Laws* in Volume 1, Chapter 7):

1. The association in the dog's mind of satisfaction with the response we desire to encourage, and discomfort with the response we desire to inhibit.
2. The amount of satisfaction or discomfort.
3. The closeness in point of time and the preciseness of the connection between the response and the satisfaction or discomfort.
4. The frequency with which the response we desire is connected with the given situation and the duration of each such connection.
5. The readiness of the response to be connected with the situation.
6. The fact that to your dog a "situation" is at first a complex matter consisting of many elements in addition to the one element to which you are teaching him to give the desired response.
7. It is easier to obtain the response you desire de novo, than to get rid of a response already established and form a new one (184–185).

Books also began to appear during this period that were expressly written for average dog owners. For example, Lemmon (1914) published an interesting little book for dog owners detailing the various benefits of dog training and other germane topics, ranging from parlor tricks to the proper care and selection of a family dog. An early and enthusiastic dog-training authority and editor of *Dog World Magazine,* Will Judy (1927), published a book sold under the same title as Lemmon's tract, viz., *Training the Dog.* Judy's very popular version contains numerous illustrations, training tips, and ways to control common behavior problems. Although such books occasionally contain valuable insights, most of the information is passé in comparison to contemporary standards. Nonetheless, this popular dog-training literature provides a valuable cultural and historical backdrop for studying and appreciating subsequent progress in the field.

ORGANIZED COMPETITIVE OBEDIENCE

The appearance of organized obedience training and the sanctioning of competitive trials by the American Kennel Club (AKC) slowly took form during the late 1930s. The person most often attributed with the distinction of bringing obedience competition to America from Europe is Helene Whitehouse-Walker. An avid poodle breeder and exhibitor, Walker discovered that in England the poodle and the German shepherd excelled in competitive obedience work. During an extended stay in England, she studied the various methods in use and subsequently introduced the sport of competitive obedience to the American dog fancy. She was an untiring advocate for the recognition of obedience training as a dog sport. The first American obedience trial took place in 1933 at Mt. Cisco, New York (Burch and Bailey, 1999). Walker petitioned the AKC for recognition of obedience trials early in the 1930s, with full sanctioning and legitimacy being granted by the AKC in 1936. In collaboration with her assistant, Blanche Saunders (1946), and with Josef Weber, they established the official rules and obedience tests used by the AKC to judge obedience proficiency and to grant appropriate awards. In 1940, Walker and Saunders, traveling across the country in a house trailer, promoted the benefits of dog training and performed numerous obedience demonstrations. By 1941, many obedience clubs had already been organized and had started to offer public obedience classes to meet a growing interest in the new sport.

DOGS AND DEFENSE

As it turns out, this series of events was a stroke of good fortune for a country about to go to war. The pioneering efforts of Walker and Saunders provided a ready resource for a volunteer organization that would soon form to procure dogs for the war effort. Dogs for Defense (DFD) was spearheaded by Alene Erlanger, a prominent breeder and fancier, along with numerous other breeders, handlers, and trainers committed to the use of dogs for national defense. The AKC played a prominent facilitatory role in the organization and success of the DFD, which was officially launched in January 1942 and continued to serve a procurement function until March 1945. The activities of the DFD were coordinated by the Quartermaster General's Office. Interestingly, Mrs. Erlanger, a dog fancier, breeder, trainer, and judge, wrote the first major dog-training manual for the army (TM 10-396-War Dogs), as well as numerous technical bulletins and training films (Waller, 1958).

War Dogs

Prior to this time, the U.S. military had made little use of dogs (primarily sled dogs), and the DFD rapidly became the official source of dogs for military use. Although originally charged with the procurement and training of sentry dogs, the civilian instructors proved ill-prepared to train military working dogs and handlers. The responsibility for the procurement and training of sentry-dog teams was transferred to the Remount Branch in the summer of 1942. The DFD was delegated procurement responsibilities by the Remount Branch, setting up several procurement centers across the country for receiving dogs. The Quartermaster General established various training centers, including Front Royal Quartermaster Remount Depot (Virginia), Camp Rimini (Montana), Fort Robinson (Nebraska), San Carlos (California), and Cat Island (Mississippi). From 1942 to 1944, the DFD recruited 40,000 dogs. Of these, 18,000 were distributed among the various training centers. Approximately 8000 were returned to their owners as the result of some physical or temperament shortcoming detected during initial evaluations. Ultimately, some 10,000 dogs were mobilized and trained for military service during World War II. These dogs were trained to perform five primary duties: sentry, sled and pack, messenger, mine detection, and scouting. Dogs provided outstanding service in the war effort, with at least one having been awarded a Silver Star and Purple Heart for heroism—commendations that were subsequently revoked because of an army policy against the issuance of such awards to animals. Approximately 3000 dogs were *demilitarized* at the conclusion of World War II and returned to civilian life as heroes, with very few complaints regarding their behavior upon discharge from service (Waller, 1958).

After the War

At the end of the war, many handlers and trainers (civilian and enlisted) left the military to pursue civilian dog-training careers. One of these civilian trainers was William Koehler. Despite Koehler's fame (known mostly for his work at Walt Disney Studios), credentials, and achievements, no dog trainer inspires quite as much heated controversy as he does. Proponents and ardent apologists [most notably Hearne (1982)] defend his training methods with an almost irrational fervor, whereas detractors vigorously condemn them as being excessively brutal and cruel. In response to his critics, he appeared to be comforted by an apparent haughty self-estimation and an unbridled contempt for their evident lack of appreciation and understanding, exclaiming "I guess the nicest thing that could happen to you is to enjoy the enmity of the incompetent" [quoted in Lenehan (1986:43)]. Koehler had little tolerance for these "cookie people" and "humaniacs" (terms he was pleased to use when referring to his critics), whose gentle approach he eschewed as "nagging a dog into neurosis." Although many of Koehler's problem-solving methods (hanging, beating, and other abusive practices) have been repudiated, many active dog trainers still use his methods for obedience training, usually in a modified form.

As the popularity of dog training caught on during the 1950s and 1960s, many capable and humane dog trainers appeared on the scene. Of particular note in this regard are Winifred Strickland (1965) and Milo Pearsall (Pearsall and Leedham, 1958), both highly influential and successful competitive obedience trainers. In 1965, Pearsall, together with Earl Traxler, founded the National Association of Dog Obedience Instructors (NADOI) in Manassas, Virginia (Tardif, personal communication, 2000). An important goal of the organization was to encourage greater uniformity in group dog obedience instruction and to disseminate relevant information to foster that end. Pearsall emphasized the need to train dogs from a canine point of view, thereby making training more humane and easy for dogs to understand. In addition, Pearsall is remembered for pioneering puppy group classes or "kindergarten puppy training" (K.P.T.) and stressing the use of guided *play* rather than more adversarial training techniques. NADOI members are primarily group instructors training dogs in close adherence to AKC obedience regulations, often doing so in preparation for AKC-sanctioned obedience competition. Many others deserve mention, but, unfortunately, space severely limits this discussion, and the subject will need to be left for another time. One trainer active during this time, however, deserves special mention for her contributions to modern dog training and dog behavior counseling. Ramona Albert (1953) developed several key advances in our understanding of dog behavior (and misbehavior). She strove in her practice to connect with dogs on a motivational level, but avoided the moralistic and emotionally charged anthropomorphic interpretations of a dog's intentions, a pitfall that snared so many trainers of her time. In addition, she strongly emphasized the importance of *listening* to a dog's behavior as a form of subtle communication revealing its inner state. Finally, she encouraged dog owners to exercise patience and intelligence and advised them to use relatively gentle methods for gaining control. Many of her techniques anticipate more contemporary approaches in vogue today for the management of severe behavior problems, especially her approach to the treatment of aggression and separation-related problems. She appears to be the first trainer-counselor to articulate a distress-anxiety theory of destructive behavior occurring in the owner's absence.

Vietnam and Dog Training

An important influence on training theory and method occurred somewhat surreptitiously as the result of various military studies and dog-training projects contracted by the U.S. Army during the 1960s and early 1970s. Prompted by the Vietnam War, the government poured millions of dollars into basic research and development of various military-dog programs. In addition to selective breeding programs (e.g., the Biosensor Research Team or "Super Dog" Program under the command of Col. M. W. Castleberry), many behavioral studies were performed focusing on complex training objectives and a dog's ability to execute them. Contracted by the Army, Roger W. McIntire (1968) directed the Canine Behavior Laboratory at the University of Maryland, where he performed numerous studies investigating the suitability of dogs for military service. Other research activities were centralized at the U.S. Army Land Warfare Laboratory in Aberdeen, Maryland. Research objectives included the feasibility of employing remote-controlled scout dogs (Romba, 1974), mine and tunnel dogs (Breland and Bailey, 1971), multipurpose dogs (Dean, 1972a), and explosive and narcotic detection (Romba, 1971; Dean, 1972b). Most of these studies were performed by civilian behavioral psychologists in close cooperation with military-dog handlers. Naturally, this meant that many dog handlers were exposed to various classical and instrumental conditioning procedures used to modify dog behavior. Upon leaving the military, many of these handlers pursued civilian careers, applying this new knowledge of behavioral control to their public dog-training programs. [For an excellent summary of the important services performed by military working dogs in Vietnam, the reader should consult Michael Lemish's *War Dogs: Canines in Combat* (1996)].

THE MONKS OF NEW SKETE

Although many traditional dog trainers have emphasized the importance of training for attaining a satisfying relationship with dogs, the Monks of New Skete (1978, 1991) introduced a unique existential or spiritual significance and appreciation of dogs and training. For the most part, the Monks accommodated conventional dog-training methods and refined them but have also made some significant innovations of their own. An especially valuable contribution was the emphasis they placed on the human-dog relationship as something possessing value in its own right. Traditionally, *how to* books often gave considerable space to practical applications of training, such as competitive obedience and protection training, but neglected to emphasize the relationship-enhancing aspects of obedience training. The Monks specifically stress the value of training as a means for building a relationship through enhanced communication and cooperation. Ultimately, the training process is viewed as a means to intensify one's sensitivity and awareness of the self, the dog, and nature. The essence of this philosophy of training is poignantly expressed by the founder of the New Skete breeding and training project, Brother Thomas Bobush, who wrote,

> Learning the value of silence is learning to listen to, instead of screaming at, reality: opening your mind enough to find what the end of someone else's sentence sounds like, or listening to a dog until you discover what is needed instead of imposing yourself in the name of training. (1978:xiii)

In terms of technical innovations, the incorporation of massage and relaxation techniques into the training and socialization process was, perhaps, the Monks most lasting contribution to modern dog training.

NEW YORK AND THE NORTH AMERICAN SOCIETY OF DOG TRAINERS

In 1972, a youthful Job Michael Evans entered the cloistered environs of the New Skete monastery to became a monk and apprentice dog trainer under the tutelage of Brother Thomas. During the next 11 years, he helped to guide the monastery's breeding and training program and cowrote the highly successful "How to Be Your Dogs Best Friend" (1978). He left the monastery in 1983 and shortly thereafter established a dog-training and counseling service in New York City. Evans rapidly became a highly influential author, professional dog trainer, and speaker. He is credited with authoring the first books written expressly for the instruction of private dog trainers (1985, 1995). Together with other prominent New York dog trainers, he helped to found the Society of North American Dog Trainers (SNADT) in 1987. Charter members included several highly regarded trainers, such as Carol Benjamin, Arthur Haggerty, and Brian Kilcommons. The organization soon established a respected multilevel certification process and a code of ethics. SNADT promoted a positive public image of the dog-training profession and its value for society: "SNADT believes that dog training is an essential service for a humane and rational society that cherishes dogs in the human environment. Dog training is an honorable profession worthy of public respect and esteem" (Evans, 1995:47). SNADT operated out of the American Society for the Prevention of Cruelty to Animals (ASPCA) for several years, until it was brought to an untimely end in 1995.

SCIENCE AND BEHAVIOR

Mountjoy and Lewandowski (1984) have noted that most of the basic concepts and principles of modern behavior modification (e.g., shaping, chaining, positive and negative reinforcement, time-out, stimulus fading, and response prevention) were in steady use long before they were named and systematically studied in the laboratory. By way of illustrating these observations, they describe an animal act [performed in 1799 and reported by J. Strutt (1876)] consisting of a dozen little birds carrying toy muskets and wearing paper caps on their heads. A soldier bird marched a "deserter" bird up to a toy canon, when

> Another bird was immediately produced, and a lighted match being put into one of his claws, he hopped boldly on the other [to]. . . the cannon, and applying the match to the priming, discharged the piece without the least appearance of fear or agitation. The moment the explosion took place, the deserter fell down, and lay apparently motionless, like a dead bird but at the command of his tutor he rose again; and the cages being brought, the feathered soldiers were stripped of their ornaments, and returned into them in perfect order. (1801/1876:341)

The complexity and sequential order of this performance clearly suggest that the bird trainer was intimately familiar with many of the basic principles of learning (including systematic desensitization) and various sophisticated behavior-organizing procedures (such as shaping and chaining). It was not until animal behavior became the subject of experimental study that the familiar scientific terms would be applied to these practical techniques and procedures.

A pronounced influence on the study of dog behavior and psychology was the publication of the seminal research of the Russian physiologist Ivan Pavlov and his coworkers (1927/1960). Credited with the discovery of classical conditioning (see *Classical Conditioning* in Volume 1, Chapter 6), Pavlov clearly recognized the significance of animal training for a science of behavior:

> It is evident that many striking instances of animal training belong to the same category as some of our phenomena, and they have borne witness for a long time to a constant lawfulness in some of the psychical manifestations in animals. It is to be regretted that science has so long overlooked these facts. (1928:55)

The result of his revolutionary research was a detailed and exhaustive inventory of functional relations controlling the acquisition and extinction of conditioned reflexive behavior. In the wake of Pavlov's discoveries, progress in the science of behavior and learning was extremely energetic and productive, resulting in thousands of studies over the course of the 20th century.

In America, at about the same time Pavlov was making his mark on the history of psychology in Russia, Edward Thorndike (1911/1965) was systematically studying voluntary or instrumental behavior at Columbia University (see *Instrumental Learning* in Volume 1, Chapter 7). Thorndike and coworkers made numerous detailed observations on how animals learned to escape from puzzle boxes by manipulating various ropes and levers. Whereas Pavlov's work focused on the effects of antecedent stimuli on reflexive behavior, Thorndike was more interested in how instrumental behavior was affected by its consequences. In short, Thorndike believed that animals learned how to escape from puzzle boxes through a process of *trial and error* (perhaps more precisely stated as *trial and success* and *trial and failure*) in which successful (rewarded) behaviors are *stamped in,* whereas unsuccessful (punished) behaviors are *stamped out.* Thorndike referred to this general principle as the *law of effect.*

According to Thorndike, all "learning is connecting." Trial-and-error learning is dependent neither on deliberate reasoning (insight) nor on the exercise of some specialized instinct but depends entirely on the selective stamping in or stamping out of relevant stimulus-response connections. Together, Pavlov and Thorndike formed the intellectual and methodological foundations for the experimental study of animal behavior and learning.

Another major contributor to the history of behaviorism was B. F. Skinner, whose efforts resulted in the development of a formal training theory based on the work of Pavlov and Thorndike. In 1951, Skinner wrote an important short article directed toward a lay readership concerning behaviorism and its relevance for animal training, entitled "How to Teach Animals." To my knowledge, this was the first time that the process of explicitly *shaping* dog behavior by using conditioned reinforcement was systematically described. The method involved using a toy cricket (clicker) to selectively reinforce successive approximations of free-operant behavior in the direction of a desired response (e.g., the dog touching the handle of a cabinet with its nose). In this same article, Skinner also discusses various other operant procedures (e.g., backward chaining) used to organize complex behavioral sequences. This is an important article for novice trainers to study and absorb. In that same year, Keller and Marian Breland—early students of Skinner—announced that they had founded a new psychological discipline, using Skinnerian principles, devoted to the training of animals. Referring to this new field as "applied animal psychology" or "behavioral engineering," the behaviorists boasted that they were "in a position to outstrip old-time professional animal trainers" (Breland and Breland, 1951:202).

Despite the Brelands' energetic efforts and enthusiasm, their behavioral enterprises failed to advance much beyond the operant conditioning of a series of commercial animal exhibits (e.g., dancing chickens, rabbits playing a piano, and pigs placing wooden coins into a "piggy" bank) used to advertise animal feeds. In addition to their commercial efforts, the Brelands were also contracted to perform military feasibility studies (e.g., mine detection). Early in their career, they assisted Skinner in Project Pigeon and ORCON—an acronym for *organic control systems* (Skinner, 1960). Project Pigeon involved training a multiple-pigeon crew to guide a winged bomb (called a Pelican) by pecking rapidly at a target image displayed before them on a plastic disc. A very high rate of pecking kept the bomb on target, with each peck producing an electrical signal regulating a set of servomechanisms controlling the wings. Although the laboratory work was reportedly successful, the feasibility project failed to convince military officials of its suitability for actual deployment.

Despite the Brelands' early commercial success, operant conditioning (i.e., automated training) proved problematic as a practical means for controlling animal behavior. Several conceptual flaws and shortcomings proved distressing and humbling for these early pioneers of operant technology. In their influential article, "The Misbehavior of Organisms" (obvious wordplay on the title of Skinner's seminal text "The Behavior of Organisms"), they had to concede that the strict behavioristic account of learning proposed by Skinner was not adequate to explain many of their practical observations and training difficulties:

> Three of the most important of these tacit assumptions [held by behavior analysts] seem to us to be: that the animal comes to the laboratory as a virtual *tabula rasa,* that species differences are insignificant, and that all responses are about equally conditionable to all stimuli.
>
> It is obvious, we feel, from the foregoing account, that these assumptions are no longer tenable. After 14 years of continuous conditioning and observation of thousands of animals, it is our reluctant conclusion that the behavior of any species cannot be adequately understood, predicted, or controlled without knowledge of its instinctive patterns, evolutionary history, and ecological niche.
>
> In spite of our early successes with the application of behavioristically oriented conditioning theory, we readily admit now that ethological facts and attitudes in recent years have done more to advance our practical control of animal behavior than recent reports from American "learning labs" (1961:684).

More recently, Marian Breland (now Bailey), together with Bob Bailey, an ex-Navy dolphin trainer and associate at Animal Behavior Enterprises, have come out of retirement to give seminars and workshops for an enthusiastic following of "clicker" trainers. They have teamed together to stage a traveling chicken-training show, during which trainers are challenged to test their timing skills to shape chicken behavior.

APPLIED DOG BEHAVIOR

The momentum behind the "ethological facts and attitudes" alluded to by the Brelands was forged by the pioneering efforts of such ethologists as Konrad Lorenz and Niko Tinbergen. The origins of ethology, however, are rooted in the work of Charles Darwin. *The Expression of the Emotions in Man and Animals* (1872/1965) was especially influential in this regard. In this book, Darwin described and cataloged many of the common social displays exhibited by dogs. He argued that social animals, including dogs, evolve innate species-typical communication systems to meet habitual social demands placed upon them. Following in the example set by Darwin, Georges Romanes collected a variety of dog-related anecdotes and used them to support the notion of a continuity in the evolution of human and animal behavior. Romanes argued that dogs had evolved a high level of intelligence and other humanlike abilities. These highly interesting reports were obtained from a variety of correspondents and published as a collection in *Animal Intelligence* (1888). Another early figure of considerable importance in this regard is William James (1890/1950). Like Darwin and Romanes, James illustrated many of his psychological principles and theories with stories and examples taken from observations of dog behavior. Similarly, C. Lloyd Morgan, the author of several books on animal behavior and learning, performed hundreds of experiments with his personal dogs. He has been credited with introducing the concept of *trial-and-error learning* to describe the way his fox terrier, Tony, learned how to open a latched gate with his head (Gregory, 1987). In one of his texts, *An Introduction to Comparative Psychology* (1903), Morgan extensively illustrates and amplifies various psychological concepts and principles with numerous experiments and interesting observations of dog behavior and learning.

The application of comparative psychology, learning theory, and ethology in the treatment of behavior problems has only slowly taken form. An early effort to organize the available scientific information about dogs was made by F. J. J. Buytendijk (1936), whose book, *The Mind of the Dog,* contains especially interesting material on olfaction and other sensory abilities exhibited by dogs. In 1955, Konrad Lorenz published *Man Meets Dog,* a popular examination of dog evolution and behavior from the viewpoint of ethology. Many of Lorenz's ideas are dated, but his evident love and appreciation for dogs is an inspiration that continues to exert a profound influence. In that same year, Heini Hediger (1955/1968) published a valuable contribu-

tion to animal-training literature. In *The Psychology and Behaviour of Animals in Zoos and Circuses,* he describes animal training in terms of its ethological and scientific significance. Hediger emphasized the importance of animal training as a means for achieving a more complete understanding of animal behavior and maximally intensifying the human-animal relationship.

An important advance in the study of applied dog behavior and genetics occurred with the founding of Fortunate Fields in Switzerland by Dorothy Harrison Eustis. The large project, under the scientific directorship of E. Humphrey, aimed at developing an ideal working dog through selective breeding and training (Humphrey and Warner, 1934). Pioneering efforts in the study of dog behavior and genetics were also carried out by L. V. Krushinskii (1960) in Russia. In the United States, J. P. Scott and J. L. Fuller at the Jackson Laboratory (Bar Harbor, Maine) directed basic research into the genetics and ontogeny of social behavior in the dog. Their studies lasted over a decade and culminated in the publication of their highly influential text *Genetics and the Social Behavior of the Dog* (1965). Finally, as previously mentioned, in 1967 the Biosensor Research Program brought together numerous consultants and advisors (e.g., Michael Fox) to breed, socialize, and train an improved military working dog.

An early veterinary effort to apply the findings of experimental psychology to dog behavior and training was pioneered by L. F. Whitney (1961, 1963). In his book *Dog Psychology: The Basis of Dog Training,* he describes and illustrates many of the basic learning principles promulgated by Pavlov and Skinner. Whitney's effort was significant in terms of introducing modern behaviorism and training theory to the dog-fancy culture and bringing lure and clicker training to the attention of dog owners, thereby providing an alternative to the more force-oriented methods prevalent at the time. Unfortunately, Whitney was not well versed in the finer points of behavior analysis and its application.

During the 1970s, a number of historically significant texts were published. Prominent among these authors was Michael L. Fox, a veterinarian and psychologist. Fox was an energetic experimentalist who published numerous articles and books on the normal and abnormal behavior of dogs and wolves. He was particularly interested in developmental processes and the comparative study of domestic and wild canids (Fox, 1971). Another respected contributor to the dog behavior literature of the time was Eberhard Trumler (1973), a student of Lorenz. Trumler brought the benefit of scientific training in ethology together with many years of close observation of dog behavior. Trumler's book provided a valuable source of information for many dog trainers and counselors. Finally, F. J. Sautter and J. A. Glover (1978) wrote a useful introduction to learning theory and the experimental study of dog behavior. Their book, subtitled appropriately, *A Primer of Canine Psychology,* neatly brought together an impressive body of scientific literature relevant to dog behavior, training, and development.

In the early 1960s, Dare Miller (1966), founder of the Canine Behavior Center in Los Angeles (Brentwood), California, began to employ various behavioral techniques to manage and control dog behavior complaints. Miller, who referred to his training and counseling practice as *dog psychology,* emphasized the role of frustration and anxiety in the development of behavior problems. Miller also appears to have believed that dog behavior maladjustment reflected human psychiatric problems: "One can only be sure of curing a dog if one has first psychoanalyzed its owner" [quoted in Mery (1970)]. In the early 1970s, W. E. Campbell (a protégé of Miller at the Canine Behavior Center) wrote a series of controversial articles concerning dog behavior for the journal *Modern Veterinary Practice.* Subsequently, a spate of articles written by veterinarians specializing in the treatment of companion animal behavior problems began to appear in professional veterinary journals.

Since then, a handful of veterinary behaviorists have written hundreds of articles, as well as several books, on the subject of animal behavior, including one text devoted to clinical behavioral medicine. Although noteworthy and stellar exceptions exist, the vast majority of these reports and studies involve case histories and the description of various treatment protocols. In addition, because the findings of most of these reports are based on very small samples, frequently involving just one animal, validation through statistical analysis is not possible. Until recently, few studies incorporated adequate experimental controls and none (to my knowledge) used blinded trials or reversals. As a result of these shortcomings, the veterinary behavior literature lacks convincing scientific authority, being largely the accumulation of anecdotal evidence, clinical impressions, and untested hypotheses (Appleby and Heath, 1997). In recent years, a trend in the direction of more careful research (including blinded trials) and the collection of statistically analyzable data has become more fashionable in the field. To some extent, this change of emphasis in veterinary behavioral research has been the result of pressures (and money) from pharmaceutical companies seeking quality scientific data with which to convince governmental authorities to license drugs for the treatment of animal behavior problems. Another likely incentive explaining this promising change was the American Veterinary Medical Association's decision in 1993 to recognize behavioral medicine as a veterinary specialty. With the advent of such recognition and respectability came the attached responsibility of situating this emerging field upon more scientifically responsible foundations.

While behavioral counseling and training have long been provided by professional dog trainers, the explicit application of psychological principles to such problems was heralded by the publication of a brief article entitled "Animal Clinical Psychology: A Modest Proposal" (Tuber et al., 1974) and a similar one written for a broader readership in *Psychology Today* published the following year (Tuber and Hothersall, 1975). In these articles, the authors (comparative psychologists and a veterinarian from Ohio State University) described several case histories and behavioral protocols used to treat problems such as thunder phobias and separation anxiety. The authors urged their colleagues to take up the banner of applied animal psychology and turn their skills and knowledge to the treatment of animal behavior problems. Unfortunately, only a scant few actually responded to their challenge by offering their professional services to owners with problem pets. Apparently, graduate students at Michigan State University (MSU) got the message, with three of them going on to make major contributions to the field of applied animal behavior after obtaining their doctorate degrees: Henry Askew, Peter Borchelt, and Daniel Tortora. All attended MSU during the late 1960s and early 1970s while studying comparative and experimental psychology under the tutelage of M. Ray Denny and Stanley Ratner (Nitschke, personal communication, 2000).

Given its auspicious beginnings and favorable media attention, the field has attracted only modest interest and support from the academic community outside of veterinary schools, with very few accredited programs currently offering professional training in applied animal behavior science. The field has developed more or less independently of applied behavior analysis and other scientific disciplines that could have offered valuable conceptual principles, research tools, and behavioral techniques for its advancement and wider academic acceptance. Currently, very little funding is allocated to applied animal behavior research, placing strong constraints on its competitive viability and thwarting its ability to produce quality research. One result of these circumstances is that very few of the current therapies used by applied animal behaviorists have received rigorous scientific validation. In 1991, the Animal Behavior Society (ABS) formed an accreditation committee with the authority to certify applied animal behaviorists. ABS certification is based on academic qualifications and experience but does not require qualifying examinations.

In 1998, the American College of Applied Animal Behavior Sciences (ACAABS) announced its intent to certify applied animal behaviorists based on academic credentials, practical experience, and a qualifying examination. A subsidiary of the American Registry of Professional Animal Scientists (ARPAS), the college was formed to enhance the level of professionalism in applied animal behavior and to increase the competency of practitioners providing services in the field. Objectives of the college include establishing postgraduate education and experience requirements for certification, examining and certifying applied

animal behaviorists, promoting continuing education, stimulating relevant research, and facilitating the dissemination of knowledge of applied animal behavior. In addition to educational and experiential requirements, certification depends on the candidate successfully passing a Diplomate Certification Examination. Currently, the ACAABS is primarily composed of animal behaviorists working with large animals, but will likely become more attractive to applied animal behaviorists working with family dogs and cats in the future.

CONTEMPORARY TRENDS IN DOG TRAINING

Operant techniques have been widely employed in the animal entertainment industry. In addition to the Brelands already discussed, animal trainers like Ray Berwick (1977) of Universal Studios employed operant procedures to train a variety of animals to perform on screen and television. Berwick's film credits include *The Birds* and *Birdman of Alcatraz*. Berwick's popular animal-training book outlines various clicker training procedures and included a tin clicker for use by the reader. Operant training paradigms have also been employed in the training of sea mammals. A noted sea-mammal trainer who has attracted considerable public attention for her work is Karen Pryor. In her autobiography *Lads Before the Wind* (1975), Pryor recounts her development as an animal trainer, describing in close detail the application of operant technology to the training of dolphins. She has written an influential self-help text (Pryor, 1985) in which she outlines the basic behavior analytical methods used for controlling human and animal behavior. However, Pryor is mostly recognized in the dog world for having championed and refined the clicker training method first introduced to dog owners by Whitney in the early 1960s. Squier (1993) has written a valuable review of Pryor's contribution as an animal trainer, outlining and discussing the major points of her training system. Another influential contemporary figure is Ian Dunbar (1979), a veterinarian and psychologist. A popular and charismatic speaker, he has presented numerous seminars over the years, reaching thousands of listeners with his dog-training philosophy. Following in the tradition set out by Pearsall, he has been a strong advocate of early puppy training and socialization classes.

Finally, the American Humane Association (AHA) has facilitated efforts to develop humane guidelines for the dog-training profession. In March 1998, a task force of 22 dog trainers and behaviorists, animal care professionals, and humane workers was convened by the AHA in Denver, Colorado. In November 1998, several advisory working committees met together in Valley Forge, Pennsylvania, for the purpose of producing humane dog-training guidelines. While embraced by many dog-training and dog-related organizations, the project has recently attracted significant controversy following the publication of an article in *DVM Newsmagazine* in which a portion of the unpublished humane guidelines document was released to the public (Brakeman, 2000). The document is currently undergoing a final review and revision process that will hopefully succeed in making it more acceptable to the dog-training community.

Over the years, numerous popular books and magazine articles have been written by professional dog trainers in an effort to educate the dog-owning public about general obedience training and the management of common behavior problems. By necessity, much of importance in this regard has been left out of this brief history. My hope is that this chapter has provided the readers with a broad overview of some important contributions leading up to current practices and theory employed by professional dog trainers and behaviorists. A comprehensive and thorough treatment of the history of dog training and behavioral counseling remains to be written.

REFERENCES

Albert R (1953). *Living Your Dog's Life.* New York: Harper and Brothers.

Allman JM (1999). *Evolving Brains.* New York: Scientific American Library.

Animal Behavior Society (ABS) (1999). Executive committee meeting [Minutes]. *Anim Behav Soc Newsl,* 44(3):10.

Appleby D and Heath S (1997). Behavior therapy techniques: A need for critical evaluation. In DS Mills, SE Heath, and LJ Harrington (Eds), *Proceedings of the First International Conference on Veterinary Behavioural Medicine.* Potters Bar, Great Britain: Universities Federation for Animal Welfare.

Berwick R (1978). *How to Train Your Pet Like a Television Star.* Los Angeles: Armstrong.

Blaine DP (1858). *An Encyclopedia of Rural Sports.* London: Longman, Brown, Green, Longmans, and Roberts.

Boone JA (1939). *Letters to Strongheart.* New York: Prentice-Hall.

Boone JA (1954). *Kinship with All Life.* New York: Harper and Row.

Brakeman L (2000). AHA publishes new humane dog training guidelines: Two years of consultation yields document for use by pet owners, DVMs, and legal system. *DVM Newsmagazine,* May:2S, 12S.

Breland K and Breland M (1951). A field of applied animal psychology. *Am Psychol,* 6:202–204.

Breland K and Breland M (1961). The misbehavior of organisms. *Am Psychol,* 16:681–684.

Breland M and Bailey R (1971). *Specialized Mine Detector Dog: Interim Report.* Aberdeen Proving Grounds, MD: U.S. Army Land Warfare Laboratory.

Burch MR and Bailey JS (1999). *How Dogs Learn.* New York: Howell.

Burch MR and Pickel D (1990). A toast to Most: Konrad Most, a 1910 pioneer in animal training. *J Appl Behav Anal,* 23:263–264.

Buytendijk FJJ (1936). *The Mind of the Dog.* Boston: Houghton Mifflin.

Campbell WE (1975/1985). *Behavior Problems in Dogs.* Santa Barbara, CA: American Veterinary Publications.

Carlton HW (1915). *Spaniels: Their Breaking for Sport and Field Trials.* London: Field House.

Coon N (1959). *A Brief History of Dog Guides for the Blind.* Morristown, NJ: The Seeing Eye.

Darwin C (1872/1965). *The Expression of the Emotions in Man and Animals.* Chicago: University of Chicago Press (reprint).

Dawkins R (1976). *The Selfish Gene.* New York: Oxford University Press.

Dean EE (1972a). *A Feasibility Study on Training Infantry Multipurpose Dogs.* Aberdeen Proving Grounds, MD: U.S. Army Land Warfare Laboratory.

Dean EE (1972b). *Training Dogs for Narcotics Detection: Final Report.* Aberdeen Proving Grounds, MD: U.S. Army Land Warfare Laboratory.

Dunbar I (1979). *Dog Behavior: Why Dogs Do What They Do.* Neptune, NJ: TFH.

Duncan L (1958). *The Rin-Tin-Tin Book of Dog Care.* Englewood Cliffs, NJ: Prentice-Hall.

Eccles JC (1989). *Evolution of the Brain: Creation of the Self.* London: Routledge.

Evans JM (1985). *The Evans Guide for Counseling Dog Owners.* New York: Howell.

Evans JM (1995). *Training and Explaining: How to Be the Dog Trainer You Want to Be.* New York: Howell.

Fox MW (1971). *Integrative Development of Brain and Behavior in the Dog.* Chicago: University of Chicago Press.

Gregory RL (1987). *The Oxford Companion to the Mind.* New York: Oxford University Press.

Griffith BF (1952). *Historic Dogs.* Haverford, PA: Clinton L Mellor.

Halliday WR (1922). Animal pets in ancient Greece. *Discovery,* 3:151–154.

Hammond TS (1894). *Practical Dog Training: Training vs Breaking.* Forest and Stream.

Hearne V (1982). *Adam's Task: Calling Animal's by Name.* New York: Alfred A Knopf.

Hediger H (1955/1968). *The Psychology and Behaviour of Animals in Zoos and Circuses,* G Sircom (Trans). New York: Dover (reprint).

Horlock KW (1852). *Letters on the Management of Hounds.* London: Office of *Bell's Life in London,* Strand.

Hull DB (1964). *Hounds and Hunting in Ancient Greece.* Chicago: University of Chicago Press.

Humphrey E and Warner L (1934). *Working Dogs.* Baltimore: Johns Hopkins University Press.

Jackson F (1997). *Faithful Friends: Dogs in Life and Literature.* New York: Carrol and Graf Publishers, Inc.

James W (1890/1950). *The Principles of Psychology,* Vols 1 and 2. New York: Dover (reprint).

Jansen HW (1974). *History of Art.* Englewood Cliffs, NJ: Prentice-Hall.

Judy W (1927). *Training the Dog.* Chicago: Judy.

Krushinskii LV (1960). *Animal Behavior: Its Normal and Abnormal Development.* New York: Consultants Bureau.

Lemish MG (1996). *War Dog: Canines in Combat.* Washington, DC: Brassey's.

Lemmon RS (1914). *Training the Dog.* New York: McBride, Nast.

Lenehan M (1986). Four ways to walk a dog. *Atlantic Monthly,* 257(April):35–48, 89–99.

Lorenz K (1955). *Man Meets Dog.* Boston: Houghton Mifflin.

Lytle H (1927). *How to Train a Bird Dog.* Dayton, OH: AF Hochwalt.

McIntire RW (1968). *A Final Report on the Behavioral Evaluation and Selection of Breeding.* College Park, MD: Canine Behavior Dogs for Army Training and Laboratory, University of Maryland.

Merlin RHA (1971). *De Canibus: Dog and Hound in Antiquity.* London: JA Allen.

Mery F (1968). *The Life, History, and Magic of the Dog.* New York: Grosset and Dunlap.

Miller D (1966). *The Secret of Canine Communication: HI-FIDO.* Brentwood, CA: Canine Behavior Center.

Monks of New Skete (1978). *How to Be Your Dog's Best Friend.* Boston: Little, Brown.

Monks of New Skete (1991). *The Art of Raising a Puppy.* Boston: Little, Brown.

Morgan CL (1903). *An Introduction to Comparative Psychology.* London: Walter Scott.

Most K (1910/1955). *Training Dogs.* New York: Coward-McCann (reprint).

Mountjoy PT and Lewandowski AG (1984). The dancing horse, a learned pig, and muscle twitches. *Psychol Rec,* 34:25–38.

Pavlov IP (1928/1967). *Lectures on Conditioned Reinforcement,* Vol 1, WH Gantt (Trans). New York: International.

Pearsall MD and Leedham CG (1958). *Dog Obedience Training.* New York: Charles Scribner's Sons.

Plutarch (1914). *Plutarch's Lives, Pericles,* B Perrin (Trans). Cambridge: Harvard University Press.

Premack D (1962). Reversibility of the reinforcement relation. *Science,* 136:255–257.

Pryor K (1975). *Lads Before the Wind.* New York: Harper and Row.

Pryor K (1985). *Don't Shoot the Dog: The New Art of Teaching and Training.* New York: Bantam.

Richardson EH (1910). *War, Police, and Watch Dogs.* London: William Blackwood and Sons.

Riddle M (1987). *Dogs Through History.* Fairfax, VA: Denlinger's.

Romanes GJ (1888). *Animal Intelligence.* New York: D Appleton.

Romba JJ (1971). *Training Dogs for Heroin Detection: Interim Report.* Aberdeen Proving Grounds, MD: U.S. Army Land Warfare Laboratory.

Romba JJ (1974). *Remote Control of War Dogs (Remotely Controlled Scout Dogs): Final Report.* Aberdeen Proving Grounds, MD: U.S. Army Land Warfare Laboratory.

Saunders B (1946). *Training You to Train Your Dog.* New York: Doubleday.

Sautter FJ and Glover JA (1978). *Behavior, Development, and Training of the Dog: A Primer of Canine Psychology.* New York: Arco.

Scott JP and Fuller JL (1965). *Genetics and the Social Behavior of the Dog.* Chicago: University of Chicago Press.

Skinner BF (1951). How to teach animals. *Sci Am,* 185:26–29.

Skinner BF (1960). Pigeons in a pelican. *Am Psychol,* 15:28–37.

Spitz C (1938). *Training Your Dog.* Boston: Marshall Jones.

Squier LH (1993). The science and art of training: A review of Pryor's *Lads Before the Wind. J Exp Anal Behav,* 59:423–431.

Strickland WG (1965). *Expert Obedience Training for Dogs.* New York: Macmillan.

Strutt J (1801/1876). *The Sports and Pastimes of the People of England.* London: Chatto and Windus.

Thorndike EL (1911/1965). *Animal Intelligence.* New York: Macmillan (reprint).

Trimble L (1926). *Strongheart: The Story of a Wonder Dog.* Racine, WI: Whitman.

Trumler E (1973) *Your Dog and You.* New York: Seabury.

Tuber DS and Hothersall D (1975). Behavior modification hath charms to soothe the savage beast. *Psychol Today,* 8:30, 82.

Tuber DS, Hothersall D, and Voith VL (1974). Animal clinical psychology: A modest proposal. *Am Psychol,* 29:762–766.

Tossutti H (1942). *Companion Dog Training.* New York: Orange Judd.

Varner JG and Varner JJ (1983). *Dogs of the Conquest.* Norman: University of Oklahoma Press.

Von Stephanitz M (1925). *The German Shepherd Dog in Word and Picture,* 2nd Am Ed. Jena, Germany: Anton Kampfe.

Waller A (1958). *Dogs and National Defense: A Study on the History of War Dog Training and Utilization During World War II.* Washington, DC: Department of the Army, Office of the Quartermaster General.

Warden CJ and Warner LH (1928). The sensory capacity and intelligence of dogs, with a report on the ability of the noted dog "Fellow" to respond to verbal stimuli. *Q Rev Biol,* 3:1–28.

Wayne RK and Ostrander EA (1999). Origin, genetic diversity, and genome structure of the dog. *Bioessays,* 21:247–257.

Weber J (1939). *The Dog in Training.* New York: McGraw-Hill.

Whitford CB (1928). *Training the Bird Dog.* New York: Macmillan.

Whitney LF (1961). *Dog Psychology: The Basis of Dog Training.* New York: Howell.

Whitney LF (1963). *The Natural Method of Dog Training.* New York: M Evans.

Xenophon (1925/1984a). Cynegeticus (On hunting). In EC Marchant (Trans), *Xenophon: VII Scripta Minora.* Cambridge: Harvard University Press (reprint).

Xenophon (1925/1984b). On the art of horsemanship. In EC Marchant (Trans), *Xenophon: VII Scripta Minora.* Cambridge: Harvard University Press (reprint).

2

Behavioral Assessment

Faust:

Thou'rt right indeed; no traces now I see

Whatever of a spirit's agency.

'Tis training—nothing more.

Wagner:

A dog well taught

E'en by the wisest of us may be sought.

Ay, to your favour he's entitled too,

Apt scholar of the students, 'tis his due!

JOHANN W. VON GOETHE, FAUST (1808)

BEHAVIOR ADJUSTMENT problems occur at all ages and involve practically every major canine behavior system. Naturally, given the evolutionary divergence between humans and dogs, one would expect significant tensions and conflicts to arise from time to time resulting in development of behavior problems. Although some of these problems can be quite serious and difficult to resolve, the vast majority are relatively innocuous and highly responsive to remedial training. Unfortunately, though, even minor adjustment

BEHAVIORAL ASSESSMENT

Descriptive	Functional
• What?	• How?
• When?	• Why?
• Where?	

FIG. 2.1. Behavioral assessment involves both careful description and functional analysis.

problems can be life threatening for a dog. Every year, approximately 2 million dogs are killed in U.S. shelters, many of them dying unnecessarily as the direct result of an unresolved behavior problem (Patronek, 1996). In addition, large numbers of otherwise healthy companion dogs are euthanized by veterinarians because of an intractable behavior problem (see *When the Bond Fails* in Volume 1, Chapter 10).

Understanding how dog behavior problems develop is central to designing effective prevention and training programs. Behavior problems develop under the influence of a complex web of biological and experiential influences. Accurately determining what these causal factors are has a direct bearing on the ultimate success or failure of behavior modification and therapy; acquisition and organization of pertinent information is vital to this process (Danneman and Chodrow, 1982). Broadly speaking, such information falls into one of two broad categories (Figure 2.1): descriptive (what, when, and where) and functional (how and why). As will be reiterated throughout this text, failure to appreciate fully the complex etiology of behavior problems adversely affects both the quality of assessment efforts and the efficacy of training recommendations. A thorough descriptive and functional assessment includes interviews, direct observations, and detailed medical and behavioral information obtained through questionnaires.

PART 1: DESCRIPTIVE AND FUNCTIONAL ASSESSMENT

BEHAVIORAL FACT-FINDING

An important source of behavioral information is the questionnaire (see the samples below). Relevant questionnaires are generally sent to the client, completed, and returned in advance of the first session with a dog. In addition to questionnaires, behavioral fact-finding involves both *interviewing* and *observing* techniques, with the most adequate picture being obtained by employing all three strategies. Interviewing techniques typically involve asking relevant questions over the telephone and in person. Observing techniques usually involve noting how a dog interacts with its owner and the home surroundings, as well as assessing how it responds to the trainer, unfamiliar people, animals, and other environments away from the home. Additional observing techniques include photographs, audio recordings, and videotapes. Finally, although not always practical, whenever possible, it is highly desirable to observe the dog engaging in the unwanted behavior.

Telephone Interview

The initial telephone call is important for both clients and dog behavior consultants. For clients, seeking help is often the culmination of a rather involved process. A safe assumption is that a client has already given considerable thought to the dog's problem and has probably tried many things in a haphazard sort of way, perhaps already trying professional advice that may not have worked. Picking up the phone and making the call is a major commitment to do something constructive about the dog's behavior. Unfortunately, poorly skilled counselors may take this opportunity to shame and criticize clients for their shortcomings and ignorance, rather than giving them the support and encouragement that they need to succeed. As the result of personal feelings of guilt and embarrassment, dog owners may be highly sensitive and vulnerable to such treatment. Effective counselors maintain a "relaxed, congenial, and non-judgmental" atmosphere during the interview process (Voith, 1980). Finally, the initial conversation leaves the client with a lasting impression of the counselor's professionalism and attitude—an impression that can facilitate or impede future counseling and training efforts.

The telephone interview offers a valuable opportunity to obtain candid information about the client, the dog, and the problem situation. From this initial contact information, tentative diagnostic and prognostic hypotheses can be formed. Perhaps the most important aspect of the telephone interview is the opportunity it gives a dog behavior consultant to assess the situation and to decide whether to accept or to decline a case. The decision to accept or decline is a professional and ethical prerogative based on numerous factors, but such decisions especially depend on the trainer's qualifications to deliver the required information and skills needed to resolve the problem successfully. *The ability to recognize the limits of one's craft is a true sign of professionalism.* In addition to an ethical responsibility toward their clients and the dogs, trainers also have an ethical responsibility to public safety and should decline cases in which there exists doubt about the possibility of success or where significant danger outweighs the potential benefits of intervention. For example, an owner calls reporting a situation in which a recently adopted dog, without much warning or provocation, attacked a visiting child, biting the child severely in the face (leaving several deep lacerations and puncture wounds). In response to such information, the behavior counselor should outline the legal and public safety risks associated with owning such a dog. In addition, care should be taken to emphasize the limited state of current knowledge about dog behavior, especially with respect to the prediction and control of aggression. The proper disposition of such a case will depend on the client receiving reliable information and direction from various professionals, including the trainer, veterinarian, and attorney. Although the telephone interview may provide sufficient information to form such decisions, it is preferable in most cases to meet with the family and the dog in person to assess the situation and evaluate the risks properly.

In another hypothetical situation, the initial call may involve a dog exhibiting destructive behavior and excessive barking when left alone. As the conversation moves along, however, the client may confide in passing, "Oh yeah, Sparky is sometimes a little unpredictable with strangers, especially when they first enter the house." The client may go on to describe how the dog is usually friendly, but only after he has had a chance to calm down and "make friends on his own terms." Obviously, without such information, the behavioral counselor might very well become Sparky's next victim, without ever knowing that a danger even existed.

When clients describe their dog's behavior problem, it is often expressed in subjective terms, for example, "The dog becomes spiteful when I leave him alone;" "He is so sweet most of the time, but then all of sudden—wham;" "He likes most people, but sometimes he just goes ballistic." Surprisingly, although tainted by anthropomorphism and sentimentality, clients' assessments are often very useful and well considered (demonstrating that they have thought a lot about the problem before calling), and they are often able to remember and express the finest detail—if they are given a fair chance to do so. Although the interview must be structured and guided to get the most out of the process, unnecessarily interrupting or interjecting opinions and comments that might wait should be avoided, at least during the early stages of the conversation. It is of utmost importance to allow clients to express their opinions fully and to feel comfortable while doing so. To accomplish this, counselors should remain open-minded and avoid counterproductive criticism and moralizing. One way to be supportive over the phone is to acknowledge the client's insights and efforts with brief comments of understanding and active interest in what they are saying. Remaining distant and quiet while on the phone only serves to alienate clients, make them nervous, and increase their awkwardness and embarrassment, perhaps causing them to withhold vital information. Finally, the quality of information obtained from interviews is strongly influenced by the way in which questions are asked (Hunthausen, 1994). Questions charged with judgmental innuendo should be avoided. Once clients have expressed the problem in their own terms, counselors can restate the details in more objective behavioral terms.

During the telephone interview, basic information about the dog can be recorded on a worksheet, including such items as signalment (age, sex, sexual status, and breed/mix), origin (breeder, pet store, friend, shelter, etc.), and age at adoption. Information about the presenting complaint should include the three W's (*what* happens, *when* does it happen, and *where* does it happen) and the three H's (*how* long, *how* frequent, and *how* severe). It is useful to emphasize the most recent occurrence of the behavior problem and, from there, organize contributory information around it as the interview develops. Of course, these various questions are preliminary to the private meeting in the home, at which time more detailed information can be obtained.

Another important function of the telephone interview is client education. Most dog owners seeking help for a behavior problem have little knowledge about what to expect and may have many concerns or fears about the training process and its likelihood of success. Sometimes a client is concerned that the dog will be physically hurt or its spirit broken by training. More recently, a growing number of clients want to be reassured that aversives *will* be used, having had exposure to previous training efforts in which a trainer refrained from the use of such procedures. Trainers should briefly explain how behavior modification works and the type and extent of aversives that are typically used, thereby allaying some of these worries and fears. Misleading or exaggerated statements about the relative role of rewards versus aversives may only serve to plant a seed of mistrust in the client toward the trainer-counselor, especially if the trainer ultimately needs to resort to aversive techniques to resolve a behavior problem. Besides providing some general information about the training process, trainers can also give clients a few useful preliminary tips in advance of the first meeting. Such information can be very helpful, plus everyone likes getting something for free.

Lastly, clients may also want some information about what to expect as the result of training. Although giving guarantees about behavioral change or boasting about one's successes is inappropriate, it is reasonable to discuss the likelihood of success in terms of past experience. Most consumers of behavioral advice are not looking for miracles; they are, however, looking for an honest assessment

and a professional effort. A sure sign of professional incompetence and insensitivity is casually recommending euthanasia, over the phone, as a trivial matter. In cases involving aggressive dogs where training is not likely to be successful, the trainer should advise the client to contact a veterinarian for additional diagnostic evaluation and other possible options—options that may or may not include euthanasia. Ultimately, the option to euthanize a dog is a joint decision made by the client and the veterinarian, under the advisement of the trainer. The recommendation of euthanasia, if and when it is made, should be the outcome of a thorough behavioral and veterinary assessment of the dog.

Despite obvious limitations, under some circumstances, either because of travel distances involved or monetary constraints, the behavioral assessment and counseling process may need to be carried out over the phone or the Internet. In such cases, it is useful to provide the client with a detailed behavioral questionnaire and to set up a series of telephone appointments once the questionnaire has been returned and studied. Supportive information like videotapes, audiotapes, photographs, charts, and a behavioral journal are all very useful tools in the analysis of behavior problems at a distance.

Home Interview

Whenever possible, the counselor should interview family members and make direct observations of the dog's behavior in the home. The home interview is a continuation and refinement of the process initiated during the telephone interview. During the home interview, additional information is obtained that may not have been offered by the client during the telephone interview or not provided by the questionnaire. It is crucial to obtain detailed information about all previous efforts to resolve the behavior problem in advance of making specific recommendations. Once such information is in hand, the counselor may explore a variety of working hypotheses, more fully discuss treatment rationales, and establish realistic expectations about the likelihood of success. Of utmost importance is the counselor's ability to convince the client that the counselor is able help. If the client-owner lacks confidence in the counselor's abilities and expertise, the process is bound to fail. Perhaps the single most important function of the home interview is to *prepare* a client family emotionally and psychologically to work through the behavior problem successfully. This process involves much more than simply informing clients about dog behavior and learning; it includes a great deal of sensitivity about their fears, disappointments, and attitudes about the process itself (Askew, 1996). In addition, clients must be made fully aware that behavioral change is not a magical nostrum, but a systematic and logical process that sometimes demands personal commitment, self-sacrifice, and a readiness to change one's own behavior in order to modify the dog's behavior. Without pointing fingers or resorting to shaming tactics, counselors should carefully explain that behavior is a dynamic reflection of the interaction between the dog and the environment, especially the social interaction between the client family and the dog. To change a dog's behavior, the behavior of people interacting with the dog may also need to change. Although changing a dog's behavior is the ultimate goal (and many means are provided to clients to achieve that end), to obtain lasting change, consistent with cynopraxic goals (see Chapter 10), a client's perception and behavior toward a dog may also require significant modification. Finally, the physical environment may also require alteration. Consequently, the home interview involves asking questions about where the dog spends most of its time: where it eats, sleeps, plays, and is exercised and trained.

Successful counselors are attentive and empathetic listeners who exhibit a sincere interest and caring attitude about clients' difficulties in controlling their dog or failure to form a satisfying relationship. Such understanding and accommodation helps to mediate a trusting rapport between the counselor and the dog owner. Instilling guilt or shaming an owner provides little productive incentive for the owner to change the situation. Instead of assigning guilt and shame, clients should be assigned a positive and realistic sense of responsibility for their dog's behavior and

well-being. From a cynopraxic perspective, the client family is held responsible for stewarding constructive change—not for past shortcomings.

DEFINING BEHAVIOR AS A PROBLEM

First and foremost, identifying a behavior pattern as a *problem* involves a cluster of cultural and personal preferences and normative judgments. These judgments reflect the client's attitudes and expectations, current scientific understanding, societal mores about animal behavior, and costs (economic and emotional) associated with the dog's behavior. A behavior problem is a tendency or pattern of behavior that sufficiently deviates from the owner's expectations or society's norms that efforts are prompted to change it into a more acceptable form. Behavior that fits our norms and expectations is considered normal and acceptable, whereas behavior that deviates too far from them or produces excessive costs for society or dog owners is deemed unacceptable or abnormal. Of course, there is considerable room for debate with respect to what clients may consider abnormal and unacceptable versus what society considers abnormal and unacceptable.

This general model accommodates problems ranging from minor adjustment issues and nuisances to major behavioral maladaptation such as aggression and compulsive habits. According to this model, some behavior problems may simply stem from a client's idiosyncratic preferences or misunderstandings of normal dog behavior, rather than from a behavioral symptom of a disorder or pathological state. What may be agreeable to one client and situation may be unacceptable to another person living under different circumstances. In some cases, an owner may view a particular behavior as being highly objectionable and unacceptable, until its ethological or functional significance is explained. In this case, the owner misinterpreted a normal behavior as representing a problem. At the other extreme, a highly unacceptable behavior may be defended by a client (a common situation involving aggression cases) until its characteristics and implications are properly

---

Before Training

Prefers aggressive   X   O   Likes petting
play and chase games   • • • • •/• • • • •   and gentle play
                    0   0.5   1.0

Expectancy Deviation Score: 0.7

- -

After Training

Prefers aggressive   X   O   Likes petting
play and chase games   • • • • •/• • • • •   and gentle play
                    0   0.5   1.0

Expectancy Deviation Score: 0.2

FIG. 2.2. Expectancy deviation scores can be used to identify and quantify problem areas, as well as to provide a measure of behavioral change and improvement resulting from counseling and training.

interpreted and understood. Consequently, an important aspect of cynopraxic intervention involves educating clients about normal dog behavior, adjusting their perceptions and misunderstandings, and, when necessary, facilitating more realistic expectations about the dog's behavior.

Assessing behavior problems includes objectively evaluating how the unwanted behavior affects a dog's quality of life, the client's needs (including bonding issues, safety, and preserving personal belongings and surroundings), and society's prerogatives (especially safety and health). One way to quantify a behavior problem that reflects the foregoing parameters is by identifying and assigning a value to a client's dog-behavior ideal and then identifying on the same behavioral continuum or trait what best represents the dog's actual behavior. Behavioral profiles measuring expectancy convergence/divergence provide a valuable means for assessing interactive conflict (see the *Puppy Behavior Profile*). The *Puppy Behavior Profile* is an especially useful tool for assessing puppy adjustment problems. Figure 2.2 shows a sample pretraining and posttraining profile. Clients are instructed to place an X over the point on the continuum that best describes their puppy's behavior and an O over the point that best represents their ideal. The upper half of the sample profile indicates at the outset of training the existence of a significant deviation between what the client expects from the puppy and what the puppy actually does. In the lower half of the sample, posttraining measures show a strong shift and convergence between the client's expectations and puppy's actual behavior. These changes can be quantified by assigning numerical values to the owner's ideal and their perception of the puppy's actual behavior. In the case of the pretraining profile, subtracting the larger value (0.9) from the smaller value (0.2) yields an expectancy deviation of 0.7. A similar calculation applied to the posttraining sample yields an expectancy deviation of 0.2. By comparing assessment data from the outset of training with data obtained at the conclusion of training, a quantified measure of change can be obtained to demonstrate the benefits of cynopraxic intervention. When a dog's behavior closely converges with its owner's expectations, the level of conflict between the owner and dog is obviously reduced, and presumably the social bond is more secure. Conversely, if the owner's expectancies strongly diverge from the dog's behavior, the bond may be threatened or, perhaps, destroyed over time by serious and unresolved conflict.

In addition to obtaining a behavioral expectancy profile, detailed questionnaires and direct interviews (both over the telephone and in-home) give a dog behavior consultant a fuller picture of the client's perception and understanding of the situation. Of course, nothing can take the place of directly observing a dog's behavior and the controlling environment. Furthermore, since a client's judgment is often clouded by the influence of

BEHAVIOR

ANTECEDENTS	CONSEQUENTS
Establishing operations Discriminative stimuli	Reinforcement Punishment

FIG. 2.3. Behavior is functionally dependent on controlling antecedents and consequents.

various factors such as anthropomorphism, inexperience with dogs, hearsay opinions, and cultural biases, the cynopraxic counselor is well advised to observe the dog in the home whenever possible.

FUNCTIONAL ANALYSIS AND WORKING HYPOTHESES

To organize and mediate behavioral change, a dog's problem behavior must be objectified and assessed in terms of its biological and adaptive significance (Voith and Borchelt, 1996). Most behavior problems develop within a context of complex influences involving both biological (nature) and experiential (nurture) factors. Identifying the antecedents and consequences controlling the expression of unwanted behavior is a major consideration in the assessment of any behavioral complaint (Figure 2.3). A guiding principle here is the notion that behavior functions under the control of antecedent variables (e.g., eliciting stimuli, discriminative stimuli, and establishing operations) and the influence of consequences produced by the unwanted behavior (e.g., marking events, positive and negative reinforcement, and punishment). Table 2.1 shows the various steps taken to perform a functional analysis of unwanted behavior. Objectively speaking, behavior problems present one or more of three general failings: (1) not enough (a deficiency in some pattern of behavior), (2) too much (an excess of some behavior), or (3) intrusion (behavior expressed under inappropriate circumstances).

Forming a working hypotheses about the functional significance of the unwanted behavior provides counselors with a rational foundation for behavioral intervention. From the working hypothesis, a training plan is designed, implemented, and tested. The training plan should include a functional evaluation of the various contributing instrumental and Pavlovian factors involved (obtained from the history, interview, and direct observation of the dog's behavior), as well as any significant ethological considerations believed to play a role in the expression of the unwanted behavior. It is often useful to search the literature for updated scientific information relevant to the problem before formulating a training plan. Finally, specific criteria should be decided upon in advance for assessing the general success or failure of the training plan. Although moving haphazardly from hypothesis to hypothesis is not appropriate or very constructive, it is often necessary to adjust assumptions about a dog's behavior based on its response to behavior modification and training. In fact, a dog's response to training serves either to confirm or to disconfirm the working hypothesis or behavioral diagnosis.

DEAD-DOG RULE

Ogden Lindsley (1991) has argued that behavioral assessment is properly limited to the occurrence of some activity or accomplishment, rather than specifying the absence of behavior, that is, something that a dead man is able to do. He argues that something a dead man can *do* is not behavior at all in the proper or analytical sense of the word. The "dead-man test" was proposed by him as a litmus test for determining whether some target represented a proper objective for behavior modification. Putting aside some questionable theoretical implications, the dead-man test offers a practical means for identifying behavioral goals and assessing change. The dead-dog rule is a hybrid variant of Lindsley's test, but departs somewhat from it in terms of emphasis and application. For one thing, the absence of behavior is not always an improper object of assessment, especially in the case of punitive contingencies, where the primary goal is to suppress behavior, that is, to render absent some behavior. According to Lindsley's test, however, the absence of responding is something a dead man or dog can do and, therefore, is not behavior. Also, some limits

TABLE 2.1. Steps in performing a functional assessment

1. Obtain a detailed history of the problem together with various contributing factors such as general health and nutrition.

2. The stimuli and situations under which the unwanted behavior occurs or does not occur are identified. These include motivational considerations (e.g., establishing operations), discriminative stimuli, and classically conditioned triggers. Contextual factors should also be given careful consideration, since many behavior problems are highly contextualized.

3. Identify biological predispositions (e.g., temperament) and ethological considerations that contribute to the expression of the target behavior.

4. Identify and compile antecedents (see item #2) and consequences (e.g., inadvertent or bootleg reinforcement) and other potentially aggravating influences (e.g., competitive tensions and attention-seeking behavior) existing between the owner and the dog. This list should include both current contingencies of behavior reinforcement as well past behavioral influences controlling the behavior.

5. Obtain a baseline of the unwanted behavior (estimated frequency and magnitude—both informal and formal, as needed).

6. Whenever possible, directly observe the unwanted target behavior.

7. Discuss all past efforts to change the behavior.

8. Develop a working hypothesis or set of hypotheses about the functional antecedents and consequences presumed to be operationally significant with respect to the occurrence of the undesirable behavior.

9. Develop a training plan or strategy of intervention based on a working or *diagnostic* hypothesis.

10. Assess the training plan or strategy in terms of the effect it has on the occurrence of the unwanted behavior.

set on behavior imply the absence of behavior without necessarily specifying an alternative behavior: the unwanted behavior is simply blocked (response prevention), suppressed (punishment), or extinguished (the reinforcing contingency is discontinued). Further, a dog can learn to lay quite still as though dead, something an actual dead dog *does*, but in the former case staying still is certainly an active behavior that is controlled by reinforcement. Perhaps, more properly stated, the objective should not be to train the dog *not to move* (something a dead dog can do), but to train the dog to stay for some limited duration of time—something a dead dog cannot do. The dead-dog rule is used as prescriptive measure and means to specify training goals in affirmative terms, rather than serving as a litmus test or theoretical position regarding behavior per se.

In contrast to punishment training, the goal of reinforcement training is either to increase or produce some target behavior, not

eliminate it. For example, according to the dead-dog rule, the objective of training a dog not to jump on guests is better stated in terms of alternative behavior incompatible with jumping up, that is, sitting, standing, or walking about in the presence of guests. When using a reinforcement contingency (positive or negative), defining the behavioral objective in negative terms (that is, no jumping) violates the dead-dog rule, since *not jumping* is something a dead-dog can do. In the case of reinforcement training, the dead-dog rule holds that behavioral objectives should be described in affirmative terms rather then negative ones, that is, in terms of an absence of behavior. Punishment, extinction, and response prevention result in a reduction or elimination of behavior, whereas reinforcement results in an increase or production of behavior. In some cases, the absence of behavior is not an adequate or reliable objective for behavior modification. This is especially true in the case of aggression. Remembering that reinforcement training results in an increase or production of some behavior, it makes little sense to define behavioral objectives occurring as the result of reinforcement in terms of an absence of behavior. Reinforcement cannot eliminate behavior, except in a secondary way; reinforcement is productive of behavior and, consequently, behavior operating under the control of reinforcement contingencies should be assessed in affirmative behavioral terms. Consequently, the goal of reinforcement training is not to suppress aggression but to facilitate and reinforce behavior incompatible with aggression—arguably the most successful means for modifying such behavior problems. Therefore, successful intervention should be assessed in terms of affirmative changes in behavior, such as increased levels of affectionate interaction, friendly displays, and cooperation—not the absence of threats and aggressive episodes. The dead-dog rule is applicable here since a dead dog neither threatens nor bites. What a dead dog cannot do is to exhibit increased affection, friendliness, and cooperative behavior. In general, the absence of aggression is an inadequate criterion for measuring treatment success, although it is commonly used for such purposes. Instead, the objective of training should be to identify and strengthen behavioral tendencies and activities that are incompatible with aggression. Although punishment may be able to suppress aggression temporarily, it will probably not alter the motivational pressures causing aggression and may make the problem much worse and more difficult to resolve in the long run. Consequently, success should not be gauged by the absence of aggression, but by an increase of target activities that are motivationally and behaviorally incompatible with aggression.

Many other undesirable behaviors undergoing modification through positive and negative reinforcement procedures are often improperly assessed in violation of the dead-dog rule. For example, the goal of house training is most frequently described in terms of an absence of household elimination rather than the objective of training a dog to eliminate exclusively outdoors. The former violates the dead-dog rule (a dead dog does not eliminate indoors), but the latter formulation is in agreement with the dead-dog rule, that is, a dead dog cannot be expected to eliminate exclusively outdoors. Certainly, it is useful to count elimination incidents indoors and prevent or discourage their occurrence, but the primary focus of assessment and modification should be directed toward training the dog to eliminate outdoors.

TRAINING PLAN

The training plan addresses both antecedents as well as consequences believed to control the expression of unwanted behavior. In addition to assessing and altering unwanted behavior, trainers are also concerned with using antecedents and consequences to shape and control more desirable alternative behavior.

Evaluating the Training Plan

Obtaining baseline information is vital for evaluating the effectiveness of the training plan selected. The most common measures of behavioral change are rather informal. Initially, the client is asked such questions as how often, when, and where the target behavior occurs. Then, over the course of the intervention, various measures of change are taken, relying primarily on the client's impressions about the strength and frequency of the unwanted behavior. As previously discussed, a valuable baseline measure can be obtained by assessing the amount of deviation or dissonance between the owner's expectations of the dog's behavior and what the dog actually does. In general, a high degree of expectancy dissonance is correlated with client expressions of distress and disapproval, whereas a low degree of expectancy dissonance is reflected in expressions of pleasure and acceptance of the dog. Instruments used to assess expectancy dissonance also offer an objective means to quantify subtle interactive shifts between the owner and dog—changes that may otherwise pass undetected by other methods of quantification.

Methods of Measuring Behavior

These approaches are often adequate for practical purposes, but sometimes more detailed and careful measures and analyses are needed. Behavioral change can be quantified by directly measuring behavior. Five methods for measuring behavior are employed: event recording, emission duration, absence duration, interval recording, and response strength. Event recording refers to the continuous counting of every occurrence and duration of the target behavior over the course of some fixed period of time. For example, before a specific training plan is implemented to reduce pulling on the leash, the trainer might count the number of times the dog pulls and record the duration of each pulling episode during a 15-minute walk. If the dog pulls a great deal, however, such measurements of discrete pulling episodes might not be very useful. In this case, the overall time spent pulling might provide more practical information about the target behavior. The target behavior can be expressed in terms of the percentage of time spent pulling. A trainer might not find either of these measures very convenient but instead choose to measure the amount of time during which the dog does not pull.

In cases where a target behavior occurs at a high rate, making counting impractical, or when several target behaviors need to be recorded at the same time, the trainer may prefer to employ an interval-recording strategy. Interval recording involves noting whether the target behavior occurs during a set (often very brief) period. Interval recording does not involve counting actual responses but only records whether the target response(s) occurred during the time interval under observation. In addition to rate and duration, the strength of the target behavior can also be obtained in some cases. For instance, the strength of pulling can be directly measured by attaching a pull-type scale to the leash. After every minute of walking, the trainer can record the amount of pounds of pull pressure exerted by the dog on the leash and then average the results. Such pretraining measurements give trainers an objective baseline of data with which to assess the benefits of the training plan, especially in cases in which such precise recording is needed to document a study evaluating the training procedure. Unless collecting data for

specific research or testing an unproven procedure, most such measurements are roughly recorded in the form of journal notes or impressions that assist in evaluating or adjusting the working hypothesis and training plan.

In contrast to the typical *free-operant* methodology used in the learning laboratory, many dog-training activities involve *discrete-operant* training procedures. In discrete-operant training, a dog's behavior is brought under the control of a specific stimulus event (e.g., cue or command) that sets the occasion for the occurrence of some response and reinforcement. Once the target response is emitted and reinforced, the dog must wait to be released or signaled to perform some other task. Most obedience exercises are trained by using a discrete-trial methodology. In the case of free-operant training, the animal is free to respond at any time before or after reinforcement is delivered, although in practice the pattern of responding is strongly influenced by the schedule of reinforcement employed by the experimenter. Free-operant responding is measured in terms of frequency or rate. Rate of response is determined by recording the number of times the response occurs within a given period. Discrete-trial behavior is quantified in terms of a probability relationship based on the number of opportunities the dog has to respond and the number of times the appropriate response occurs. For example, if a dog responds 6 of 12 times it is signaled to sit, the probability of sitting is estimated by dividing 12 into 6, or 0.5 (i.e., he sits 50% of the time). In everyday practice, such calculations are rarely made regarding the performance of obedience exercises, but this method is useful for quantifying obedience training when a stringent measure is required.

Single-subject Designs for Assessing Behavioral Change

In addition to expectancy-dissonance measures, there are several general strategies for estimating the benefits of training and the efficacy of the procedures used to control behavior, but all require some careful baseline measurements in order to generate a valid comparison between pretraining behavior and posttraining behavior. Once a baseline is established, the training plan can be implemented and its influence measured at various points. In other words, the target behavior (dependent variable) is measured prior to the implementation of the training plan and then, again, after the training procedure (independent variable) under consideration has been employed. Changes in the strength or frequency of the target behavior presumably reflect an effect produced by the training procedure.

The single-subject design utilizes a dog's behavior as its own control for evaluating the benefits of training and counseling. In the single-subject design, baseline measures or A phase of the target response are compared with a training or B phase. Under conditions in which the effect of the training procedure is being stringently evaluated, the B phase is followed by the withdrawal of the training procedure (extinction or test A phase) or A-B-A (Figure 2.4). However, removing an effective training procedure is not an acceptable option when working with a family dog,

especially in cases involving a serious behavior problem. Under normal training conditions, involving week-to-week sessions, each training session involves a distinct A phase and B phase, followed by a week interval during which the client practices the procedures with the dog—an extended B phase (EXT-B). The following week, a second assessment or A phase and another treatment or B phase is carried out. Finally, a third assessment and treatment phase is added to the process with the final session. The overall training program takes the form: A-B-(B-EXT)-A-B (EXT-B)-A-B-(EXT-B). . . Follow-up (Figure 2.5).

If the training plan is working effectively, each successive baseline measure should show significant improvement over the prior week. If improvement does not appear from week to week, then the training hypothesis and plan should be appropriately adjusted and reevaluated. Over the course of 3 weeks of training, a dog's behavior should exhibit a consistent trend toward improvement, that is, show

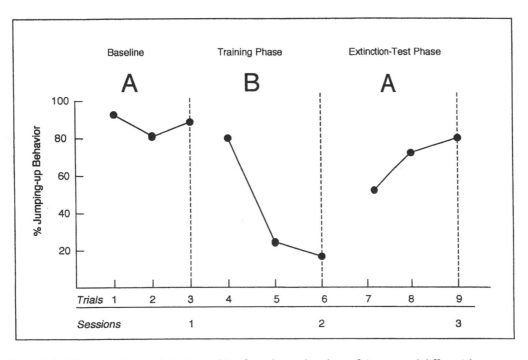

FIG. 2.4. Changes in jumping behavior resulting from the combined use of time-out and differential reinforcement of other behavior. The B or training phase indicates a strong reduction in jumping relative to baseline levels, whereas the test-extinction phase shows that jumping behavior recovers when the training procedures are discontinued.

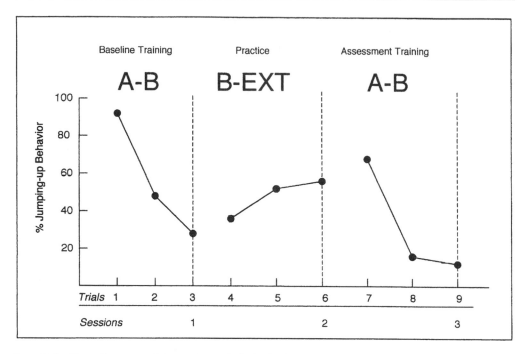

F IG. 2.5. Normally, every training session includes both a baseline phase and a training phase, with an extended B or practice phase between sessions.

evidence of less unwanted behavior and more desirable alternative behavior. Ideally, a monotonic learning curve climbs most steeply from week 1 to week 2 (acquisition phase), and more modest improvement continues between weeks 2 and 3 (adaptation phase), with gradual progress toward asymptotic levels (steady phase) after week 3 (Figure 2.6). The working hypothesis and the efficacy of the training procedures used are further validated by applying them to a larger sample of dogs exhibiting similar presenting signs. If a similar benefit is observed, then there is a high likelihood that the working hypothesis and training plan are producing an effect that is generalizable to other dogs with similar problems.

Although single-subject experimental designs [e.g., AB/AB reversal, multiple baseline, and alternating treatments—see Chance (1998) and Bellack and Hersen (1977)] and related assessment techniques are frowned upon by some researchers who demand a stringent statistical analysis of data, the techniques do offer a relatively simple way for dog behavior counselors and trainers to get a gen-

eral picture of the effectiveness of an untested or questionable methodology. Such assessment techniques can be usefully employed to collect, evaluate, and report such behavioral data. From such information, reasonable hypotheses may then be formulated and, perhaps, tested in a more rigorous fashion.

The foregoing assessment techniques can be applied in a formal or informal manner, depending on the trainer's purposes or needs for collecting such data. These experimental methods and others are absolutely indispensable in canine behavioral research conducted to evaluate and compare the relative efficacy of various training and behavior therapy procedures. Unfortunately, very little such data and validation currently exists in the applied animal behavior literature. Most available reports to date consist of case studies in which complex behavioral interventions, involving a number of procedural elements (e.g., various behavior modification procedures or drugs), are assessed by obtaining clients' impressions of their dog's improvement. Such reports are typically descriptive narratives that include signalment,

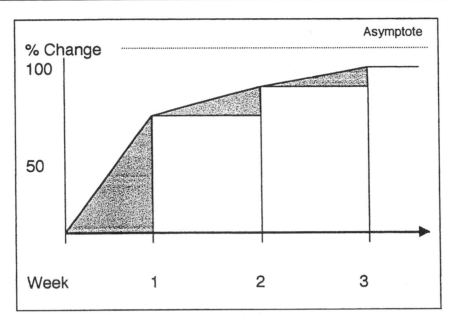

FIG. 2.6. The typical learning curve shows rapid acquisition, followed by more gradual adaptation and steady phases of learning.

the presenting behavior, diagnosis, treatment, and results—with virtually no supporting data. Further, few efforts have been made to control the obvious risks of placebo effects or a client's desire to please the experimenter with positive results. Although such information can be useful for stimulating further research, thus far case studies have not accomplished much more than to stimulate the publication of more case studies. The paucity of data is a serious problem for the field of applied animal behavior. Carefully employed single-subject assessment methods offer an excellent starting point for important data-based research.

Compliance

Client compliance depends on a number of factors, including the counselor's ability to convey a confident and knowledgeable attitude, to develop an accurate and convincing assessment of the presenting complaint, and to provide the client family with a treatment program that is minimally intrusive and disruptive. Further, all training recommendations should be realistic for the nonbehaviorist client to perform. *The training plan should be fully understood by the client and involve procedures that are within the ability of family members to apply.* Asking clients to do something that they consider cruel is not likely to be carried out when the counselor leaves the home. Also, recommendations that are impractical in terms of their daily schedule, skills, or knowledge will not result in effective intervention. This imperative for compliance is particularly important when working with children.

To be effective, the training plan must be sensitive to the family's needs and philosophy of discipline. No matter how brilliant and considered the plan, it will inevitably fall on deaf ears and fail if it is not accepted and followed by family members. For example, recommending that all family members withhold all sources of positive reinforcement and social interaction from their dog for the rest of its life, except, and only if, the dog sits on command and remains in a sit-stay for some period of time, would represent for many dog owners a rather bizarre, extreme, and unacceptable intrusion upon their autonomy and ability to enjoy their dog. For many owners of problem dogs, the above cure would be significantly harder to live with than the problem itself. Treatment protocols recommending highly restrictive, arbitrary, and unnatural interaction between the owner and dog should be cautiously evaluated. Highly intrusive or aversive recommendations should only be implemented when scientific evidence both supports the treatment's rationale and its efficaciousness and, then, only under circumstances in which less intrusive or aversive means are unlikely to work. Under the protective veil of professional authority and pseudoscience, dog behavior advice having little therapeutic value may succeed in capturing the public's imagination and become widely dispersed. Unfortunately, as a result, more-effective methods may be overshadowed, leaving serious behavior problems untreated or worsened by neglect or mismanagement. Richard Dawkins (1976) has referred to such ideas and practices as *memes:*

> Just as genes propagate themselves in the gene pool by leaping from body to body via sperms or eggs, so memes propagate themselves in the meme pool by leaping from brain to brain via a process which, in the broad sense, can be called imitation. If a scientist hears, or reads about, a good idea, he passes it on to his colleagues and students. He mentions it in his articles and his lectures. If the idea catches on, it can be said to propagate itself, spreading from brain to brain. . . . When you plant a fertile meme in my mind you literally parasitize my brain, turning it into a vehicle for the meme's propagation in just the way that a virus my parasitize the genetic mechanism of a host cell. (192)

Memes are viruslike ideational contagions that seem to survive solely for the sake of their replication and perpetuation by infecting others. Although of questionable value, memes, when sanctioned by authority, can be surprisingly resistant to rational argument and persist despite the absence of scientific merit or proof of efficacy. Unproven, but highly popular, memetic protocols are common in dog training and may function on the level of magical incantations or rituals that may make people feel better with the illusion of accomplishing something. Memetic protocols may make people feel better with the illusion of accomplishing something (placebo effect) but probably do little to change the dog's behavior or to improve the human-dog bond. Whatever con-

ceivable benefits (e.g., establishing deference, enhancing attentional abilities, or increasing impulse control) that might be achieved by the aforementioned sit-stay protocol, such benefits can be obtained by more creative and enjoyable means, including techniques that the average family might be expected to willingly perform. For example, Voith and Borchelt (1982) describe a sit-stay protocol that has enjoyed significant popularity over the years. Although their so-called "nothing in life is free" (NILIF) program emphasizes a sit-stay contingency to promote behavioral compliance, the NILIF program is not promulgated as an absolute or lifelong imperative to ensure the remission of the problem behavior. In general, the significant issue at stake is not sitting and staying per se, but the development of a rule-based structure for facilitating harmonious interaction between the owner and dog. By ensuring that the dog attends to and consistently defers to the owner's directives, the owner's leadership is enhanced while interactive tensions and conflicts are minimized. Compliance training can be accomplished without excessively intruding upon the human-dog bond; in fact, when properly introduced, such training can produce a lasting beneficial effect on the relationship.

In addition to avoiding recommendations that may potentially harm the relationship between family and dog, training recommendations should not present risks of injury to the owner or dog. Although well-timed corrections can be highly effective and expedient, recommendations involving the hitting and hanging of aggressive dogs (Koehler, 1962; Hart and Hart, 1985a) should be avoided. Not only are such methods of questionable efficacy, they may actually significantly worsen the situation if improperly performed and, perhaps, cause the owner to be bitten or cause physical injuries to the dog.

In conclusion, both excessively intrusive and aversive techniques may adversely affect owner compliance or violate humane standards of practice. Cynopraxic trainers should make an effort to conform their training interventions to the LIMA (least intrusive and minimally aversive) principle by employing procedures that represent the least necessary intrusion upon the human-dog bond and cause the dog a minimal amount of discomfort, as necessary to achieve the behavioral objective. Further, training recommendations should do no harm to the human-dog relationship, to the dog, or to the owner in the process of implementing them.

Rather than dictating a one-sided program that cannot be realistically implemented by the family, the cynopraxic counselor should work with the family in a spirit of teamwork to find a common solution. Toward achieving this aim, the counselor should listen to the family's needs and be creative. Just as it is certainly true of dogs, people are individuals possessing unique strengths and weaknesses that need to be recognized and integrated into the training plan. Good cynopraxic counselors know how to work well with both people and dogs.

Follow-up

The last step in the training process is follow-up. Follow-up assessment helps to further confirm or disconfirm the working hypothesis and the training plan, with respect to short- and long-term benefits. Typically, follow-up is neglected by busy trainer-counselors unless clients call for additional help—no news is good news. Mailing a brief follow-up questionnaire 6 months after the last session can be very useful in evaluating the lasting benefits of the intervention, as well as maintaining a good working relationship with clients. When possible, cases involving serious aggression should include a follow-up session after 3–6 months to detect and counter recidivist tendencies. Research efforts designed to evaluate the effectiveness of specific training interventions should always include an assessment of both short-term (3 to 6 months) and long-term (1 to 3 years) benefits.

DESCRIBING AND CLASSIFYING BEHAVIOR PROBLEMS

Rational assessment and intervention require that a dog's behavior problem or disorder be described and classified in scientific terms. Canine behavior problems can be classified according to precipitating etiology, descriptive features, or function, that is, controlling antecedents and consequences. However, as

Medawar [1967, quoted in Tinbergen (1974)] points out, "It is not informative to study variations of behaviour unless we know beforehand the norm from which the variants depart" (1967:109). To assess a dog's behavior properly, an ethogram of normal behavior is a necessary foundation. A dog ethogram is an orderly compilation of what a dog does. Table 2.2 does not pretend to be exhaustive in this regard but serves to provide an abbreviated catalog of significant functional systems and species-typical behavior patterns that are associated with most common behavior problems and disorders. The ethogram borrows from an earlier system devised by Scott (1950).

Significant controversy exists surrounding the notion of abnormal or dysfunctional behavior. Some behavioral practitioners (e.g., applied behavior analysts) eschew the notion of abnormal behavior, asserting that all behavior (normal or otherwise) is foremost a reflection of environmental contingencies (Burch, personal communication, 2000). If behavior appears abnormal, it is not because of some flaw or other cause lurking within the organism, but is the result of "abnormal" contingencies upon which the organism is forced to act and adjust. Many dog behavior consultants and therapists, however, do espouse the view that behavior itself may be abnormal to the extent that it has lost its adaptive function. According to this view, abnormal behavior is characteristically rigid and unresponsive to environmental contingencies, that is, it has lost its adaptive plasticity and efficiency. From a biological perspective, behavior may become abnormal when it is unable to achieve homeostatic equilibrium in response to internal or external stressors (Fraser, 1980). Others describe abnormal behavior in terms of maladaptive behavioral excesses and deficits in which species-typical actions appear under- or overresponsive to environmental stimuli. According to this viewpoint, the animal's abnormal behavior is the result of a complex constellation of adverse cognitive and motivational factors impeding its ability to function properly. Proponents of this perspective are apt to view abnormal behavior as stemming from the disruptive influences of anxiety and fear,

TABLE 2.2. Dog Ethogram

Category and Activity	Problems
Affiliative behavior: All behaviors involved in the formation and maintenance of the human-dog bond [e.g., separation distress, attention seeking, proximity seeking, contact seeking, following, cooperative behavior, social facilitation, staying close (going out and returning back to handler), and obedience to command].	*Excesses:* Overattachment, excessive separtion distress, demanding attention-seeking behavior. *Deficits:* Aloofness, uncooperative, independent.
Appetitive behavior: All patterns of foraging and ingestive activity (e.g., eating and drinking). Caching (burying food and toys).	*Excesses:* Obesity, pica, coprophagy, destructive behavior, digging, compulsion (licking, sucking, air snapping). *Deficits:* Anorexia.
Caregiving (epimeletic behavior): Licking, nursing (standing and laying), anogenital stimulation for elimination, scruff carrying, severing umbilical cord, discipline, regurgitation, protection.	*Excesses:* Pseudopregnancy, excessive care giving (grooming, licking). *Deficits:* Failure to groom, nurse, or otherwise care for young.
Care seeking (et-epimeletic behavior): Jumping up, mouth licking (regurgitation), attention seeking, whining and whimpering, begging, petting demands, pawing, hand and face licking (directed towards humans), submissive crawling up, nuzzling.	*Excesses:* Social instrusiveness, contact dependency, jumping up, begging, excessive attention seeking. *Deficits:* Withdrawn, disinterested, failure to bond.
Competitive ritualization (agonistic behavior): Agonistic pucker, alpha T, standing over, piloerection (hackles), pupillary constriction, stiff-leggedness, direct stare (sometimes with red glow), upright ears, tail cocked above the back line, standing over, pawing, mouthing, jumping up with threat, fang baring. Other behaviors under this heading include growling, snarling, biting (hard and inhibited), snapping, fang whacking, jaw punching, redirected attacks.	*Excesses:* Inappropriate dominance displays toward owner. Aggression in a variety of forms, especially involving attacks during competitive conflicts. Inappropriate reactions to physical control and restraint. *Deficits:* Overly inhibited, shy of contact, difficult to train.
Play: • Agonistic: Mouthing, biting clothing, jumping up • Predatory: Ball play, toy shaking, pouncing • Sexual: Mounting, riding up, pawing • Social: Chase and evade, play bow, tug lay • Solitary: Carrying toy, throwing toy, chase and pouncing, rolling, cynosoliloquy (self-play ritual).	*Excesses:* Uncontrollable or disruptive play involving provocative mouthing and biting, jumping up, and chase games. Excessive exploratory interest in environment, resulting in destructive behavior. *Deficits:* Absence of appropriate play behavior , curiosity and exploratory interest in the environment (*see Exploratory behavior*).
Predatory behavior: Hunting (sniffing, tracking, scanning), stalking, and predatory attack sequence (chasing, catching, shaking kill, choking kill, and other behavior aimed at securing and devouring prey).	*Excesses:* Attacking and killing other animals. *Deficits:* No interest in hunting or pursuing game (hunting dogs).

TABLE 2.2. Dog Ethogram—*continued*

Category and Activity	Problems
Resting and sleeping (shelter seeking): Sprawling, sleeping on back, bow and humpback stretch, curl rest, lateral recumbent, sphinx rest, yawning. Resting and sleeping include various shelter-seeking behaviors and efforts to secure a favorable place to rest (e.g., turning about several times before lying down).	*Excesses:* Sleeping problems, narcolepsy. *Deficits:* Unable to sleep through the night, pacing, vocalization.
Urine marking and identification: Raised-leg urination, squatting, over-marking, scratching.	*Excesses:* Urine marking in the house, excessive raised-leg marking on walks. *Deficits:* Unable to eliminate away from familiar odors, locations, and substrates.
Sexual behavior (courtship): Licking and sniffing ears, mouth, and genitals; mounting, harassing, pawing, riding up, female snapping, roaming, intermale aggression, scent marking, standing with tail averted to the side, intromission and tie.	*Excesses:* Sexual interest directed toward inanimate objects. Mounting exhibited toward humans. *Deficits:* Failure to engage in sexual behavior with conspecifics.
Elimination behavior: Various postures (squatting, standing, leg lifting), defecation, submissive urination, fear-induced defecation and anal release.	*Excesses:* Inappropriate elimination, excitment-submissive urination during greetings, separation-related elimination. *Deficits:* Inhibited eliminating in strange areas, constipation, urinary retention, interfering placement preferences.
Exploratory behavior: Sniffing, digging, chewing, scent rolling, vomeronasal response. Includes all investigative and inquisitive interactions directed toward the physical, biological, and social environment.	*Excesses:* Distractibility, scavenging, boredom-related excesses, searching trash bins, inappropriate social investigation toward humans. *Deficits:* Disinterest, depression (boredom), fear of novelty and unfamiliar situations, reduced play and curiosity.
Fearful behavior: Shaking, pupillary dilation, panting, salivation, urination, ears back, corners of the mouth retracted down and back, tail between the legs, running away, possible antecedent to aggression when escape blocked.	*Excesses:* Panic, phobias, generalized anxiety, psychosomatic disorders, social flight and avoidance. *Deficits:* Lack of appropriate fear (e.g., toward cars or electrical cords).
General motor activity: Walking, running, trotting, loping run, jumping, hopping, "observation jumping," crawling, stalking.	*Excesses:* Hyperactivity, motor stereotypies (whirling, fence running, pacing). *Deficits:* Hypoactivity (depression).
Greeting and departure rituals (active submission, et-epimeletic): Jumping-up, licking, tail wagging, wiggle-waggle display, spinning, play face, sniffing, bringing comfort item, excitement urination, moan howl.	*Excesses:* Intrusive behavior, jumping on guests, excitement urination, interfering with departures. *Deficits:* Disinterest at greetings/departures.

TABLE 2.2. Dog Ethogram—*continued*

Category and Activity	Problems
Packing behavior (allelomimetic): Running together, group defense, rallying around the owner, leader-follower behavior, social-facilitated eating and various other forms of "contagious" behavior.	*Excesses:* Proximity and contact-seeking behavior, overprotective of the group. *Deficits:* Failure to develop appropriate following behavior, aloof, disinterested in coordinated activity (*see Affiliative behavior*).
Submissive ritualization (active): Jumping up (greeting behavior), licking, tail wagging, rubbing against, grabbing with muzzle (see *Care-seeking (et-epimeletic behavior* and *Greeting and departure rituals*).	*Excesses:* Overly submissive and fearful toward people. *Deficits:* Inability to defer to owner or show appropriate appeasement gestures to other dogs.
Submissive ritualization (passive): Licking, lowering of body, averting eye contact, ears back, submissive pucker (corner of mouth), grinning (baring front teeth), lateral recumbency, exposure of inguinal area, yelp, nuzzling, crawling, tail low or between the legs.	*Excesses:* Excessive greeting behavior, obnoxious submission, attention-seeking compulsions. *Deficits:* Reduced social interaction, reserved, distant.
Territorial behavior: Barking, threat and attack, scent marking.	*Excesses:* Threatening and attacking guests and passersby, aggressive toward other dogs, fence fighting, excessive barking. *Deficits:* Lacks normal protective response, reduced alarm barking.
Vocalization: Barking, whining, howling, mewing, "purring," moaning, shrieking, squealing, whimpering, yowling.	*Excesses:* Barking at minimum provocation, barking to control attention, barking and howling at separation. *Deficits:* Mute.

frustration, and irritability. In contrast to the behavior analytical approach, practitioners embracing the cognitive-motivational perspective view the source of dysfunction to reside both within the organism itself and the environment. Finally, some forms of abnormal behavior are clearly the result of pathological conditions operating within the organism (e.g., nervous pointer dogs). Generally, the position held throughout this text is eclectic, combining the strengths of the above orientations as appropriate for pragmatic explanatory purposes. Emphasis, however, is placed on the disruptive influences of unpredictable and uncontrollable environmental conditions on the etiology of dysfunctional or maladaptive behavior.

Adverse environmental conditions exert a disruptive and disorganizing influence on behavior in several ways. First, a routine lack of environmental predictability and controllability is believed to be a significant source of anxiety, frustration, and depression (helplessness). Second, unpredictable and uncontrollable environmental conditions may precipitate persistent and problematic conflict, irritability, and stress, thereby impeding the dog's ability to adapt successfully, perhaps, continuing to exert an adverse influence even after environmental conditions are normalized (autokinesis). Third, a lack of consistent, predictable, and controllable interaction between the owner and dog promotes distrust and exerts a damaging influence on the bonding process.

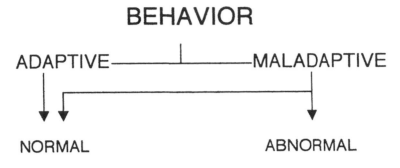

FIG. 2.7. Behavior is broadly categorized as being adaptive or maladaptive. Maladaptive behavior can be either normal or abnormal, depending on its etiology.

Behavioral Diagnostics and Classification

Behavioral diagnostics and the classification of behavior problems involves placing the results of descriptive and functional assessment into the context of specific diagnostic categories. In some cases, classification entails identifying an ethological functional system (or systems) that is adversely affected and expressed in a disorganized, dysfunctional, or maladaptive way (Figure 2.7). This process is impeded by the lack of a uniform and standardized system for classifying dog behavior problems, an especially problematic situation in the case of aggression- and separation-related problems. Some strides have been made toward formalizing such a classification system (Borchelt and Voith, 1981; Odendaal, 1997) but much remains to be done in this critical area.

The functional analysis and classification of behavior problems as diagnostic entities can provide a valuable frame of reference and functional link to relevant intervention strategies and working hypotheses. Behavioral diagnostics can also help one to form reasonable prognostic expectations about treatment outcomes. Despite these potential benefits, caution should be exercised to avoid the intrusion of anthropomorphism and the language of

human psychodiagnostics when classifying dog behavior problems. Superficially, it may help an owner to possess an authoritative-sounding name to refer to his or her dog's behavior problem, but paraphrasing Kierkegaard's words, "To label me is to negate me." *Naming* is a *framing* process, and the act of naming may consequently place the behavioral specifics into a misleading etiological context, thereby potentially impeding effective treatment. Counselors should take extreme care when applying diagnostic terms to dog behavior complaints and to avoid terms possessing vague or anthropomorphic associations borrowed from the lexicon of human psychiatry. In addition to mislabeling and confusion, some diagnoses carry a stigma or connotation that can be very problematic and counterproductive with respect to treatment activities. For example, the label of *dominance aggression* may result in a greater risk that the dog will be euthanized rather than treated, simply because there is no reliable or permanent cure for the problem—an especially sad outcome since no one seems to agree on what is meant by the term *dominance* or how it causes a dog to become aggressive (see Chapter 8). Finally, naming and classifying behavior problems as diagnostic entities may generate the illusion that the behaviors in question are better known or understood than is actually the case. This can be a serious source of confusion. Not only do the causes of many behavior problems remain to be elucidated, most of the behavioral protocols commonly used to treat them have not been scientifically tested or validated.

COMMON ETIOLOGICAL FACTORS UNDERLYING BEHAVIOR PROBLEMS

Biological and Physiological Factors

Many behavior problems surface as the result of underlying disease processes (Parker, 1990; Reisner, 1991). Abrupt mood changes, including heightened irritability and despondency, disorientation, and loss of appetite are possible symptoms of physical disease and should be reported to a veterinarian. Discomfort and physical pain are often associated with depressed affect, increased irritability, and aggressive behavior. Chronic ear infections, hip osteoarthritis, dental conditions, a variety of physical injuries, hypothyroidism, and a great many other medical conditions have been associated with aggressive behavior. It is of great importance, therefore, that a veterinary examination be performed as part of the diagnostic evaluation of unusual or acute displays of aggression. Normal hormonal influences may facilitate the expression of some undesirable sexually dimorphic behavior patterns, such as household micturition, mounting, roaming, and intermale aggression. Elimination problems involving inexplicable loss of control, increased frequency, or "leaking" may indicate the existence of a hormonal imbalance or disease rather than a failure to learn. Under the influence of persistent stress and anxiety, various pathological changes involving the hypothalamic-pituitary-adrenocortical (HPA) system may occur (see *Fear and Biological Stress* in Volume 1, Chapter 3). Besides the release of corticoid hormones, stressful stimulation of the adrenal cortex also stimulates the release of sex hormones. Under chronic anxiety and other stressful conditions, the adrenal glands may become enlarged (adrenal hypertrophy), producing excessive amounts of these various

hormones, perhaps contributing to increased irritability and heightened aggressive tendencies. Bizarre atypical behavior and seizures are often symptomatic of neurological conditions. Severe parasitic infestations have been associated with the development of many behavior problems ranging from heightened irritability to destructiveness. Coprophagia may be associated with advanced pancreatic disease and various nutritional disorders, such as thiamine and other vitamin-B-complex deficiencies. Hyperactivity may result from neurological impairment. Occasionally, the failure of a dog to learn may be due to sensory deficits such as deafness, especially in breeds prone to such ailments. Interestingly, Chapman and Voith (1990) have found little support for the opinion that behavior problems in geriatric dogs are primarily attributable to physical conditions. Geriatric behavior problems are often new and unrelated to previous problems. They found no correlation between a lack of early "appropriate training" and the development of behavior problems in older dogs. Since organic disease may reflect itself in behavioral changes, it is imperative in cases involving severe or unusual behavior problems that appropriate diagnostic testing and thorough veterinary examination precede the initiation of behavioral assessment and training.

A biological factor of considerable importance is genetic predisposition (see *Genetic Predisposition and Temperament* in Volume 1, Chapter 5). Although biological predisposition may incline some dogs to develop abnormal behavior (e.g., nervous pointers), most behavior adjustment problems are a composite of nature (biology) and nurture (experience) influences. So-called clinically abnormal dogs that are unresponsive to training and other management strategies are rather rare. Both normal and abnormal behavior develop within a biological and environmental context. Some severe behavior problems are under a powerful biological influence, which may prove very difficult to control through behavioral means alone. Although these behavior problems may not be fully cured, nearly all of them can be controlled by appropriate behavior modification, training, and appropriate veterinary support. The critical factor is client commitment and compliance.

Dysfunctional Social and Environmental Influences

Although biology most certainly plays a significant role in the development of normal and abnormal behavior, the vast majority of behavior adjustment problems are social (human-dog relationship) problems or environmental (home adaptation) problems. In addition to the predisposing influences of biology, behavior problems develop under the influence of numerous contributory factors, such as environmental stressors, unpredictable and uncontrollable aversive or attractive events, sensory and physiological privations (e.g., boredom and excessive confinement), socialization and environment-exposure deficits, and mistreatment. Under the influence of such adverse conditions, adjustment anomalies can hardly be described as pathological or abnormal. Such dysfunctional behavior, presenting under the influence of destructive or disorganized antecedents and consequences, would be better characterized as normal behavior operating under abnormal or dysfunctional conditions. In short, disorganized contingencies of reinforcement and punishment result in disorganized and dysfunctional behavior.

Most behavior problems respond exceedingly well to cynopraxic and behavioral intervention alone. Such intervention frames and organizes the problem situation so that disorganized antecedents and consequences are reorganized in a way that results in the development of more effective and adaptive behavior. Consequently, unwanted behavior is either modified or replaced with more acceptable behavior.

Deprivation and Trauma

Early socialization and environmental exposure play important roles in the development and mastery of basic social skills, confidence, and health. Inadequate access to experience of this kind or emotional trauma occurring during these early sensitive weeks may lead to the precipitation of persistent emotional effects and behavior deficits. Puppies are most prone to develop phobic reactions early in life, especially during the period running roughly between 8 and 10 weeks of age (see *Learning and Trainability* in Volume 1, Chapter 3). Puppies exposed to intense startle or trauma during this sensitive period for the acquisition of conditioned fear are at risk of developing lifelong phobias. For example, a single bee sting may have far-reaching impacts on an adult dog's comfort and quality of life. Puppies commonly play with bees, some even catching and eating them, apparently oblivious to their prey's painful objections. Yet, under the right conditions (e.g., the stress of being left alone), a puppy who is stung in an especially sensitive area may develop a pronounced fear of bees that is easily generalized to the fluttering sounds and movements of other flying insects as well, perhaps, in addition, precipitating a pattern of excessive worry and anxiety when left alone. Such fear can be emotionally crippling and detrimental to the dog's future as a working dog or companion, with the generalized fear of insects becoming an almost constant source of fearful discomfort, sympathetic arousal, and anxious vigilance during spring and summer months.

Such naturally occurring traumatic events are hard to entirely guard against, but many of the traumas that produce lasting negative behavioral effects are preventable. Just as many children are abused with physical punishment, puppies are often subjected to brutal punitive actions by the hand of angry owners. Crushing beatings followed by long hours of isolation in the name of behavioral control are not only cruel but totally unjustifiable. Dogs exposed to such treatment may present behavioral signs indicative of post-traumatic stress disorder (PTSD) and learned helplessness (LH), but some dogs, even despite the most abusive treatment, are extraordinarily resilient and may not show any significant signs of detriment as the result of abuse (Fisher, 1955). Temperament appears to play a significant protective or facilitatory role in the expression of disturbed behavior (see *Learning and Behavioral Disturbances* in Volume 1, Chapter 9). Behavioral signs of PTSD and LH include increased irritability and reactivity, anxious vigilance (increased sensitivity to startle), irrational fearful reactions, explosive-impulsive behavior (aggression occurring under minimal provocation), hypoactivity or hyperactivity, social withdrawal and avoidance, depressed mood, decreased motivation, learning and training deficits, and lack of normal responsiveness to routine discipline. These symptoms often worsen with the passage of time, with affected dogs appearing hyperactive and distracted but at the same time remaining socially withdrawn and insular. Some dogs may exhibit exaggerated and compulsive efforts to make physical contact but overshoot the mark and fail to obtain what they appear to so desperately need. Consequently, even though they may be socially demanding and demonstrative, their efforts never connect with their owners in a satisfying way. Paradoxically, such intrusive excesses appear to reflect a dysfunctional coping mechanism designed to maintain social distance and avoidance rather than to maximize social contact and comfort.

Social isolation and sensory deprivation have been frequently implicated in the development of various emotional and cognitive disorders (Scott and Fuller, 1965). Many dogs spend long dreary days and nights locked in basements or confined to empty crates. Under such conditions, dogs may be stressed and inclined to develop a variety of behavior problems. Further, crate confinement is often used to control dogs that are the most incompatible with restraint by crating. For active and curious young dogs, crate confinement may produce significant frustration and distress, leading to compensatory excesses when they are released. In such cases, the crate provides a hub for a daily round of frustration and distress, followed by heightened excitability and hyperactivity, leading to punishment and more confinement, isolation, and so on. Long periods of solitary confinement to an unsocialized part of the house (e.g., in the basement or garage) should be avoided. As a rule, if a dog needs to be crated, it should be done in a part of the house where it normally spends time with people when not confined, usually the kitchen or bedroom. In addition, dogs that by necessity must be routinely left alone for long periods should be provided with a dog companion. Clark and colleagues (1997) reported that although the provision of out-of-cage exercise had little effect on

immune function and cortisol measures of stress, behavioral measures indicated that single housing may adversely affect canine well-being. Finally, single housing may promote nonsocial repetitive behavior (e.g., pacing and circling) and sustained efforts to increase sensory input, perhaps in an effort to stave off boredom (Hubrecht et al, 1992).

Although a crate can be a useful training tool, it is too often used as an alternative to proper training and may become a way of life for problem dogs—a steel straitjacket! The use of crate confinement should always signify that some active and purposeful training is being accomplished by its implementation and, further, a plan is in place to ensure that the dog is eventually released from such close quarters—a philosophy of crate confinement referred to as *constructive confinement*. Admittedly, some dogs appear to adjust well to life in a crate, and, in other cases, it is justified as a means to control an ongoing behavior problem, especially in cases involving destructive behavior or house-training difficulties. In such cases, it may be necessary to confine the dog by crating to prevent injury or damage to household belongings. In general, though, a crate should not be used in a cavalier manner or employed for everyday confinement without good reason.

Dogs need daily attention. They thrive on the variety and stimulation provided by social contact, long walks, and structured activities like obedience training and ball play. Dogs are first and foremost social animals whose primary identity is experienced in their immediate social relations and cooperative activities. If they need to be left alone for long periods during the day, then efforts should be made to ensure that they obtain sufficient social attention, exercise, and environmental stimulation when the family returns home from school or work. Unfortunately, this rather obvious obligation is often forgotten in the busy modern family, and the dog's needs are neglected. This passive neglect can exert a very destructive effect on a dog's behavior and cause it to become marginalized over time. The combination of crate confinement and neglect may adversely affect the bond between the owner and the dog. Patronek and colleagues (1996) found that dogs confined to crates were at an increased risk of relinquishment to animal shelters:

> Dogs that spent most of the day in the yard or in a crate were at an increased risk for relinquishment. Because of the retrospective nature of this study, it was not possible to determine whether dogs were relegated to the yard or a crate as a result of behavioral problems or whether keeping dogs in these situations resulted in isolation from the family, less attachment, and less training, thereby increasing the risk of relinquishment. Because crates are commonly recommended to the novice dog owner as a training or behavior management device, determining whether crates are being use appropriately in specific situations is important. (579)

In approximately a third of cases in which dogs were relinquished, owners commented that keeping a dog was much more work than they had expected. Other significant risk factors identified by the study include

- Failure to participate in obedience classes after acquisition
- Lack of routine veterinary care
- Sexually intact status
- Inappropriate care expectations
- Dogs obtained from a shelter
- Dogs acquired after 6 months of age

Interestingly, with respect to dogs with behavior problems, getting good advice appears to make a big difference. Owners who received helpful advice were 94% less likely to give up their dogs than were owners who had received bad advice. The study should give one pause to consider the potential consequences of recommendations, knowing that bad advice may have life-threatening implications.

Excessive Indulgence

Just as neglect and isolation may exert an adverse influence, excessive or inappropriate contact and indulgence can also contribute to the development of maladaptive behavior. Although the role of anthropomorphic attitudes and spoiling activities in the etiology of behavior problems is controversial (Voith et al., 1992; O'Farrell, 1995; Jagoe and Serpell, 1996), given the robust effects of learning and socialization on behavior, it is reasonable to assume that noncontingent reinforcement

(spoiling) and dependency-enhancing activities (pampering) would lead to some problematical long-term cognitive and behavioral effects. In fact, Vilmos Csányi and colleagues (Topál et al., 1997; Douglas, 2000), at Eötvos Lóránd University in Budapest, have reported evidence suggesting that heightened social dependency may impede a dog's ability to function independently, thereby impairing its problem-solving abilities. They found that anthropomorphic attitudes as measured by questionnaires were highly correlated with a dog's relative success at solving problems without help. When performing a simple problem-solving test, dogs most closely bonded with their owners tended to perform worse than dogs having a less intimate bond. Although moderate amounts of spoiling and pampering are probably not detrimental, excessive dependency-enhancing interaction may adversely affect a puppy's development, perhaps facilitating the development of certain behavioral deficiencies and problems. Overly dependent dogs appear to fixate developmentally and remain "perpetual puppies": they may fail to develop adultlike attentional and impulse control abilities, lack appropriate skills (e.g., delay of gratification) needed to cope with frustrative situations, respond maladaptively to anxious arousal, and, finally, are often prone to exhibit disruptive separation-related behavior when left alone. Since overly indulgent owners may fail to address assertive or threatening behavior properly, these incipient signs of developing aggression may be allowed to develop into a more serious and intractable problem.

Unfortunately, the dearth and quality of relevant research makes it difficult to make any hard and fast statements about the role of rearing practices on the development of behavior problems; however, it is reasonable to assume that excessive indulgence (spoiling and pampering) does exert some adverse influence on development and should be avoided. One is inclined to conclude that indulgent excesses in the direction of social permissiveness, on the one hand, and excessive dependency-enhancing activities, on the other, may contribute to the development of dominance- and separation-related problems in susceptible dogs—problems that tend to appear as they reach adulthood. Although indulgent and permissive rearing practices may not represent the *sufficient conditions* under which serious behavior problems develop, such practices may represent significant *necessary conditions* influencing the incubation and expression of such problems in genetically predisposed dogs. Further, given that such problems do occur, a history of permissiveness may make such problems more difficult to manage or control through behavioral means. Conversely, the presence of good rearing practices may be *necessary* for the development of well-adjusted dogs, but good rearing practices alone may not be *sufficient* to prevent the development of a serious behavior problem. In addition to avoiding indulgent excesses, the owner should be encouraged to incorporate sound rearing practices, including integrated compliance training, handling and desensitization activities (e.g., massage), and exposing the puppy to varied environments involving different people and other dogs.

Inappropriate Play and Bootleg Reinforcement

Many behavior problems can be traced to inappropriate play. Permissiveness toward undesirable puppy excesses like mouthing, jumping up, and teasing displays often lead to persistent problems later. Although there appears to exist a significant independence between aggressive play (e.g., tug games) and serious aggression (Podberscek and Serpell, 1997; Goodloe and Borchelt, 1998), excessive and aggressive tug-of-war and chase games may inadvertently elevate a puppy's relative competitiveness, increase its aggressive readiness, and gradually cultivate its confidence to act out aggressively toward humans (Netto et al., 1992). Hard agitational tug games not only develop aggressive readiness and confidence, they also encourage puppies to bite hard and to struggle with a human opponent. Puppies being raised for bite work as police or military working dogs are routinely agitated with rag play, thereby promoting aggression that is gradually and systematically shaped through various stages into a full attack response. Essentially, such efforts are designed

to facilitate aggression toward people through the confidence-building safety of play.

Despite the risk associated with excesses, not all competitive play should be discouraged, however. Structured and pacifying tug games can perform a useful role in the control of playful aggression, the promotion of bite inhibition, and control over aggressive impulses. To make such play constructive and avoid untoward side effects, the owner should always initiate play, control the direction and intensity of play, and teach the puppy to release the tug object (usually a ball with length of rope) on command, thereby promoting impulse control and deference. Once the object is released, the competitive phase of the play is concluded and is immediately followed by the cooperative phase of the game. The cooperative phase consists of tossing the ball a short distance and encouraging the dog to return with it. The owner either proceeds to initiate additional tug activity or trades a piece of food for the ball. Signs of excessive aggressive effort or unwillingness to release the toy should be appropriately discouraged.

Chase games are also notorious for establishing competitive interaction and serving as a staging ground for more serious problems later. Problems deriving from chase-and-catch games often begin innocently as part of routine play in which the owner chases the puppy while the latter has a toy. Gradually, the innovative puppy discovers that its owner becomes even more excited and "fun" when a sock or stocking is lifted. In time, the puppy discovers that it can outrun its exasperated owner. Perhaps, under the facilitative influence of rag play and other competitive activities that give the puppy permission to bite, combined with species-typical defensive mechanisms, the puppy may at some point growl or snap. This is especially likely to occur from behind a piece of furniture or other similar situations producing a feeling of entrapment. Both agitational tug and chase games tend to increase competitiveness and narrow relative dominance between puppies and owners. It is important to remember in all cases involving competition: *only near equals compete*. Excessive or unstructured competitive play may blur important social boundaries and set into action a chain of events and lasting effects that may predispose puppies to exhibit more problematical behavior as adults. For example, dogs exposed to excessive chase interaction may prove very difficult to train to come when called, and dogs whose primary interaction with humans is playful may not appropriately limit social excesses when required to do so.

Early learning strongly impacts on how puppies will behave as adults. Many behaviors that are considered cute tend to be perpetuated and may take on unwanted dimensions as a dog matures. Puppies are often allowed to bark manipulatively or to jump on countertops while their owners are preparing food. Although such behavior may initially present itself as an affirmation of a puppy's good appetite and enthusiasm, the owner often realizes too late how much a nuisance such demanding behavior can be in adult dogs. Occasionally, an owner (or children) may pity the soulful drooping eyes and beckoning drool of a begging puppy at dinnertime, only to establish a persistent habit and nuisance.

Often owners are actually very diligent to reward only desirable behavior and to punish undesirable behavior, but problems still arise in spite of their best efforts. Many factors could be at work in such cases, but inadvertent reinforcement should be considered first. Frequently, a consequence that an owner believes to be aversive is not actually punitive for a puppy or dog. This is also the case with many ostensible rewards that fail to strengthen behavior; simply because we think a puppy or dog should like something does not necessarily mean that it will. Most puppies appear to enjoy petting and praise, but they may not be very willing to work hard for it as a reward. To some extent, the value of petting and praise as a reward may stem from its being paired with the emotional relief produced by the termination of an aversive event (negative reinforcement) or with reassurance that the avoided event is not forthcoming. Romba (1984) has suggested that the primary benefit of petting and praise during avoidance training is to reduce fear and anxiety associated with the process. Although social rewards can be effectively used as positive reinforcers

in their own right (see *Motivation, Learning, and Performance* in Volume 1, Chapter 7), their reliability is enhanced when they are presented in conjunction with tangible rewards, such as food and play. Finally, dogs appear to respond innately to high, repeated tones as attractive sounds and tend to become excited by their presentation, whereas abrupt or drawn-out guttural sounds may be perceived as threatening signals, causing behavioral inhibition (see *Sensory Preparedness* in Volume 1, Chapter 5). As a result, repeated high tones (praise) may be biologically prepared for association with rewarding events, whereas abrupt (reprimand) or low drawn-out (warning) tones may be preferentially associated with punitive outcomes. Properly manipulated, tonal variations of voice can be used very effectively in the control of behavior.

Punitive events can be especially problematic. A puppy's social behavior is driven by two complementary motivations: competition and affiliation. The social impact of these motivational variables is simultaneously to distance the puppy while at the same time enhancing its need for social contact. Most attention-seeking behavior appears to be related to active submission. Because of the motivational connection between attention-seeking and active submission, punishment of excessive attention-seeking behavior may actually frustratingly amplify it, especially if it falls short of evoking passive submission. The synchronic dynamics of attraction and repulsion are consistent with adaptations needed in order to maintain a stable pack organization, where a dominance hierarchy stratifies social relations (a distancing factor) but at the same time minimizes the risk of social disintegration (attraction factor). Problems arise when these variables are present in unbalanced proportions. A puppy driven by excessive dominance testing is independent and prone to develop behavior patterns that threaten social cohesion (the owner rejects it). On the other hand, the attention seeker (actively submissive) is often overly dependent, hyperactive, and prone to become excessively attached and cope poorly when left alone.

A puppy's reliance on attention seeking (active-submission behavior) and dominance testing (competitive interaction) is precisely what it is biologically inclined to do in order to maximize its survival and success in a pack community. Many puppies come into the home with an established social status—hard earned and often vigorously defended. Such *dominant* puppies respond to their owners *provocative* discipline efforts as challenges and react competitively, sometimes exhibiting precocious aggressive reactions together with hard biting. It is very easy for a puppy to slip into a faulty perception of the owner's intentions during punitive interaction. When discipline fails to reach a sufficient threshold, it may be interpreted as a weak challenge by the dominant puppy and countered with oppositional defiance. Other puppies appear to confuse the owner's inadequate disciplinary efforts as an invitation to play and compete. The edge of discipline may be so blunt and ineffectual that puppies may misinterpret its intended meaning. Care must be taken to guard against such frustrating and counterproductive interaction. Such puppies are most effectively managed with a combination of time-outs and instrumental counterconditioning.

Another source of unintentional maintenance of undesirable behavior involves intermittent reinforcement. Many behavior problems are supported by an intermittent schedule of reinforcement occurring concurrently with other training efforts being applied to suppress the unwanted behavior. This is a very common situation, possibly perpetuating a continuous cycle of unnecessary and escalating punishment. For example, most owners of large dogs recognize the need to train them not to jump up. For the most part, such training efforts are carried out conscientiously by owners, but, on some special occasions of affectionate significance, an owner may allow the dog just one exception to the rule. As is the case with any disconfirmed generalization (behavioral or otherwise), the counterexample defines the rule or, at least, undermines the intended rule. Further, if a dog has a strong inclination to jump up, such periodic reinforcement will progressively make it more difficult to extinguish fully. Such dogs are often intermittently reinforced for jumping up by well-meaning but misguided guests who actually encourage and evoke such behavior, leading the dogs to experiment on guests not so inviting of bad canine manners.

Finally, inadvertent or bootleg reinforcement is a frequent problem in family situations where differences of opinion exist regarding an unwanted behavior. For instance, one family member may feel strongly that the dog should not be allowed on furniture while other members enjoy such behavior and allow it in the objector's absence. Occasionally, a dog's behavior becomes a serious source of family tension and disagreement, with the dog suffering inconsistent and abusive treatment. Training requires a united front with a shared sense of purpose and agreement on the behavior being modified. It is for this reason (and many others) that counseling and training are best carried out in the context of the home in the presence of the entire family whenever possible. Behavior counselors should establish a consensus among family members before training proceeds.

CONTROL AND MANAGEMENT OF BEHAVIOR PROBLEMS VERSUS *CURE*

Behavior problems cannot always be cured, but most can be effectively managed and controlled by applying appropriate behavior modification and training efforts. Although the vast majority of behavior problems are responsive to treatment, some problems are *untreatable*. For example, dogs that occasionally bite guests or children without giving recognizable warning signals beforehand pose many difficulties. Such behavior problems are designated untreatable because the results of behavior modification cannot be adequately tested and evaluated without exposing some person to the potential danger of being bitten. Although dogs exhibiting such problems may be managed through careful handling and preventive restraint measures, the absence of other relevant behavior (e.g., threats) with which to infer a dog's level of aggressive arousal and likelihood of attack precludes the possibility of making reliable judgments about the relative effectiveness of treatment efforts.

One is left only with the absence of aggressive episodes or reduced magnitude of aggression (behavior that may still do significant damage) to judge progress. In both cases, assessment of treatment success depends on exposing the dog to potential victims (without possessing a reliable indicator of attack likelihood) and assessing success by the absence of attack during such potentially aggressive contacts. Obviously, the mere absence of aggressive behavior is not an adequate assessment measure (see *Dead-dog Rule*) and should not be used in isolation to evaluate the benefit of training efforts or to predict the future likelihood of attacks. Therapeutic benefit is objectively assessed by the presence of prosocial behavior correlated with safety from aggression. In the case of aggression problems designated as *treatable,* past episodes of aggression present on a highly predictable basis and are regularly preceded by recognizable threat displays or other clear signs of impending attack. Progress in such cases can be more safely inferred by the reduction of active threat displays, by an increase of incompatible affiliative behavior, or other behavioral changes indicating reduced aggressive arousal and a decreased probability of attack.

Most behavior problems can be controlled or managed through a variety of interventions (e.g., training, exercise, nutrition, or medication), environmental alterations, and the manipulation of antecedent variables and reinforcement contingencies controlling the unwanted behavior. Although behavior problems are highly responsive to training, they should not be construed as *curable* in the same sense as an infection might be cured by an antibiotic. Further, behavioral change obtained through behavior modification is reliably maintained only as long as the critical control and management efforts are maintained. Perhaps the greatest obstacle to success is too much improvement occurring too early and rapidly in the training process—a circumstance that may cause the client to become overly complacent and toy with disaster. While there is a strong temptation for both the counselor and client to prematurely congratulate each other on their achievements, it is incumbent upon responsible dog behavior consultants to remind their clients that problems (especially those involving aggression or fear) demand lifelong vigilance and commitment. There are no miracles or magic cures.

The counselor's goal is to educate clients, assess and place the behavior problem into an objective framework, instruct clients in appropriate management and training techniques, establish realistic expectations, and *do no harm.* These general considerations are particularly important when evaluating and making recommendations regarding serious aggression problems. Behavioral counseling and training may help to reduce the likelihood of aggression in the future, but clients should never be misled into believing that their dog's aggression problem can be cured by behavior modification. Although such dogs may never bite again after training, their status remains indeterminate and their recovery a lifelong process of careful management and training. Aggression problems are never cured—even if they are cured!

PART 2: EVALUATION FORMS

CLIENT WORKSHEET

Client Information

Name:

Address:

Phone: H (   )   W (   )   Fax (   )

Appointment: Date   /   /   Time: :

Veterinarian: Ph (   )

Directions:

Signalment

Name: Breed/Mix: Age:

Sex   M ❑   F ❑   Status: Intact ❑   Spayed ❑   Neutered ❑

Other:

Interviews

Telephone:

Home:

DOG BEHAVIOR QUESTIONNAIRE

Date: /   /

Client Information

Name:

Address:

Phone: H (   )   W (   )   Fax (   )

Appointment: Date   /   /   Time: :

Veterinarian: Ph (   )

Directions:

Dog Information

Name: Breed/Mix: Age:

Sex   M ❑   F ❑   Status: Intact ❑   Spayed ❑   Neutered ❑

Age when altered:

Did you notice any short- or long-term changes in your dog's behavior after altering? Was your dog altered because of a behavior problem? If yes, explain:

Are your dog's vaccinations up to date?	Yes ❑	No ❑
Does your dog have any medical conditions? If, yes, please explain?	Yes ❑	No ❑
Is your dog currently given any medications? If, yes, what medications?	Yes ❑	No ❑

Please answer the following questions. All information that you provide is confidential. It is important to answer carefully since the information will be used to help assess your dog's behavior. Please add any additional information as you see fit. If a particular question is not relevant to your dog, mark it N/A.

▶Section 1

How old was your dog when you acquired it?

Has the dog had previous owners?   If yes, explain:

Where did you get your dog? Breeder ❑   Pet store ❑   Animal shelter ❑   Friend ❑   Other ❑

How does your dog spend the majority of its time?

Where is your dog kept outdoors?

How often is your dog exercised?

How long?   More than... 10 minutes ❑   45 minutes ❑   1 hour ❑   2 hours ❑

Briefly describe your dog's daily exercise routine:

When is your dog fed?   AM ❑   PM ❑   Both ❑

What do you feed your dog?   Canned ❑   Dry ❑   Table Scraps ❑   Treats ❑

Describe your dog's feeding habits?   Finicky ❑   Good appetite ❑   Voracious ❑

What are your dog's favorite toys?

What sort of play does your dog enjoy most?   Ball play ❑ Chase games ❑ Tug ❑ Other ❑

Where does your dog sleep?   Bedroom ❑   Kennel ❑   Kitchen ❑   Other ❑

▶Section 2

Please describe the general social layout of the family (e.g., children, other adults,
and animals) and the dog's place in it?

Has your household changed since acquiring your dog?   Yes ❑   No ❑

If yes, please describe:

Does your dog enjoy children: If not, please explain:

Please describe your dog's interaction with other animals in the household:

Describe how your dog reacts to guests and strangers:

Describe your dog's behavior around other dogs:

▶Section 3

Why did you decide to acquire a dog?   Companion ❑   For child ❑   Protection ❑

Describe your dog's behavior as a puppy. Anything unusual?

Why did you choose the breed?

Have you owned other dogs in the past?

▶Section 4

Describe your dog's reaction to being left alone?

Describe your dog's behavior when you return home:

Do you use a crate?   If yes, when did you begin to crate your dog?

How many hours a day is your dog kept in the crate?

Less than... 5 hours ❑   10 hours ❑   15 hours ❑

▶Section 5

Has your dog ever been to obedience school?   Private ❑   Group ❑

How many weeks of training?

What training school or professional trainer/behaviorist did you use?

What training methods or philosophy did the trainer emphasize?

Briefly describe your impressions and benefits from training?

Does your dog come when called?

Will your dog lie down on command?

Does your dog pull when being walked?

Please describe your dog's general attitude and response to obedience training:

▶Section 6

What do you consider to be your dog's most undesirable behavior?

When did you first notice the problem?

Rank the severity of the dog's problem: Mild ❑   Moderate ❑   Severe ❑

How often does the problem occur?   Frequently ❑   Occasionally ❑   Rarely ❑

Has there been a recent change in frequency or severity?   Yes ❑   No ❑

Have there been any changes in the household that could help to explain the appearance of the problem?

What have you done so far to correct your dog's behavior problem?

Why do you think the dog is exhibiting the behavior problem?

▶Section 7

Does your dog exhibit any of the following behavior problems? *(Please circle relevant behaviors and check approximate frequency.)*

	Never	Occasionally	Often
• House soiling (urination, defecation, marking, submissive urination):	❑	❑	❑
• Excessive barking or howling:	❑	❑	❑
• Coprophagia (stool eating, other animal's feces):	❑	❑	❑
• Destructiveness (scratching, chewing, digging):	❑	❑	❑
• Jumping up (on guests or owners):	❑	❑	❑
• Mouthing on hands or clothing:	❑	❑	❑
• Chases (cars, people, other dogs):	❑	❑	❑
• Object and food stealing:	❑	❑	❑
Does the dog attempt to run away when caught?		Yes ❑	No ❑
• Dominance testing (pushy behavior):	❑	❑	❑
• Sexual behaviors (thrusting against humans, inanimate objects, roaming):	❑	❑	❑
• Compulsive habits (paw licking, flank sucking, cloth sucking, whirling, other):	❑	❑	❑
• Overly submissive behavior:	❑	❑	❑
• Fearfulness (shy or phobic reactions):	❑	❑	❑
• Excessive excitability and impulse-control deficits:	❑	❑	❑
• Sleep problems:	❑	❑	❑

Any problems not listed?

1.

2.

3.

▶**Section 8**

Does your dog threaten or exhibit aggression toward family members?   Yes ❏   No ❏

Describe all episodes of aggression (including threats) toward family members:

Does your dog ever react aggressively to grooming and other handling efforts?
(e.g., lifting, moving off furniture)?   Yes ❏   No ❏

Does your dog ever growl while being petted or hugged?   Yes ❏   No ❏

Is your dog aggressive toward nonfamily members?   Yes ❏   No ❏

If yes, please describe all episodes.

Describe your dog's reaction (growls, glares, bares teeth, snaps, barks, bites) under the
following conditions:

	Never	Occasionally	Often
• When eating:	❏	❏	❏
• When playing:	❏	❏	❏
• When chewing on a toy:	❏	❏	❏
• When approached while sleeping:	❏	❏	❏
• When punished:	❏	❏	❏
• When people visit:	❏	❏	❏
• When visitors enter yard:	❏	❏	❏
• When reached for or touched:	❏	❏	❏
• While being put into crate:	❏	❏	❏

Explain:

How old was your dog when it exhibited the first signs of aggressiveness?

Is there anyone who the dog is never aggressive toward?

Does your dog suffer from any physical condition that might explain its aggressiveness?

Is your dog more aggressive toward males or females?

Has your dog ever killed any animals?

Does your dog show signs of fear prior to becoming aggressive?

Describe the severity of past bites:

Describe in detail the last bite incident (what, when, where, why?):

Any additional comments or information that you think I should know?

PUPPY BEHAVIOR PROFILE

Client's name:

Puppy's name: Breed/Mix: Age:

Sex   M ❑   F ❑

Date:

Please respond to the following items by placing an X over the point that most accurately describes your puppy's behavior. In order to give me a clearer picture of what you would like to gain from puppy training, please place an O over the point on the continuum that best represents your ideal.

For example:

                             O   X

NEVER PLAYS   • • • • • / • • • • • TOO PLAYFUL, NEVER STOPS

A. VERY STUBBORN
AND WILLFUL   • • • • • / • • • • •   EXTREMELY
COOPERATIVE

B. CONSTANTLY
BITES   • • • • • / • • • • •   NEVER BITES

C. HARDLY PAYS
ANY ATTENTION   • • • • • / • • • • •   FOLLOWS ME
TO ME   EVERYWHERE

D. AFRAID OF
EVERYONE   • • • • • / • • • • •   LOVES EVERYONE
TO A FAULT

E. NERVOUS
AROUND OTHER   • • • • • / • • • • •   ENJOYS PLAYING
DOGS AND PUPPIES   WITH OTHER DOGS
AND PUPPIES

F. CANNOT WAIT
OR CONTROL   • • • • • / • • • • •   CAN WAIT FOR
ITSELF   PERMISSION IN
MOST SITUATIONS

G. EATS SLOWLY
AND IS FINICKY   • • • • • / • • • • •   GULPS DOWN FOOD
AND WATER

H. CANNOT KEEP
FOCUSED ON   • • • • • / • • • • •   VERY ATTENTIVE IN
ONE THING   MOST SITUATIONS
INSIDE OR OUT

I. CANNOT SIT
STILL   • • • • • / • • • • •   VERY QUIET AND
SLEEPS A LOT

J. EXCITED AND   • • • • • / • • • • •   FRIENDLY BUT
    JUMPS UP ON   NEVER JUMPS UP
    GUESTS   ON GUESTS

K. FEARFUL OF   • • • • • / • • • • •   CONFIDENT IN ALL
    EVERYTHING   SITUATIONS

L. FRETS AND   • • • • • / • • • • •   GOES TO SLEEP
    WHINES EVERY   WITHOUT EVER
    NIGHT   COMPLAINING

M. BECOMES VERY   • • • • • / • • • • •   SHOWS NO
    ANXIOUS WHEN   CONCERN WHEN
    LEFT ALONE   LEFT ALONE

N. GROWLS OR SNAPS   • • • • • / • • • • •   GIVES UP TOYS AND
    WHEN TAKING FOOD   FOOD WITHOUT
    OR TOYS   ANY STRUGGLE

O. PREFERS   • • • • • / • • • • •   LIKES PETTING
    AGGRESSIVE PLAY   AND GENTLE PLAY
    AND CHASE GAMES

P. APPEARS TO   • • • • • / • • • • •   APPEARS VERY
    LEARN VERY   BRIGHT AND
    SLOWLY   LEARNS QUICKLY

Q. ALWAYS RESISTS   • • • • • / • • • • •   ENJOYS LEARNING
    LEARNING   AND APPEARS TO
    ANYTHING NEW   WANT TO PLEASE

R. COMPLETELY OUT   • • • • • / • • • • •   WALKS CALMLY AT
    OF CONTROL,   MY SIDE AND
    PULLS HARD   NEVER PULLS

S. URINATES AND   • • • • • / • • • • •   NEVER HAS ANY
    DEFECATES   ACCIDENTS INSIDE
    EVERYWHERE   THE HOUSE

T. CHEWS EVERYTHING   • • • • • / • • • • •   LIMITS CHEWING
    IN SIGHT   TO TOYS

U. ALWAYS NEEDS TO   • • • • • / • • • • •   LIKES ATTENTION
    BE THE CENTER   BUT CAN DO
    OF ATTENTION   WITHOUT IT

V. COMES ONLY   • • • • • / • • • • •   COMES WHEN
    WHEN FORCED   CALLED

W. RUNS AWAY WHEN   • • • • • / • • • • •   ALWAYS STAYS
    OFF LEASH   NEARBY

PROFILE SCORE SHEET

Client's name:

Puppy's name: Breed/Mix: Age:

Sex   M ❑   F ❑

Date:

The owner's responses to the above items are quantified by giving a numerical value to each of the points on the continuum between 0 and 1. In the case of playfulness:

$$O \qquad X$$

NEVER PLAYS   • • • • • / • • • • • TOO PLAYFUL, NEVER STOPS

PLAYFULNESS: 0.3/0.6, yielding an expectancy divergence of 0.3.

                                        BEFORE TRAINING   *AFTER* TRAINING

A. COMPETITIVENESS
B. MOUTHING
C. INDEPENDENCE
D. SOCIALIZATION (PEOPLE)
E. SOCIALIZATION (DOGS)
F. IMPULSE CONTROL
G. APPETITE
H. DISTRACTIBILITY
I.   ACTIVITY LEVEL
J. GREETING RITUAL
K. ADAPTABILITY
L. SEPARATION ANXIETY (NIGHT)
M. SEPARATION ANXIETY (DAY)
N. POSSESSIVENESS
O. AGONISTIC PLAY
P. LEARNING ABILITY
Q. LEARNING ATTITUDE
R. WALKING ON LEASH
S. HOUSE TRAINING
T. DESTRUCTIVENESS
U. ATTENTION SEEKING
V. RECALL
W. FOLLOWING BEHAVIOR

Evaluating the Results

Low scores tend to be characteristic of a well-adjusted, cooperative, and outgoing puppy. High scores may indicate the presence of adjustment problems. Middle-range scores reflect the behavior of the average, balanced puppy. Sharp differences between the owner's assessment of the puppy's behavior and his or her ideal provides a framework from which to develop training plans that focus on relevant target behaviors. The results can be simplified by clustering the various responses around several basic categories of behavior and averaging the scores:

1. COMPETITIVENESS: A, B, F, N, O, R
2. SOCIABILITY: C, D, E, U
3. REACTIVITY: G, H, I, K
4. TRAINABILITY: P, Q, V, W
5. ADJUSTMENT: J, L, M, S, T

PUPPY TEMPERAMENT TESTING AND EVALUATION

The purpose of puppy temperament testing is not intended so much as a tool to prognosticate adult tendencies and behaviors, but to evaluate active behavioral systems as they stand at the time of testing. Temperament tests serve an important function by isolating areas of strength and areas where additional socialization and training are needed. In conjunction with the Puppy Behavior Profile, the temperament test provides an objective means for assessing the puppy's behavioral needs. Temperament tests are carried out by a scorer and a handler (often the owner) working together.

PUPPY TEMPERAMENT TESTING PROCEDURES (HANDLER'S INSTRUCTIONS)

TEMPERAMENT TEST SCORE SHEET

Client's name:

Puppy's name: Date:

A. SOCIAL ATTRACTION (PASSIVE HANDLER)   ►►

The social attraction test determines the puppy's level of interest in people and willingness to interact with them. The passive handler stands and calls the puppy by name and may also clap hands. Further encouragement may be offered by crouching down, but as the puppy approaches, the handler should once again stand upright.

A. SOCIAL ATTRACTION (PASSIVE HANDLER)

1. Comes, jumps up, and bites hands or clothing.
2. Comes happily with tail erect, vigorous contact.
3. Comes immediately with tail down, less contact.
4. Hesitates, but comes with encouragement, little contact.
5. Puppy does not come.
6. Other: ☐

B. SOCIAL ATTRACTION (ACTIVE HANDLER)   ►►

A continuation of the above test but with the handler moving away from the puppy. The handler may encourage the puppy using his name and slapping his or her side. Further encouragement may be given by running in spurts away from the puppy. The passive handler test measure's the puppy's natural willingness to come, whereas the active handler test evaluates this puppy's willingness to follow.

B. SOCIAL ATTRACTION (ACTIVE HANDLER)

1. Follows, bumps, jumps up, bites, easily distracted.
2. Follows enthusiastically, forging out front.
3. Follows but tail lowered, sometimes lagging.
4. Follows only after hesitation, requiring encouragement.
5. Does not follow.
6. Other: ☐

C. CONTACT TOLERANCE ►►

The handler sits cross-legged on the floor and attempts to pet the puppy over its entire body. The handler should examine its ears and mouth, lift the front and rear paws, and stroke the full length of the tail.

C. CONTACT TOLERANCE

1. Vigorously jumps up, claws, and bites.
2. Jumps up, paws, licks, and sometimes bites.
3. Paws and licks, and stands ground.
4. Licks and tends to roll on side.
5. Avoids being petted.
6. Other: ☐

D. PHYSICAL CONTROLS ►►

1. *Jowl control:* The control includes direct eye contact and slight elevation for a second or two.
2. *Stand control:* The puppy is prompted into a stand and restrained in the position for 10 seconds.
3. *Sit control:* From the stand, the puppy is physically prompted into the sit and required to hold the position.
4. *Down control:* The right paw is pulled forward as the handler applies pressure to the puppy's shoulder, causing the puppy to lie down for 10 seconds.
5. *Lateral down:* The puppy is rolled over on its side and held in that position with gentle massage and eye contact for 10 seconds.

D. PHYSICAL CONTROLS (JOWL, STAND, SIT, DOWN, DOMINANT-DOWN).

1. Struggles vigorously with biting and clawing.
2. Struggles and bites.
3. Struggles but does not bite.
4. Calms down after a brief struggle.
5. Accepts control without struggle.
6. Other: ☐

Physical controls give a fairly accurate picture of the puppy's relative competitiveness. The controls are carried out in such a way that the puppy is mildly challenged and given the opportunity to react competitively or to accept the prompting with cooperation and subordination.

E. IMPULSE CONTROL ►►
(POSSESSIVENESS)

The puppy is provided with a fresh beef bone (or equally appealing alternative). After allowing the puppy to chew on it for a while, the handler (carefully) attempts to take it away.

E. IMPULSE CONTROL
(POSSESSIVENESS)

1. Sustained growling and snapping.
2. Protects object with growling.
3. Holds object but releases with muzzle hold.
4. Releases object on verbal request.
5. Shows no interest in object.
6. Other: ☐

F. IMPULSE CONTROL ►►
(DELAY OF GRATIFICATION)

The puppy is observed while required to stand quietly waiting for the presentation of a treat. Next, the puppy is required to take the treat gently.

F. IMPULSE CONTROL
(DELAY OF GRATIFICATION)

1. Sustained lunging and jumping.
2. Lunging and jumping but soon controls impulse.
3. Jumps but quickly settles and waits.
4. Sits or stands quietly for the treat.
5. Will not take the treat.
6. Other: ☐

G. BALL PLAY ▶▶

The puppy is briefly teased with a tennis ball before it is tossed. Each puppy is given three opportunities and graded on the best outcome.

G. BALL PLAY

1. Fetches the ball, but runs away or teases with it.
2. Fetches the ball, but does not bring it back.
3. Fetches the ball, and brings it straight back.
4. Runs after the ball, but does not pick it up.
5. Ignores the ball.
6. Other: ☐

H. RAG PLAY ▶▶

A strip of burlap is wiggled and dragged away from the puppy. If the puppy takes the rag, it is engaged in a brief tug game. The puppy is offered a treat in exchange for releasing the rag.

H. RAG PLAY

1. Takes rag with aggressive growling and will not let go.
2. Takes rag immediately, sustained growling and tugging.
3. Takes rag and tugs, releases on verbal request.
4. Follows the rag but does not take it.
5. Ignores the rag.
6. Other: ☐

I. SEPARATION REACTION ▶▶

The puppy is put in a separate room for 1 minute. The puppy is distracted from barking before being let out.

I. SEPARATION REACTION

1. After _____ seconds, intense distress vocalization and sustained and frantic efforts to escape.
2. After _____ seconds, vocalizes with scratching or digging to escape.
3. After _____ seconds, whines and paws but calms down after _____ seconds.
4. After brief distress, quickly calms down.
5. No reaction.
6. Other: ☐

J. REACTIVITY AND PROBLEM SOLVING (BARRIER FRUSTRATION) ▶▶

The puppy is placed behind a wire barrier that it must go around in order to obtain a highly desirable treat placed in its view and to make contact with the handler.

J. REACTIVITY AND PROBLEM SOLVING (BARRIER FRUSTRATION)

1. Intense distress followed by futile efforts to go through the barrier.
2. Distress followed by several unsuccessful attempts to solve the problem.
3. Some initial distress, but calms down and solves the problem.
4. Shows little distress and solves the problem quickly.
5. No reaction.
6. Other: ☐

K. STARTLE REFLEX

►►

K. STARTLE REACTION

The handler drops a shaker can behind the puppy about 5 feet away. The puppy is reassured afterward and observed for its initial reaction as well as its speed of recovery.

1. Barks at the handler.
2. Holds ground and stares at the handler.
3. Crouches down but quickly recovers and approaches.
4. Cowers, recovers slowly and retreats.
5. Frightened and runs away.
6. Other: ☐

Notes and comments:

Recommendations:

REFERENCES

Askew HR (1996). *Treatment of Behavior Problems in Dogs and Cats: A Guide for the Small Animal Veterinarian.* Cambridge, MA: Blackwell Science.

Bellack AS and Hersen M (1977). *Behavior Modification: An Introductory Textbook.* New York: Oxford University Press.

Borchelt PL and Voith VL (1982). Classification of animal behavior problems. *Vet Clin North Am Symp Anim Behav,* 12:625–635.

Chance P (1998). *First Course in Applied Behavior Analysis.* New York: Brooks/Cole.

Chapman BL and Voith VL (1990). Behavioral problems in old dogs: 26 cases (1984–1987). *JAVMA,* 196:944–946.

Clark JD, Rager DR, Crowell-Davis S, and Davis DL (1997). Housing and exercise of dogs: Effects on behavior, immune function, and cortisol concentration. *Lab Anim Sci,* 47:500–510.

Danneman PJ and Chodrow RE (1982). History-taking and interviewing techniques. *Vet Clin North Am Symp Anim Behav,* 12:587–592.

Dawkins R (1976). *The Selfish Gene.* New York: Oxford University Press.

Douglas K (2000). Mind of a dog. *New Scientist,* http://www.newscientist.com/features.jsp?id=ns 22281.

Fraser AF (1980). *Farm Animal Behaviour.* London: Bailliere Tindall.

Goodloe LP and Borchelt PL (1998). Companion dog temperament traits. *J Appl Anim Welfare Sci,* 1:303–338.

Fisher AE (1955). The effects of early differential treatment on the social and exploratory behavior of puppies [Unpublished doctoral dissertation]. University Park: Penn State University.

Hart BL and Hart LA (1985). *Canine and Feline Behavioral Therapy.* Philadelphia: Lea and Febiger.

Hubrecht RC, Serpell JA, and Poole TB (1992). Correlates of pen size and housing conditions on the behaviour of kennelled dogs. *Appl Anim Behav Sci,* 34:365–383.

Hunthausen W (1994). Collecting the history of a pet with a behavior problem. *Vet Med,* 89:954–959.

Jagoe JA and Serpell JA (1996). Owner characteristics and interactions and the prevalence of canine behaviour problems. *Appl Anim Behav Sci,* 47:31–42.

Koehler W (1962) *The Koehler Method of Dog Training.* New York: Howell.

Lindsley OR (1991). From technical jargon to plain English for application. *J Appl Behav Anal,* 24:449–458.

Medawar PB (1967). *The Art of the Soluble.* London: Methuen.

Netto WJ, Van der Borg JAM, and Sleger JF (1992). The establishment of dominance relationships in a dog pack and its relevance for the man-dog relationship. *Tijdschr Diergeneeskd,* 117(Suppl 1):51S–53S.

Odendaal JSJ (1997). A diagnostic classification of problem behavior in dogs and cats. *Vet Clin North Am Prog Companion Anim Behav,* 27:427–443.

O'Farrell V (1995). The effect of owner attitudes on behaviour. In J Serpell (Ed), *The Domestic Dog.* New York: Cambridge University Press.

Parker JP (1990). Behavioral changes of organic neurologic origin. *Prog Vet Neurol,* 1:123–131.

Patronek GJ, Glickman LT, Beck AM, et al. (1996). Special report: Risk factors for relinquishment of dogs to an animal shelter. *JAVMA,* 209:572–581.

Podberscek AL and Serpell JA (1997). Environmental influences on the expression of aggressive behaviour in English cocker spaniels. *Appl Anim Behav Sci,* 52:215–227.

Reisner I (1991). The pathophysiologic basis of behavior problems. *Vet Clin North Am Adv Companion Anim Behav,* 21:207–224.

Romba JL (1984). *Controlling Your Dog Away from You.* Aberdeen, MD: Abmor.

Scott JP (1950). The social behavior of dogs and wolves: An illustration of sociobiological systematics. *Ann NY Acad Sci,* 51:1009–1021.

Scott JP and Fuller JL (1965). *Genetics and the Social Behavior of the Dog.* Chicago: University of Chicago Press.

Serpell JA (1996). Evidence for an association between pet behaviour and owner attachment levels. *Appl Anim Behav Sci,* 47:49–60.

Tinbergen N (1974). Ethology and stress diseases. *Science,* 185:20–27.

Topál J, Miklósi A, and Csányi V (1997). Dog-human relationship affects problem solving behavior in the dog. *Anthrozoös,* 10:214–224.

Voith VL (1980). Anamnesis. *Mod Vet Pract,* 61:460–462.

Voith VL and Borchelt PL (1982). Diagnosis and treatment of dominance aggression in dogs. *Vet Clin North Am Small Anim Pract,* 12:655–663.

Voith VL and Borchelt PL (1985). Separation anxiety in dogs. *Compend Continuing Educ Pract Vet,* 7:42–53.

Voith VL and Borchelt PL (1996). History taking and interviewing. In VL Voith and PL Borchelt (Eds), *Readings in Companion Animal Behavior.* Trenton, NJ: Veterinary Learning Systems.

Voith VL, Wright JC, Danneman PJ, et al. (1992). Is there a relationship between canine behavior problems and spoiling activities, anthropomorphism, and obedience training? *Appl Anim Behav Sci,* 34:263–272.

Von Goethe, J W (1901). *The Tragedy of Faust, Works of Johann Wolfgang Von Goethe.* Anna Swanwick (Trans). New York: WI Squire.

Fears and Phobias

"Fear of" is generally "fear about" something. Since fear has this characteristic limitation—"of" and "about"—the man who is afraid, the nervous man, is always bound by the thing he is afraid of or by the state in which he finds himself. In his efforts to save himself from this "something" he becomes uncertain in relation to other things; in fact, he "loses his bearings" generally.

MARTIN HEIDEGGER, *What Is Metaphysics?* (1945)

INCIDENCE OF FEAR-RELATED BEHAVIOR PROBLEMS

Behavior problems often present with some collateral element of aversive emotional arousal, especially fear, anger, anxiety, or frustration. A national survey performed by Goodloe and Borchelt (unpublished data— see Voith and Borchelt, 1996) found that fear is a common emotional factor motivating dog behavior. The dog-owner respondents were asked to indicate whether their dog exhibited signs of fear "sometimes, often, or always" in various social and nonsocial situations. Of the 2018 dog-owning respondents, 38% indicated that their dog exhibited some amount of fear toward loud noises, 22% reported observing fear toward unfamiliar adults, 33% of the dogs were fearful toward unfamiliar children, and 14% exhibited fear toward unfamiliar (nonthreatening) dogs. Previously, Campbell (1986) surveyed 1422 dog owners about their dog's behavior. The information was obtained from a questionnaire provided to clients at various veterinary hospitals in California. His findings indicated that 20.2% of the respondents observed some degree of fear toward noises, especially in dogs who were over 3 years of age. Statistical reports from animal behavior clinics show considerable variation in the incidence of fear as a behavioral complaint. For example, records from the Animal Behavior Clinic at the University of Pennsylvania (1984 to 1987), indicate that 7% of 489 dogs presenting a behavioral problem exhibited a fear of noises, with 4.3% of the group exhibiting fear toward people (Voith et al., 1993). At the University of Tennessee, Shull-Selcer and Stagg (1991) reported that 30% of the cases they treated at the animal behavior clinic were fear related. Approximately 20% (N = 154 consecutive cases) of the dogs treated by Askew (1996) exhibited fear as a major behavior problem. These figures are in sharp contrast to those reported by Beaver (1994), who found that fear presented in only 1.4% of 855 cases seen at the Texas A&M veterinary behavior clinic.

ASSESSMENT AND EVALUATION OF FEAR-RELATED PROBLEMS

A thorough behavioral history should be recorded and appropriate questionnaires completed by the dog owner. Assessment profiles generally indicate the involvement of one or more of the following etiological factors: (1) genetic or neurobiological predisposition, (2) early socialization or environmental exposure deficits, or (3) aversive or dysfunctional learning. Also, since a variety

of underlying medical conditions [e.g., hypothyroidism (Aronson, 1998)] can present symptoms that include apprehensiveness and fear, dogs presenting with fear-related problems suspected of being associated with a physical cause should be referred for veterinary examination. Dogs that are affected by a genetic predisposition are distinguished by a chronic, lifelong, and generalized fearfulness. Such dogs often suffer heightened or extreme sensitivity to sensory input and may habitually overreact to unfamiliar situations. Differentiating a genetic predisposition from socialization or exposure deficits is not always easy, since these etiological factors often present with very similar signs. Temperament information about a dog's sire and dam can be helpful in making such determinations. A history of inadequate socialization or environmental exposure is often associated with persistent fears toward strangers (xenophobia), fear of children (pedophobia), fear of novelty (neophobia), or fear of the outdoors and new places (agoraphobia). In cases where fearfulness is the result of a specific learning event (e.g., startle, trauma, or abuse), a dog's fearful behavior may be limited to a small number of eliciting stimuli and situations or widely generalized. Such dogs are often otherwise very outgoing and confident. Of the aforementioned etiologies, fearfulness stemming from some identifiable learning event is usually the most responsive to behavior modification, followed by problems associated with socialization or exposure deficits. Problems stemming from a genetic predisposition or neurobiological disorder are the most difficult to resolve through behavioral means alone. The resolution of fear problems depends on sorting out fear-eliciting situations and events. The dog behavior consultant must carefully identify the stimuli that evoke fear and the situations in which fearful behavior is likely to occur. Detailed information is collected about the behavior and the locations in which it has occurred in the past. Whenever possible, a functional analysis and assessment should be performed. The results of such analysis are very useful in terms of accurately describing the problem, developing an appropriate plan of behavior modification, and forming a realistic prognosis.

CONTRIBUTIONS OF LEARNING

Fear problems involve both instrumental behaviors (escape and avoidance) and underlying motivational states (fear, anxiety, and panic) operating under the influence of classical conditioning. In the laboratory, instrumental and classical learning are often studied separately. Under natural conditions, there is a great deal of interaction and overlap between instrumental and classical conditioning in the learning and unlearning of fearful behavior. Unlike in the laboratory, natural behavior is not arbitrarily divided into distinct voluntary and reflexive categories but is the unified expression of complementary instrumental, cognitive, and motivational factors. Behavior operates under the influence of an animal's *disposition to learn,* including various innate and acquired expectancies and the pressure of numerous motivational imperatives (see *An Alternative Theory of Reinforcement* in Volume 1, Chapter 7). In addition, regulatory feedback mechanisms or *cognitive analyzers* guide behavior according to the relative success or failure of an animal's behavior to achieve intended goals. The relevant motivational substrates operate under the influence of two general constraints:

1. Both attractive (appetitive) and aversive emotional arousal are reflexive in nature and can be altered (amplified or attenuated) only by appropriate procedures involving sensitization-habituation or classical conditioning.
2. Attractive and aversive motivational states can be influenced only by the elicitation of complementary or antagonistic attractive or aversive motivational states.

In other words, motivational states cannot be reinforced or punished by the manipulation of consequences as one finds in the case of instrumental behavior. This observation is not intended to suggest that rewards and punishment have no effect on motivational substrates. In fact, the acquisition of food or the avoidance/escape from aversive stimulation may produce very significant motivational effects via satiation or relief, respectively. The critical issue at stake here is that underlying emotional arousal is not responsive to rewards and punishers in the same way that overt voluntary behavior is affected by instrumental consequences—one cannot punish or reward an emotion.

Classical and Instrumental Interactions

Undoubtedly, cognitive and motivational substrates bring classical behavior and instrumental behavior together into a functional unity. Despite their mutual dependency, however, instrumental behavior and reflexive behavior perform relatively distinct functions. For example, although one can choose not to act in some way or other, one cannot arbitrarily decide to experience or not to experience some emotion. Given the presence of a sufficiently salient stimulus, the emotion will occur and continue to occur until (1) it has run its course (habituation), (2) the eliciting stimulus is terminated (stimulus change), or (3) an antagonistic emotional state is aroused by another stimulus (counterconditioning). In contrast to the constraints associated with reflexive emotional arousal, instrumental behavior exhibits considerable independence from stimulus determinants. Although instrumental behavior operates in conformity with motivational incentives such as fear or hunger, it is not entirely controlled by such incentives. Dogs have at their disposal a great deal of latitude and "choice" about motivationally significant courses of action present at any given moment. This is a very important aspect of how motivational incentives affect instrumental behavior; they do not drive or direct the animal into action—they provide options. Motivational incentives present as a menu of options for action. This feature gives instrumental behavior and learning considerable freedom from biological and emotional pressures, that is, it is characterized by a high degree of voluntary initiative and purposiveness.

Fear and Instrumental Reinforcement

A further distinction should be drawn with respect to the relationship between motivational influences and instrumental reinforcement. Although instrumental behavior may heed motivational pressures to take some course of action, sometimes to the extent of blurring instrumental and reflexive distinctions, the reduction of an aversive drive state does not appear to be the most important factor involved in the reinforcement of instrumental behavior. The common view that reinforcement is the result of a response-produced drive reduction has been largely repudiated in the learning laboratory. This is not to say that a drive-reducing outcome (that is, an event that satisfies some need) might not play a significant role in reinforcement. Certainly, the reduction or induction of drive may play a vital motivational role by lowering or raising thresholds for arousal and activity (that is, the disposition to learn); however, these changes in motivational state appear to exercise only a secondary influence on instrumental reinforcement. Reinforcement of instrumental behavior appears to hinge more directly on the recognition that some behavior successfully controlled the occurrence of a motivationally significant outcome. The central idea being developed here is that reinforcement is based more on the exercise of successful control over some attractive or aversive outcome than it is on the reduction of a drive or motivational state. The reduction of motivational arousal may alter a dog's disposition to act, but it is a secondary or collateral effect associated with the successful control of attractive or aversive outcomes.

In contrast, classical conditioning depends on the formation of a predictive relationship between the occurrence of two stimulus events such that, given that S1 occurs, S2 will probably follow. Classical conditioning provides predictive information about the occurrence of significant events, thereby motivationally preparing dogs to act in an adaptive and effective manner. Such conditioned associations require the presentation of an antecedent conditioned stimulus (CS) occurring in close temporal and spatial proximity with the occurrence of a biologically significant unconditioned stimulus (US). As already noted, there is a close interdependent relationship between classical learning and instrumental learning: *Successful control depends on adequate prediction, and adequate prediction depends on successful control.* Adaptation to the changing environment depends on an animal's ability to predict and control appetitive and aversive events (see

A Brief Critique of Traditional Learning Theory in Volume 1, Chapter 7).

The foregoing general observations have considerable relevance for the modification of behavior associated with fear. The mere reduction of some aversive emotional state (e.g., counterconditioning) may not be sufficient in itself to alter associated instrumental avoidance/escape behavior. Although counterconditioning can be a very useful preliminary step in the management of intense fear, the ultimate goal is to "convince" dogs that they can control or cope with the feared situation. Fear is overcome by confidence building. Demonstrating to fearful dogs that they can control the feared situation is often a very effective treatment approach. Consequently, a critical concern in behavior modification is that the animal learn to control feared events in a constructive and purposive way. Many common fears appear to be related to a lack of competency in the face of some unfamiliar or potentially dangerous situation. For example, dogs that are fearful of water will probably not become much better when being taken near water, unless they are also taught through gradual steps how to swim or otherwise enjoy it. As a dog's confidence improves, activities such as retrieving games can be added to the experience, showing the dog that being in the water can be fun, as well. Obviously, simply reducing the aversive emotional arousal associated with such situations would not go very far in permanently resolving a dog's fear of water. Similarly, a dog that is fearful of climbing stair steps is best treated by gradually teaching it the necessary motor skills needed to climb steps.

A relatively complex interface between instrumental and classical conditioning exists in the relationship between fear and aggression (see Chapter 7). Although some degree of directive training (e.g., response prevention and attention control) is often needed for the resolution of fear-related behavior problems, excessive reliance on inhibitory techniques is not useful and should be avoided. The risk of exacerbating undesirable emotional arousal through punishment is particularly problematic in the case of fear-related aggressive behavior. Punishment may partially or temporarily suppress aggressive behavior but will not reduce underlying aversive emotional tensions driving the behavior. Under such circumstances, any hope for a permanent solution is highly doubtful. Such treatment, if it succeeds at all, may only train a dog to avoid behaving aggressively under circumstances in which punishment is likely to occur. Unfortunately, since the provocative stimuli and the underlying aversive tensions involved have not been properly identified or addressed, they will likely persist over time, ultimately producing an even more difficult and dangerous situation. Similarly, while avoidance behavior can often be temporarily suppressed by punishment, the underlying fear motivating such behavior is not reduced by punitive treatment. Fear-related behavior problems are the result of a composite of instrumental and classical conditioning elements, each requiring specific behavior modification efforts.

WHAT IS FEAR?

Freeze, Flight, and Fight Reactions

Fear is a normal self-protective response to potentially injurious stimulation. There are three broad ways in which adaptive fear is expressed: freeze, flight, and fight. Freezing is an inhibitory response to fearful arousal that is typically elicited by low levels of stimulation or a distant threat. Fleeing, on the other hand, is an excitatory response to fearful arousal that is elicited by high levels of fear or the close presence of an intrusive threat. Fear-elicited fighting occurs in situations involving intense fearful arousal and where flight is blocked by the threatening target. Normal fear is adaptive and transient. In addition to freeze-flight-fight responses, fear drives the expression of a wide range of preparatory physiological changes and overt species-specific defensive reactions (Bolles, 1970).

Signs of Fear

Outward signs of fear include a variety of distinctive body postures, facial expressions, and physiological indicators (see *ANS-mediated Concomitants of Fear* in Volume 1, Chapter 3). Depending on the fear-eliciting situation, dogs will freeze, attempt to escape (e.g., strain away,

hide, or cower), or attack. Postural signs of fear include lowering and arching of the body, tucking the tail tightly between the legs, raised hackles (piloerection), intense muscular stiffening (flexor dominance), and thigmotactic reactions that frequently involve efforts to lean on the owner or against some other object (including the floor), apparently seeking security and support. A fearful dog will often lower its head and avert eye contact, fasten its ears back, and retract the corners of its mouth. Other signs of fear include pupillary dilation (mydriasis), restlessness, panting, nervous licking, shivering and trembling, decreased and thick salivation (sympathetic arousal), and, in some cases, profuse watery salivation (parasympathetic rebound). In the case of extreme fear arousal, dogs may exhibit tonic immobility (catalepsy), lose bowel and bladder control, or evacuate anal glands. Fearful dogs may scramble frantically to escape or evade a feared object while loudly whining, yelping, yipping, or shrieking. In addition, depending on the dog's temperament and past experience, fearful stimulation may evoke a defensive attack, especially in situations where the dog is restrained or prevented from escaping.

INNATE AND ACQUIRED FEAR

Phylogenic Sources of Fear

Adaptive fear is often evoked by unconditioned aversive stimuli that have evolutionary significance for dogs. These phylogenic sources of fear include such triggers as pain, rapid stimulus change, loud noises, sudden movements, heights, strangers, isolation, fire, water, and unfamiliar social and environmental situations. Phylogenic or *natural triggers* of fear are associated with imminent threat and evoke preparatory physiological arousal mediating species-typical escape responses.

Although natural triggers of fear such as pain and loud noises are correlated with fear, they are not fear itself. What an animal strives to control by escape and avoidance is fearful arousal, and only secondarily loud noises or pain insofar as they elicit fear. For example, storm-phobic dogs treated with an appropriate medication will more calmly tolerate thunder and lightning going on around it.

While under the influence of medication, fear is reduced, and dogs no longer exhibit an urgent need to escape. Thunder and lightning are still present in the situation—what is absent under the influence of medication is fearful arousal.

Ontogenic Sources of Fear

Ontogenic sources of fear are largely the result of learning and experience. Motivationally neutral stimuli that happen to occur in close association with unconditioned fear may become predictive signals that help an animal anticipate an impending threat. These learned sources of fear evoke apprehensive arousal and corresponding purposive behavior aimed at avoiding the phylogenic trigger of fear. Successful avoidance occurs when anticipated *fear* arousal is prevented or postponed by appropriate behavior. Fear asserts itself when the CS no longer adequately predicts the US or when a previously effective avoidance response no longer adequately controls the occurrence evoking the aversive US.

Early experiences appear to be vital for the development of social confidence and competence. Scott and Fuller (1965) and others (see below) have demonstrated that puppies that are isolated from social contact early in life develop pronounced fear-related deficits that persistently interfere with their ability to engage in normal social transactions with other dogs and humans. Similarly, puppies not exposed to sufficiently varied environments and stimuli become progressively fearful of novel stimulation as they mature.

Pathogenic Sources of Fear

Pathogenic fear (generalized anxiety and phobia) occurs when the evoking aversive US can be neither predicted nor controlled, that is, when fearful arousal cannot be avoided or escaped. Pathologically anxious or phobic dogs are unable adaptively to escape or avoid fearful arousal. Since fear arousal persists in spite of their best efforts, these dogs labor futilely under the influence of escalating fear and anxiety. Overt fearful behavior in the presence of fear-eliciting stimuli continues unabated and becomes progressively disorgan-

ized and maladaptive. The fear may become *free floating* and uncontrollable; it can be neither avoided nor escaped, but these dogs are obliged to keep trying. Such pathological or abnormal fear may persist across contexts and interfere with a variety of adaptive social and environmental transactions.

Acquisition and Persistence of Fear

Phylogenic fears do not depend on associative conditioning, although the magnitude of their expression is strongly influenced by the opposing influences of habituation and sensitization. Further, even when natural triggers do not evoke significant fear, they are influenced by a fear-expectancy bias or preparedness that facilitates rapid acquisition following aversive stimulation (sensitization). Many phylogenic elicitors of fear are highly prepared and effective in the absence of conditioning or sensitization. Pain, for example, is a powerful source of fear and is commonly used in the laboratory for studying fear. However, the fear associated with pain is not only affected by sensitization; it can also be reduced through habituation or counterconditioning. For example, recall Pavlov's experiment in which a dog was gradually exposed to increasing levels of shock followed by the presentation of food (see *Counterconditioning* in Volume 1, Chapter 6). As a result of the gradual intensification of shock and the presence of countervailing appetitive stimulation, the dog learned to tolerate even intense levels of shock, showing little more than an orienting response in the direction of expected food when the shock was delivered (Pavlov, 1927/1960).

Although fearful behavior appears to be influenced by several hereditary factors, including biological expectancy biases and relative sensitivity to fear-eliciting triggers, thresholds for fear are strongly influenced by experience and learning, especially the modulatory effects of sensitization and habituation. Phylogenic elicitors of fear may undergo significant ontogenic modification as the result of habituation (decreased sensitivity) and sensitization (increased sensitivity) to the evoking fear trigger. In addition, aversive classical conditioning may cause neutral stimuli, not normally capable of eliciting fear arousal, to become conditioned aversive stimuli by virtue of their association with unconditioned elicitors of fear. Perhaps the most important way in which fear is adaptively modulated toward phylogenic elicitors is through learning. By learning how to control and cope with natural sources of fear, animals develop confidence (incompatible with fear) around threatening situations. Many activities that are highly reinforcing for humans derive their reward value from the elation resulting from the successful control of fear-eliciting situations. Activities such as rock climbing, skiing, parachuting, and others taking place at great heights would be terrifying if it were not for the adventurer's mastery over the dangers presented by heights. The elation produced by these various activities is in proportion to the fear avoided by overcoming the dangers involved.

Other potentially viable explanations for the persistence and elaboration of fear reactions have been described. According to the James-Lange theory of emotions, the experience of fear results from a *perception* of underlying autonomic and bodily changes associated with fearful arousal. The underlying emotional substrate is different from the perceived experience felt by the animal. If this theory is accurate, the perception of fear is cognitively distinct from the original autonomic reactions. Taking this one step further, perhaps the *perception* or representation itself becomes an internal fear-eliciting CS that, in turn, triggers a specific set of autonomic fear reactions when recalled. This view could help to explain how imagining fearful experiences by human subjects results in the elicitation of fear and autonomic arousal. Gantt's theory of schizokinesis is relevant to this topic (see *Gantt: Schizokinesis, Autokinesis, and Effect of Person* in Volume 1, Chapter 9). *Schizokinesis* refers to a divergence between overt changes directly associated with classical fear conditioning and underlying visceral and autonomic concomitants. Gantt (1962) postulated that Pavlovian conditioning and extinction occur at different rates depending on the biological system involved. While overt motoric reactions associated with fear may be readily extinguished, autonomic components like heart rate and blood pressure may persist long afterward. Perhaps these perennial autonomic

traces signal fearful perceptions or prompt fearful recollections that in turn trigger broader and more intense emotional arousal.

FEAR AND CONDITIONING

Fear is elicited by a variety of unconditioned and conditioned stimuli. Like other forms of emotional arousal and reflex actions, fear can be elicited by conditioned stimuli. The conditioning of fear is the primary way in which fear irradiates to nonaversive or neutral stimuli occurring in close association with the fear-eliciting situation. The process follows the basic Pavlovian pattern: a stimulus occurring prior to the onset of a fear-eliciting event may acquire the ability to elicit similar preparatory arousal as the feared event. Conditioned emotional responses (CERs) produced in this manner are common in dog behavior and training. For instance, the reprimand "No" is conditioned by pairing the word "No" (CS) with a mildly startling or aversive event (US). After several trials in which the reprimand CS is presented in close contiguity with the aversive US, the CS will acquire startling and inhibitory properties belonging originally only to the aversive US.

Under ordinary circumstances, the ability to form fearful associations linking innocuous predictive events with impending threatening ones is highly adaptive and useful. By using environmental signals or *markers* that regularly precede the occurrence of a threatening event, animals are better equipped to anticipate danger safely and, perhaps, reduce or evade harm by prompt action. Such signals provide animals with temporal and spatial information about an aversive event, allowing them to avoid, evade, or postpone the event's occurrence. Once established, such conditioned stimuli are frequently very difficult to extinguish (see *Classical Conditioning and Fear* in Volume 1, Chapter 6).

Conditioning and Maladaptation

Although learning involving fear is normally adaptive and functional, sometimes fear learning becomes dysfunctional and maladaptive. Wolpe (1969) suggests that neuroses involving fear can be distinguished from normal responses by "their resistance to extinction in the face of their unadaptiveness" (1). Such persistent and apparently maladaptive avoidance responding often occurs following traumatic exposure to aversive stimulation. Solomon and Wynne (1953), who studied the effects of traumatic aversive conditioning on avoidance learning and extinction in dogs, trained them to jump over a hurdle separating two compartments of a shuttle box. Each compartment was separately illuminated by an overhead lamp. During the experiment, darkness became a discriminative stimulus predicting impending shock, while the light confirmed successful avoidance and predicted *safety.* The dogs quickly learned to leap over the hurdle whenever the compartment was darkened—on average, within five trials.

The resultant avoidance behavior was not only rapidly learned (often after a single occurrence), the behavior was also very resistant to extinction. The experimenters ran several hundred regular extinction trials, with one dog continuing to jump over 600 times, even though shock never occurred—the aversive CS (darkness) was sufficient to maintain the behavior. The experimenters observed that avoidance responding continued unabated with progressively shorter latencies between the presentation of the CS and avoidance response, even though overt signs of fear appeared to diminish over time. After 10 to 12 days of extinction, most of the dogs stopped resisting when prompted to go into the shuttle box, with many voluntarily hopping inside without any noticeable sign of emotional distress. These latter findings suggest that a certain degree of motivational independence exists between fear and avoidance behavior. Interestingly, with respect to compulsive behavior disorders, the authors noted that overt signs of fear were most reduced in dogs that had adopted some preliminary stereotypic pattern (superstition) that occurred just before and after the avoidance response was emitted.

Conditioned Fear and Extinction

In a follow-up study, Solomon and coworkers (1953) used several methods to extinguish traumatic avoidance behavior. They found that a combination of procedures, including response prevention (blocking) and punishment, offered the most effective means for extinguishing (or suppressing) avoidance responding. The term *punishment* in this case denotes the discontinuation of the avoidance contingency; that is, the avoidance response no longer successfully avoids or escapes the presentation of the aversive stimulus. [There is some apparent confusion in the literature with respect to the definition of *extinction* in case of negative reinforcement. Catania (1998) comments on this problem: "In negative reinforcement (escape and avoidance), extinction has often referred to the discontinuation of aversive stimuli, although the term applies more appropriately to discontinuing the consequences of responding, so that aversive stimuli occur but responses no longer prevent them" (389).] A punishment-extinction contingency alone did not prove to be very effective; in fact, it appeared to increase the strength of the jumping response in most dogs. A response prevention (blocking) procedure was also employed. In this case, a glass panel was installed above the hurdle, thus preventing the dogs from jumping over it. This procedure helped to facilitate extinction in some dogs. However, the best extinction results were achieved by alternately employing both response blocking (what the experimenters called *reality testing*) and punishment.

One possible explanation for the slow extinction rates observed in the aforementioned experiments is that the dogs lacked sufficient information about the altered significance of the training situation; that is, they failed to learn that the avoidance response was no longer necessary or functional. By blocking some avoidance responses and punishing others, both the necessity and the functionality of the avoidance response were disconfirmed. The need to block avoidance responding in order for the animals to learn the significance of altered contingencies was also suggested by an experiment performed by Wolpe (1958), who found that cats exposed to shock in the presence of food could be induced to eat again by forcing them into close proximity to food by using a squeeze panel. Once near the food (and unable to escape), the hungry cats appeared to realize that the threat of shock was no longer present and suddenly tested the situation by taking a few quick grabs and gulps of food before relaxing enough to eat normally in the experimental setting.

Many common fears are maintained under the shielding influence of successful avoidance behavior. In effect, successful avoidance prevents animals from learning that the contingencies associated with the situation have changed and no longer represent a threat. Although the avoidance behavior is no longer adaptive, dogs may continue to respond as though it were necessary to do so. Such avoidance behavior is particularly relevant in the maintenance of some compulsive behaviors in dogs. Consequently, successful extinction of avoidance behavior may require that the behavior be prevented, forcing dogs to experience directly the *reality* that the response is no longer necessary. Response prevention procedures have been demonstrated to be highly effective for the reduction of avoidance behavior and fear. Although it is not precisely clear what mechanisms actually facilitate response prevention (Mineka, 1979), some combination of extinction, competitive learning, relaxation, or cognitive reappraisal is probably involved.

Fear, Cognition, and Avoidance Learning

Seligman and Johnston (1973), who analyzed avoidance learning from a cognitive perspective (see *A Cognitive Theory of Avoidance Learning* in Volume 1, Chapter 8), theorized that once an avoidance response is learned, fear as a motivational factor fades into the background, becoming secondary to cognitive sources of reinforcement. According to this theory, avoidance is not primarily maintained by fear reduction, as postulated by two-factor learning theorists, but by the confirmation of an expectancy that the occurrence of aversive stimulation is controlled by the avoidance response. These response expectations include what to expect as the result of responding, as well as what to expect if the response does not occur. During avoidance training, animals learn to expect that (1) shock will not occur if

the response is made and (2) shock will occur if the response is not made. Since the absence of shock is preferable to the presentation of shock, animals learn to respond. If the foregoing expectations are confirmed, then the response is reinforced. On the other hand, if one or both of these expectations are disconfirmed, the response undergoes extinction. This construct is consistent with the experiments of Solomon and colleagues. Once the dogs learned that they could safely predict and control the occurrence of the aversive event, collateral fearful arousal was gradually offset by the appearance of confidence. As a result, the dogs became progressively confident and relaxed as training went on.

The pattern of avoidance responding that follows traumatic avoidance conditioning does not depend on the repeated presentation of the feared aversive event. Each time the dogs successfully jumped over the barrier, their confidence improved. Since avoidance behavior is reinforced by the absence of aversive stimulation, it would not become apparent to the dogs that the avoidance response was no longer necessary during the extinction phase, unless, of course, they happened to stop responding and discovered that shock did not occur. In the case of traumatic avoidance learning, though, few animals stop to check whether the contingency is still in effect. In variance with Wolpes's suggestion that such behavior is "neurotic" and "unadaptive," one might instead view persistent avoidance responding as a potentially highly adaptive pattern, especially in situations involving traumatic or dangerous events. Under such circumstances, stopping to test whether a particular avoidance response was still necessary would entail taking a potentially life-threatening risk. Unlike the laboratory situation, where predictive signals may be arranged arbitrarily, in nature such predictive relations are often much more consistent and reliable. Some persistent fears and phobias in dogs may be similarly interpreted as an adaptive response misapplied. This interpretation is especially relevant in cases involving traumatic fears, where *testing* the situation might be perceived as a dangerous risk that they are not willing to take.

Safety, Relief and Relaxation

The intention of the foregoing discussion is not to suggest that *fear* does not play a significant role in avoidance learning but rather to emphasize the important role of cognitive sources of reinforcement in such learning. A cognitive-behavioral approach to avoidance learning appears to account for more of the facts than either alone can explain. That fear plays a role in the maintenance and regulation of such behavior is supported by many experiments. A good example of these numerous studies is the research performed by Rescorla and LoLordo (1965), who trained dogs to avoid shock in an arrangement similar to the one already described in the Solomon-Wynne experiment. In their experiment, however, dogs were not provided with external avoidance cues but had to learn to jump in accordance with a temporal contingency (Sidman avoidance task—see *Mowrer's Two-process Theory of Avoidance Learning* in Volume 1, Chapter 8). In addition, two stimuli had been previously conditioned, one to predict shock (fear CS), and one to predict the absence of shock (safe CS). The researchers found that the rate of jumping was differentially affected, depending on the CS presented. The fear CS increased the rate of responding when it was presented, whereas the safe CS decreased avoidance responding. These findings clearly indicate that *fear* and *safety* play significant motivational roles in the modulation of avoidance behavior.

In addition to the confirmation of relevant expectancies, the jumping response may also be reinforced by consequent relief and relaxation associated with the successful performance of each avoidance response. Denny (1983) describes the combined effects of relief and relaxation:

> Relief is conceived of as a short latency, autonomic event that lasts only 15 to 20 sec. Relaxation, on the other hand, seems to be a long latency, striate muscle event that requires at least a 2.5-min non-shock period to be effective. Both relaxation and relief are assumed to be effective in making the stimuli associated with a nonshock period positive, or safe, during the acquisition of avoidance and in providing the responses that can compete with fear and help mediate its extinction. According to the

theory, both relief and relaxation occur automatically with the extended removal of an aversive or well-conditioned aversive stimulus. Nothing else is required. (215)

In addition, Denny (1971) suggests,

> Such relief and relaxation affects produced by avoidance may backchain to the fear-eliciting CS, gradually counterconditioning it and making it into a "cue for approaching safety." (253)

In combination with Seligman and Johnston's cognitive theory, Denny's notion of safety provides a persuasive explanation for the persistence of avoidance learning and its relatively relaxed and *fearless* character.

Response Prevention, Opponent Processing, and Relaxation

Baum (1970) argues that relaxation plays an important role in the mediation of extinction by response prevention (flooding). Animals exposed to a fear-eliciting situation exhibit "abortive avoidance behavior," freezing, and increased general activity but gradually settle into a period of grooming activities. He interprets the appearance of nonfearful grooming (calming) as evidence of relaxation. According to Baum, postfear relief and relaxation are necessary affective changes for flooding or response prevention to reduce fear. In fact, premature termination of a flooding session (that is, before dogs show evidence of relaxing) may make the fearful behavior worse rather than better.

Under normal conditions, relief and relaxation help to regulate fear, perhaps by mediating affective habituation. Another possibility is that relief and relaxation are opponent processes operating in the manner described by Solomon and Corbit (1974) (see *Classically Generated Opponent Processes and Emotions* in Volume 1, Chapter 6). According to this theory, the arousal of fear is followed by hedonically opposing arousal. The course of events described by Solomon and Corbit is consistent with that outlined by Denny; however, some additional features of the opponent-process theory nicely account for the effects observed when a fear-eliciting stimulus is repeatedly presented. The assumption of the opponent-process theory is that high levels of fear are followed by proportionate "slave" responses of an opposite hedonic valence (e.g., relief/relaxation). When the fear-eliciting stimulus is discontinued, these shadowing opponent affects assert themselves. An interesting characteristic of opponent processing occurs after repeated stimulation. Gradually, fearful arousal becomes less strong, apparently subdued under the restraining influence of growing antagonistic opponent processes. As a result of the repeated termination of fear-eliciting stimulation, heightened levels of antagonistic arousal progressively exert a more pronounced and longer-lasting relaxation/relief effect. Theoretically, this arrangement would provide a powerful means for modulating fear and for promoting adaptation in fear-dense environments. In the case of phobias or generalized anxiety, opponent relief/relaxation effects may fail to develop fully, may be sluggish, or may not exert sufficient strength to offset fear. One possible explanation for the failure of opponent mechanisms in the case of extreme fear is that, during particularly traumatic events, fear arousal may exceed the capacity of the opponent-processing mechanism. Instead of restraining fear arousal toward baseline levels or below baseline levels (relief/relaxation), opponent processes may only be able to partially restrain fear arousal (phobia).

ANXIETY

Fear is an adaptive emotional response to a specific event or situation that threatens to produce injury. The elicitation of fear activates animals physiologically and behaviorally for immediate emergency action appropriate to a situation. In contrast to the acute onset and temporary duration of fear, anxiety is characterized by a chronic state of nonspecific apprehension, persistent sympathetic arousal, and vigilance. Anxious dogs appear tense and physiologically braced for a threat that they cannot adequately predict, perhaps one that does not actually exist. Chronic anxiety generates stressful sympathetic arousal and underlies the development of many behavior problems, including unpredictable aggression, generalized neophobic and xenophobic tendencies, various neurotic compulsive disorders, and psychosomatic disorders. Recently, Glickman and coworkers (2000) have reported a significant correlation between fearfulness and agitation in response to strangers and a higher incidence of gastric dilatation-volvulus. Interestingly, the authors found that dogs (N = 1914) perceived by their owners to be happy were less likely to develop this relatively common and often life-threatening disorder.

Fear, Anxiety, and Predictability

From a learning perspective, the functional difference between anxiety and fear is the degree of independence between the fear response and a specific eliciting CS or US. Fear occurs in the presence of some specific stimulus or situation. When the aversive stimulus is discontinued, fearful arousal rapidly dissipates and is replaced by relief. Adaptive fear occurs in one of two situations: (1) as the result of direct stimulation by an evoking fear US or (2) as the result of the presentation of an evoking CS that is highly correlated with a fear-eliciting US. In the first situation, the elicitation of fear facilitates withdrawal from a potentially dangerous situation (escape). In the second case, anticipatory fear enables dogs to avoid the threatening situation (avoidance). Whereas a strong connection exists between fear and some evoking CS or US, maladaptive anxiety occurs independently of specific stimulation or imminent threat.

Although often maladaptive, anxiety can serve a highly adaptive function under certain circumstances. Imagine, for example, an impending event that might occur but cannot be anticipated by any available warning sign. Anxious arousal in such cases increases an animal's vigilance and prepares it to act effectively, just in case the event happens to occur.

Rescorla's Associative Interpretation

In the case of anxiety, the threatening event is not well predicted; that is, the threatening US is apt to occur independently of predictive conditioned stimuli present at the time. Post-Pavlovian theories of associative learning offer an excellent way for understanding how some anxious states are acquired and maintained

(Rescorla, 1988). Of particular significance in this regard is Rescorla's reformulation of classical conditioning. Rescorla experimentally demonstrated that associative learning incorporates information about both the occurrence and the nonoccurrence of significant events. According to this model, excitatory conditioning (acquisition) occurs when the US is highly correlated with the presentation of the CS. On the other hand, inhibitory conditioning (extinction) occurs when the US is poorly correlated with the presentation of the CS.

When the US occurs independently of the presence or absence of the CS, the US is defined as unpredictable; that is, both the occurrence of the CS as well as its omission are equally irrelevant to the occurrence of the US. A positive predictive value is assigned to the CS if it occurs more frequently than not before the US is presented. A negative predictive value is assigned to the CS if it occurs more frequently than not when the US is omitted. Therefore, the predictive value of the CS is expressed numerically between 1.0 (certainty) and 0.0 (unpredictable). The vast majority of conditioned stimuli fall somewhere between these two opposing extremes. When faced with a potentially aversive or life-threatening event that is not adequately predicted by antecedent signals, the organism is forced to maintain a chronic state of alarm, vigilance, readiness for action. This state of hyperarousal is associated with persistent anxiety and generalized biological stress. This sort of condition is highly aversive and appears to be related to the loss of safety ensuing in situations where aversive events are unpredictable (Seligman and Binik, 1977).

Denny (1971) proposes a novel hypothesis concerning the development of generalized or free-floating anxiety. According to this theory, anxious persons or animals are unable to relax properly, and this dysfunction is relatively independent of external stimulation. Instead of external cues evoking anxiety, the source of aversive stimulation is internal. Denny has argued for the possibility that affects associated with relaxation may themselves evoke anxiety. Under situations in which relaxation is regularly paired with aversive stimulation, fear may be elicited by relaxation-produced internal cues. Because of past presentations of aversive stimulation occurring with the onset of relaxation, dogs may be unable to calm down because each time they begin to feel relaxed, they begin to become anxious. One would assume that such associations might be particularly likely in cases where aversive events occur independently of other predictive cues. Under such circumstances, the most constant predictive correlation with aversive outcomes might very well be relaxation. A somewhat similar factor might underlie other forms of excessive arousal, where calming or slowing down might become a cue predicting aversive stimulation.

PHOBIA

Phobias are distinguished from other conditioned and unconditioned fears by their maladaptive character. Given the presence of a phobic stimulus, a fearful response invariably follows. Fear associated with phobias is typically far in excess to what would be expected or appropriate in the situation. Another important distinction between most phobias and common fears is the former's persistence and failure to habituate naturally. Even after many hundreds of harmless contacts with the feared object or place, a dog may continue to exhibit a strong phobic response without showing any sign of abatement over time (Hothersall and Tuber, 1979).

Biological Predisposition and Preparedness

Understanding how phobias develop is not an easy task, and the etiology of many phobic disorders still remains a mystery. Although a specific traumatic event can occasionally be identified to help explain the appearance of some phobia, most often the cause of phobic behavior is not clearly linked to a past aversive event (Marks, 1987). Some dogs appear to be biologically predisposed to behave more fearfully or to develop phobic responses more easily than others, which may be more emotionally resilient or virtually immune to disorders resulting from fearful stimulation. Seligman (1971) proposed a *preparedness* account to explain why some fearful associations are acquired more readily than others. Preparedness affects both the classical conditioning of fear and the acquisition of instrumental defensive (escape and avoidance) responses—what Bolles (1970) refers to as species-specific defensive reactions. Seligman divides preparedness into three basic categories, depending on the relative ease with which fearful associations are learned: (1) prepared (fast—sometimes one trial), (2) unprepared (slow—requires extensive associative training), and (3) contraprepared (retarded—may occur only after extensive training or not at all).

Species-specific Objects of Fear

LoLordo and Droungas (1989) suggest that some phobic responses and their objects may be inherited as highly prepared species-specific tendencies. One example of an apparent inherited fear is a puppy's fear of heights. Most young puppies exhibit a fear of heights shortly after they are able to move about. These innate fears do not require traumatic associative learning in order to be activated but appear spontaneously as part of an animal's ontogenetic development (Menzies and Clarke, 1995). Another innate fear that is commonly associated with phobic behavior is the fear of loud noises (see *Preparedness and Selective Association* in Volume 1, Chapter 5). Finally, the most common source of aversive emotional arousal is pain. The fear of pain is a very powerful source of fear and widely distributed among animals.

Some dogs exhibit a pronounced fear of strangers (xenophobia) in spite of conscientious socialization efforts. Strong evidence suggests that a heritable biological factor influences the development and expression of tendencies for social attraction and aversion. Murphree (1973), for example, has selectively bred divergent strains of pointers. One line shows a normal attraction and social responsiveness toward human handlers. The other nervous line exhibits a persistent social aversion toward people that is transmitted from one generation to the next. The pathological pointers exhibit intense fear and withdrawal behavior whenever they are approached by human handlers, regardless of the dogs' previous socialization with humans and training.

Interestingly, the nervous dogs get along well with normal pointers (Reese, 1979) and even respond well to field training.

The appearance of phobias may be causally related to the affected dog's inability to habituate normally to feared stimuli or as the result of sensitization, that is, intense or surprising exposure to the feared object or situation. Dogs exhibiting sensitive or "weak" temperament traits or suffering hypersensitivity to touch or sound are especially prone to develop adult phobias. Such predisposed individuals frequently suffer compound fears involving a wide variety of objects and situations.

Typically, natural fears are attenuated or amplified through the mutually antagonistic influences of habituation and sensitization, respectively. For example, safe encounters with other dogs from puppyhood onward will progressively raise a dog's threshold for fear in the presence of other conspecifics. On the other hand, being attacked on some occasion by an unfamiliar dog may result in the development of a lifelong fear of other dogs. Fear can also spread to other stimuli that share some similarity with the US through generalization.

Traumatic Conditioning

Traumatic experiences occurring early in puppyhood are a major source of phobic behavior in adult dogs. Puppies between 8 and 10 weeks of age appear to be especially sensitive to the effects of fearful stimulation (Fox, 1966). A highly persistent phobia may result from a single traumatic exposure during this critical period. For example, an 8½-week-old puppy known to have been stung by a bee just above his left eye developed a lasting fear of bees and other flying insects that continued for over 10 years despite thousands of safe exposures during that time. Although the dog's response was particularly strong while indoors (the context in which he had been stung), he continued to show signs of fear arousal in response to all flying insects regardless of the situation. This particular dog was otherwise very confident, independent, and quite courageous with respect to other dogs; however, whenever a fly would alight nearby, he would jump to his feet, show "airplane" ears, pant, and seek human contact for security.

Socialization Deficits

Another common source of fearfulness stemming from puppyhood is the result of inadequate socialization and environmental exposure during appropriate sensitive periods in a puppy's development. Puppies raised in isolation from human contact become progressively fearful of human contact. Freedman and colleagues (1961) found that puppies raised in isolation until they were 3 weeks old tended to approach human handlers immediately. If not exposed to people until 7 weeks of age, however, isolated puppies began to show greater aversion and avoidance, taking an average of 2 days to finally approach a passive handler. By 14 weeks of age, the puppies who had not been previously exposed to human contact were extremely and persistently fearful toward people and made no contact with the passive handler (see *The "Critical" or Sensitive Period Hypothesis* in Volume 1, Chapter 2).

The Role of Abuse

Fear of human contact and other bizarre avoidance behavior can sometimes be traced back to abusive handling and mistreatment, although appeal to abuse as a cause of fear may be somewhat inflated (Lockwood, 1997). Potential adopters are often informed by shelter workers that a prospective adoptee had been abused, especially if the dog in question exhibits a behavior problem associated with nervousness or fear. Such unverifiable information may be based on an erroneous generalization that fearful behavior is prima facie evidence that a dog has been abused or neglected. Undoubtedly, physical and emotional abuse occurs and may be a significant cause of fear; however, it probably occurs far less often than one might expect from the frequency of such reports.

Major: A Thunder-phobic Dog

A common source of fearful behavior in dogs is loud noises. Such fears are subject to threshold modulation as the result of safe exposure (habituation) or traumatic exposure (sensitization). Dogs that are repeatedly and

safely exposed to loud noises will usually learn to cope by ignoring or tolerating their occurrence. However, if a loud noise is presented in a particularly aversive or threatening manner, especially if it occurs in conjunction with noxious stimulation, a lasting alteration of fear thresholds involving loud noises may occur. In some cases, following traumatic aversive stimulation, fear thresholds may be permanently lowered, possibly resulting in the development of a phobia. Hothersall and Tuber (1979) describe a case that dramatically exemplifies the sensitizing effects of traumatic exposure to loud noise and its role in the development of fearful behavior. The dog was a 4½-year-old Labrador retriever named Major. Up until 6 months of age, Major showed no signs of fear toward loud noises such as thunder or gunshots. The owner was an avid hunter who took the dog along into the field, where he had shot his gun directly over the dog's head without producing any apparent signs of fear. The dog's confidence toward loud noises was shattered, however, as the result of an accidental explosion. The single experience was enough to permanently alter the dog's fear threshold for loud noises:

> At the age of six months, Major was chained to a bench in a body shop while his owner did some welding work. The 220-V cable to an air compressor shorted out causing an arc welder to explode with a loud bang and a flash of light. Since that one experience Major has been afraid of loud noises, storms, and gunshots. His reaction to a storm consisted of panting, shaking, constant seeking of attention, profuse salivation, and vigorous attempts to escape from the storm. Tranquilizers had no effect upon this reaction, which the owner reported would carry over the day after the storm. (246)

Major's heightened fear of loud noises probably was the result of traumatic sensitization. Sensitization in this case was particularly dramatic, generalized, and lasting (resistant to habituation), possibly because of the combined influences of event-situational unfamiliarity and an innate fear-expectancy bias facilitating the association of fear with loud sounds and sudden movements. The resulting hypervigilance and generalized fearful arousal toward other loud noises (e.g., thunder) are consistent with such an interpretation. Being chained at the time of the explosion may have made the situation even more traumatic. The condition of restraint took away the dog's ability to control the event effectively or reduce its aversiveness by escaping. Essentially, the event was both unexpected (unpredictable) and inescapable, providing the cognitive conditions conducive for the development of lasting and generalized fear [see *Post-traumatic Stress Disorder (PTSD)* in Volume 1, Chapter 9].

Another interpretation, based on the traumatic disconfirmation of safety, is also possible. Just as a threat is anticipated by various predictive signals, safety is also associated with signals (i.e., signals that predict the absence of danger). These combined signals form the contextual framework for determining whether a threatening event is likely to occur or not. The expectancy of safety usually interferes with aversive conditioning and sensitization; that is, the dog is biased with respect to the significance of potentially aversive events—they are perceived as being less of a threat. However, under the influence of a particularly traumatic and inescapable event, as in Major's case, such expectancies, previously mediated by familiarity and safety (that is, the absence of aversive stimulation), may be suddenly disconfirmed. Consequently, in the future, signals associated with safety may not be viewed with as much confidence and reliability as they were prior to the trauma. In fact, some safety signals immediately preceding the traumatic event may be counterconditioned into predictors of aversive stimulation.

Given that Major was familiar with the workshop situation and felt safe while in it, the traumatic event may have produced a dramatic and generalized disconfirmation of *safety*, which consequently extended to other situations that he also regarded as being safe. As a result of traumatic exposure to loud noises occurring under the contrary expectancy of safety, feelings of safety may come to predict potential danger. When in other situations previously associated with safety (e.g., while at home), the occurrence of loud noises may dramatically lower fear thresholds. Finally, affects associated with safety and relaxation may not only be discom-

firmed but may have been directly paired with the intense fear elicited by the explosion. As a result, instead of predicting continued safety, such internal *safety* cues may come to predict the possibility of danger, preparing a dog emotionally to anticipate a threat. As a result, whenever the dog feels safe in the future, he may inexorably become anxious and vigilant.

A third possibility should also be considered. Even if the environment was familiar to the dog, its safety may have been momentarily compromised by various local events altering the dog's sensitivity to aversive stimulation. While restrained and subjected to the sound of tools and other forms of mild aversive stimulation going on nearby, the dog may have been motivationally put on edge and rendered more sensitive and reactive to the fear elicited by the explosion. These sorts of ambient aversive stimuli may reduce the benefit of safety expectancies normally associated with a familiar environment. Safety expectancies appear to "immunize" the dog against adverse fear reactions by interfering with aversive emotional conditioning. Finally, fear elicited by the explosion may have been added to fear elicited by ambient stimulation, thus producing an additive effect on the dog's level of fear.

EXPECTANCY BIAS

Expectancy bias appears to play a major role in the learning of fear. Positive (safety) and negative (fear) expectancy biases influence a dog's perception of the environment and mediate the formation of various preferences and aversions. Many social and place preferences appear to be acquired early on in a puppy's development, with social biases being strongly influenced by attachment and bonding processes (Scott and Fuller, 1965). For example, dogs that have been socialized exclusively with humans may form a very persistent and negative expectancy about contact with other dogs. Such dogs will likely show an equally strong, but opposite, positive expectancy about contacts with people. Similarly, limited environmental exposure, especially early in a puppy's life, will likely result in the dog becoming fearful of new places as an adult.

Bias Toward the Strange and Unfamiliar

Social and place fear-expectancy biases may extend from a biological preference for the *familiar* and aversion for the *unfamiliar.* Most dogs show divergent expectancy biases toward situations and events depending on how familiar they are with them. A familiar situation is normally perceived in advance as probably being more safe than an unfamiliar one. Unfamiliar things are often viewed with suspicion. Unfamiliar situations are approached more warily simply because it is not known whether they are safe or dangerous beforehand. Dogs tend to expect more positive things to occur in the presence of familiar people and situations. Unfamiliar people and situations may be approached with greater caution, since such encounters may present opportunity as well as danger, but one cannot know for sure in advance.

In the *Republic,* Plato (Hamilton and Cairns, 1961) viewed this canine trait as a mark of wisdom:

> This too, said I, is something that you will discover in dogs and which is worth our wonder in the creature.
>
> What?
>
> That the sight of an unknown person angers him before he has suffered any injury, but an acquaintance he will fawn upon though he has never received any kindness from him. Have you never marveled at that?
>
> I never paid any attention to the matter before now, but that he acts in some such way is obvious.
>
> But surely that is an exquisite trait of his nature and one that shows a true love of wisdom.
>
> In what respect?
>
> In respect, said I, that he distinguishes a friendly from a hostile aspect by nothing save his apprehension of the one and his failure to recognize the other. (622)

The apparent preference for the familiar and aversion for the unfamiliar may adversely bias dogs against strangers (xenophobia) and novelty (neophobia). A significant implication of familiar/unfamiliar biasing is that it may cause unfamiliar persons, places, and things to be more easily associated with fear than are familiar persons, places, and things. Aversive stimulation may result in greater fear conditioning and slower extinction when it occurs in an unfamiliar situation than if the same stimulation takes place in a familiar one. The greatest potential for adverse fear conditioning is likely to occur toward an unfamiliar event (stimulus bias) in an unfamiliar situation (context bias).

The preference for the familiar and aversion for the unfamiliar undergoes ontogenetic modification as a puppy develops. Initially, puppies are biased to maintain contact with the familiar and to avoid the unfamiliar, that is, the world existing beyond the mother, other littermates, and the immediate nesting area. As puppies mature, the familiar becomes a staging platform for exploring and exploiting the unfamiliar for the benefit of their survival. Although the unknown represents an inherent risk, it is also a source of tremendous opportunity. Whereas fearful dogs withdraw from the unfamiliar because of the potential risk it represents, confident and secure dogs are attracted to the unfamiliar because of the potential opportunities it offers. The acquisition of a fearful expectancy bias toward the unfamiliar is probably influenced by the quality and quantity of early experiences with new things, social contacts with unfamiliar people and dogs, and exposure to novel places. Puppies that learn to anticipate beneficial outcomes in association with unfamiliar situations will be more likely to view such situations as a source of opportunity rather than perceiving them as a potential threat.

Exposure to varied situations involving familiar and unfamiliar stimulation in combination with human handling appears to be highly beneficial for developing puppies. Human handling, beginning as early as 5 weeks of age, appears to help puppies develop a more confident and curious attitude toward novelty (Wright, 1983). Early social handling and exposure to novelty take advantage of a puppy's less wary and more indiscriminate approach tendencies. The strange and unfamiliar are approached through the agency of curiosity and play. These early tendencies gradually give way to growing levels of fear and the decline of playful social tendencies and exploratory curiosity. It is not surprising that overly fearful dogs typically exhibit significant deficits in both areas. Puppies appear to be particularly receptive to exploring the wider environment at about 12 weeks of age, when they begin to leave the familiar surroundings of the nesting area to make more bold excursion into the surrounding environment. However, puppies that are exposed to a traumatic experience during a sortie into an unfamiliar situation might be doubly affected by the experience, (1) developing a persistent fear of the event associated with aversive stimulation and (2) becoming more wary of unfamiliar situations in the future.

Bias Toward Loud Sounds and Sudden Movements

Loud sounds and sudden movements may be influenced by an expectancy bias, making fearful conditioning toward loud sounds or sudden movements much more rapid and permanent. Also, the threshold for fearful auditory stimulation appears to be highly responsive to sensitization, and once sensitization has occurred, the resulting increased sensitivity to the eliciting stimulus may be very resistant to habituation. Many common phobias involve sudden and loud auditory stimulation (e.g., thunder fears). Also, dogs are often nervous around noisy traffic, a situation containing a variety of startling sounds and sudden movements that may be inherently aversive. Under natural conditions, the possession of low thresholds for startling sounds and sudden movements would provide a valuable defense against many potential threats, including social ones—both loud sounds and sudden movements are present in assertive threat displays. Puppies are responsive to both forms of startling stimulation from an early age onward. Initially, puppies appear to respond to such stimulation with indiscriminant startle and fear but gradually learn to respond more selectively and adaptively. Failure to provide early exposure and opportunities to learn about the significance of loud sounds and sudden movements may cause the underlying fear bias toward them to become more pronounced, generalized, and maladaptive.

Social and Sexual Biases

Many anecdotal reports and some bits of scientific evidence suggest that dogs may exhibit differential biases toward people, based on something like *social chemistry*. Gantt and colleagues (1966), for example, observed that some people are inherently more attractive and calming to dogs, whereas others appear to be inherently more aversive and agitating. Some evidence of sex-biased preferences and aversions has also been reported. Lore and Eisenberg (1986) performed a series of social approach tests indicating that male dogs tended to approach female handlers more readily than they approached male handlers. Female dogs did not exhibit a significant bias based on the sex of the handler. Wells and Hepper (1998) have found that shelter dogs (both male and female) are more defensive-aggressive toward men than women. Perhaps one result of the male dog's preference for women is that he is more prepared to associate affection selectively with women than with men. Conversely, such a bias may cause fear to be more easily associated with men than with women.

PREDICTION AND CONTROL

Predictive Information and Safety

As already discussed, event predictability and controllability play very significant roles in the learning and unlearning of fear. Predictive information is provided by both the occurrence and the nonoccurrence of aversive conditioned stimuli. Such conditioned stimuli provide predictive information about the occurrence (threat) and nonoccurrence (safety) of unconditioned aversive events. Predicted aversive events are preferred over unpredicted aversive events. A well-predicted threat renders its occurrence more controllable and, perhaps, less aversive by giving animals a chance to prepare for its occurrence. However, the absence of a some fear-eliciting CS is also predictive; that is, its omission predicts safety from the occurrence of the threatening US. For example, thunder-phobic dogs may readily learn to anticipate the occurrence of storm activity by the occurrence of various weather-related changes, such as a sharp drop in barometric pressure, the appearance of overcast skies, or humidity changes. These various meteorologic events have occurred in the past in advance of storm activity and may evoke anticipatory anxiety in thunder-phobic dogs. In fact, many dogs show signs of distress long before any evidence of thunder or lightning appears. The absence of such signals is also informative to dogs; that is, the absence indicates that a storm is not likely to occur. In other words, the absence of barometric change and other related weather indicators predict safety from the threat of storm activity.

Wolpe (1958) performed an experiment demonstrating the safety-signal hypothesis by using an auditory signal. A cat was first trained to approach a food container and eat whenever a buzzer was sounded. Once this training was well established, a second phase of the experiment was carried out. Food pellets were placed in the container, but, now, if the cat approached the container in the absence of the buzzer, it was administered a mild shock. After a brief period of adjustment and training, the cat discovered that it was safe to eat only when the buzzer preceded the presentation of food. As the result of such conditioning, the omission of the buzzer had become equally significant as its presentation; that is, the cat learned that the buzzer's omission predicted a period when shock would result if it attempted to eat from the container. Safety signals are very useful for managing and controlling fear in dogs.

Socialization and Training

To help dogs develop a confident attitude toward people, other dogs, places, and things, they must be provided with adequately diverse and orderly training activities. The provision of training and exposure assures dogs that their surroundings are highly predictable and controllable. When there exists a lack of agreement between what dogs expect and what in fact occurs, varying degrees of psychological distress, worry, doubt, and insecurity may ensue. When such events are of a highly aversive quality, generalized anxiety and chronic stress may result. Many dogs are exposed to a daily "ritual of confusion" in which punishment is presented on a noncontingent basis. Under the adverse influence of such conditions, a variety of anxiety-related

behavior problems are prone to develop (see *Learning and Behavioral Disturbances* in Volume 1, Chapter 10). Of particular significance in this regard, is the risk of maladaptive cross-association of fear and anger. Under normal conditions, fear modulates aggression, but when fear and anger become conjoined by chronic anxiety and frustrative arousal, a maladaptive outcome is prone to occur in the form of intractable vigilance and low-threshold aggression.

Failure to provide a dog with orderly (that is, highly predictable and controllable) socialization and training activities may incline it to perceive its owner's actions as being undependable or irrelevant. Such adverse assessments of the owner's competence may cause the dog to ignore the owner. This sort of situation is undesirable in any case but is especially detrimental in the case of a fearful or insecure dog, which may depend on its owner for guidance and security. A fearful dog needs a competent leader to take charge. Without its owner's help, an insecure dog may become progressively fearful under the influence of an expectation of failure when confronting threatening or unfamiliar situations. As will be discussed momentarily, fearful or insecure dogs appear to *expect to fail* in their efforts to control potentially threatening situations.

A dog's confidence in its owner (and by extension the rest of the world) is first and foremost the result of its collective and first-hand impressions of its owner's competence as a trainer and leader. If a dog is not suitably impressed by its "master's" training abilities and intelligence as a leader, it will never believe that its owner is capable of safely managing a potentially dangerous world.

EFFICACY EXPECTANCIES

Fear is an adaptive response to the extent that it motivationally prepares dogs for appropriate action in the face of threatening situations. Whether or not fear becomes problematic or maladaptive depends on a number of interrelated behavioral, cognitive, and physiological factors. As already pointed out, a great deal hinges on whether a dog believes that it can succeed in its efforts to predict and control threatening events (Bandura, 1977). Efficacy expectancies or "beliefs" are based on past experiences with both appetitive and aversive events (see *Locus of Control and Self-efficacy* in Volume 1, Chapter 9). These expectancies are influenced by learning in at least three specific ways: (1) learning what to do and when to do it, (2) learning what outcomes to expect as the result of appropriate action, and (3) learning that one is *able* to perform the required action.

Expectancy Confirmation and Disconfirmation

Efficacious action is purposive, that is, goal directed. Since the occurrence of discriminative stimuli (S), the responses (R) required, and the various outcomes (O) produced by those actions are not present in the same moment of time, but rather distributed over the course of time, the animal must necessarily form some neural or cognitive representation of how these various events are related. The events (S-R-O) and the various expectancies derived from them provide the cognitive foundation for effective action. *All organized voluntary behavior is based on assumptions and predictions (expectancies) that are differentially confirmed (reinforced) or disconfirmed (extinguished) by the outcomes they produce.*

Behavior is organized into a purposive train of events according to accumulated S-R-O expectancies formed as the result of past experience (in the sense of the Latin *experiri*, "to try out"). When a dog acts, it does so with the intention of producing some effect, if only to move its body from one location to another. Since the intended outcome does not actually exist before the action occurs, the relation between the response and outcome is necessarily mediated by some neural representation or expectancy. The intended or hoped-for outcome is only one of many possibilities that might occur, however. Since something might occur other than the intended outcome, the actual outcome must somehow be compared with the intended outcome (comparator function). The recognition of success (expectancy confirmed) is associated with various collateral effects such as feelings of elation (reward), whereas the recognition of failure (expectancy disconfirmed) is associated with disappoint-

ment (punishment). In general, the concomitant affect associated with purposive behavior is *hope* (see *Instrumental Learning* in Volume 1, Chapter 7).

Intention and Purpose

Intention is a generalized purpose-setting cognition. In obedience training, the intention corresponds to a dog's cognition of a command (discriminative stimulus) and the various emotional and motivational responses elicited by the command (conditioned establishing operations). Under natural conditions, the intention is cued by some sign triggering underlying emotional and motivational incentives to act. The intention behind an action has direct bearing on whether the consequences produced by the action will be reinforcing or punishing. For example, one intention of aggression is to force an actual or perceived threat to retreat or submit. If the behavior succeeds in achieving the intended goal (e.g., the rival runs way), it is reinforced. On the other hand, if the behavior fails to achieve its intended goal (e.g., the aggressor is displaced or defeated), the behavior is punished. In both cases, new expectancies are formed with respect to aggression occurring under similar circumstances in the future.

Expectancy and Reinforcement

Purposive actions are expected to work. Consequently, when the result of some action exactly matches an animal's expectancy, the latter is confirmed and no additional learning is necessary (asymptote). Although further learning may not occur as the result of repeated confirmations of an expected result, the animal's sense of well-being and confidence may be enhanced by such repeated success. Additional learning and adjustment occur only if the outcome fails to match (disconfirms) the operative expectancy in one of two ways: (1) The behavior either fails to obtain the intended outcome, or the outcome obtained is less than expected (disappointment). Such behavior is modified until it either succeeds (trial and *success*) or, if the behavior continues to fail, as hope is constrained by disappointment, the ineffectual behavior is gradually extinguished. (2) The behavior produces an outcome in excess of the one expected (surprise). Behavior associated with surprise is adjusted to maximize control over an unexpected opportunity. The adjustment of expectancies helps animals to fit their behavior more accurately to the surrounding environment.

Dysfunctional Expectancies

People and animals do not set out intentionally to fail, or continue to persist in a course of behavior that is hopeless, unless they happen to be neurotic. There are two general ways in which behavior becomes maladaptive or dysfunctional: (1) The behavior operates independently of purposive regulation (e.g., compulsion). (2) The behavior is emitted without an expectation of success (e.g., helplessness). In the first case, the intention and expectancy functions guiding purposive behavior may be operational, but the animal is unable to act in accordance with them. Excessively fearful dogs, for example, may properly seek safety from some threatening situation, but finding that the strategy does not work, they may nonetheless persist in the ineffectual behavior—even though they know that it will fail! *Expecting to fail in the presence of a threat is a potent source of fear and generalized anxiety.* The expectation of failure in the presence of a threat results in escalating fear, disorganized panic, and hopelessness. On the other hand, an *expectancy of success* facilitates confident and organized behavior while simultaneously modulating and constraining collateral aversive emotional arousal. Dogs that believe (a highly confirmed expectancy of success) that they will succeed are better prepared to cope with the various threats and challenges presented by the social and physical environment.

Externals and Internals

Another influential efficacy factor present in the development of persistent generalized anxiety and phobias should be considered before leaving the topic of efficacy expectancies. Rotter (1966) notes that individuals can be divided into two types of learners, depending on where they localize the locus of control over significant events. Learners who believe that control over important events is located outside of themselves (externals) are prone to expect that their efforts will fail (pessimistic attributional style), and even when they happen to succeed, they may still attribute their success to factors outside of their control. In contrast, learners who locate the locus of control within themselves (internals) are more likely to expect to succeed and to attribute their success to their own efforts (optimistic attributional style). Fearful or excessively anxious dogs are much more likely to be *external* learners. Only through appropriate training can overly fearful dogs learn that they can control external events. By *internalizing* the locus of control, dogs can eventually learn how to cope with threatening events more constructively. However, by believing that events are outside of their influence, dogs will continue to be controlled by their fears and never shake their pessimistic expectancies regarding them.

The ability of dogs to behave adaptively is not possible unless they have some idea of what to do and what to expect as a result of what they do. However, it is not enough for a dog to know these things, unless it also possesses the necessary confidence and ability to perform the required actions. A dog's degree of confidence reflects its accumulated past successes and failures. Adaptive learners expect to succeed (hopeful), whereas maladaptive learners expect to fail (hopeless). Adaptive learning promotes confidence, well-being, and an elated mood, whereas maladaptive learning saddles dogs with apprehensiveness, worry, insecurity, and generalized anxiety. Dogs that generally *expect to fail* are constrained to exist in a small corner of life where they feel most secure and likely to succeed. Dogs that expect to fail when threatened may experience unfamiliar situations and people as powerful sources of fear. Furthermore, the potential opportunities associated with the unfamiliar are not much solace for such dogs, since they are often equally inclined to expect to fail when it comes to appetitive resources, as well. Efficacy beliefs are especially influential under adverse motivational circumstances. These considerations have tremendous relevance for the management and control of behavior problems associated with fear, anxiety, frustration, and anger.

PRIMAL SENSORY MODALITIES MEDIATING ATTRACTION AND AVERSION

Touch

The sense of touch is the most primitive sensory modality mediating attraction and aversion (see *Effects of Touch* in Volume 1, Chapter 4). Touch contact with the environment gives a dog hedonic (pleasure-pain) information about stimuli acting directly on its body. Most of what is regarded or interpreted as emotional appears to be derived from information coming from the sense of touch. Touch plays a central role in the mediation of affectionate bonding and its maintenance. Higher touch analyzers interpret tactile stimulation in terms of the primal hedonic opposites of pleasure and pain. Events and situations that are either emotionally attractive or aversive are often directly or indirectly (i.e., through conditioning or generalization) linked to past experiences with touch. If born without functional touch sensitivities, dogs would be rendered insensitive, insular, and lack the ability to interpret events emotionally. Dogs that are hypersensitive to touch are more likely to be adversely affected by fear and anxiety stemming from aversive stimulation. Through the mediation of touch, animals acquire a complex range of interpretive feelings and expectations about the persons, places, and events with which they come into close contact. In addition, the accumulated experiences of touch are codified in an animal's mood and general attitude about contact with the social and physical environment. Early experiences with touch are particularly influential since they set the emotional tone and expectancy of puppies, biasing them in a positive or negative direction with respect to how they interpret close social contact as adults.

Olfaction and Emotional Learning

The role of olfaction in emotional learning is often neglected. This neglect is probably a result of the comparatively minor role that olfaction plays in the human perceptual *Merkwelt*, a perceptual organization that places much less value on olfaction than, for example, sight and hearing. In dogs, olfactory abilities are highly developed and play an important role in social learning and sexual behavior. Olfaction, in conjunction with subtle tactile and thermal learning, appears to play a vital role in the development of early preferences and aversions (Rosenblatt, 1983) (see *Social Comfort Seeking and Distress* in Chapter 4). According to this view, early neonatal ontogenesis progresses from tactile searching and contact, to detecting and following thermal gradients, to olfactory information derived from the wider environment. Olfaction is the most primitive of various sensory means for seeking and identifying significant stimuli occurring beyond immediate touch and thermal sensations. As an animal develops, additional sensory abilities are integrated for the purpose of scanning an even wider environment and, in conjunction with developing cognitive abilities, the ability to predict and control the occurrence of significant events. Consequently, it is reasonable to believe that olfactory signals are preferentially linked with information produced by appetitive, tactile, and thermal stimulation.

The olfactory tracts project directly into areas of the limbic system that are closely associated with emotional and social learning, potentially making olfaction an ideal sensory modality for counterconditioning fears and aggressiveness. Olfactory information is readily conditioned to produce lasting avoidance behavior when contingently associated with aversive or startling events. Conversely, associations between olfactory signals and appetitive or relaxing events can also be readily established. Olfaction appears to mediate conditioning of what Pavlov called the *social reflex*. Pavlov (1928) observed that dogs selectively responded to the presence of different people in his laboratory, based largely on the quality of their previous experience with them. This observation alone is not terribly interesting, but what he subsequently discovered clearly underscores the significance of olfaction for social learning and conditioning. He found that a particular experimenter had a habit of closely and affectionately interacting with one of the dogs under his care. As a result, the dog became closely attached to the experimenter and exhibited a strong conditioned social response whenever the individual entered the room. An experiment was performed to determine how much of this conditioned social response was controlled by the experimenter's scent or by other sensory stimuli. This was accomplished by placing the experimenter's clothes in the room where the dog had been confined and observing the dog's behavior. The experimenter's scent alone produced a similar (although diminished) social response in the dog as observed when the experimenter was actually present in the room with the dog [see Pavlov (1928:368) and Gantt et al. (1966)].

PLAY AND FEAR

Panksepp and colleagues (1984) argue that specific circuits in the brain are uniquely dedicated to the elaboration and expression of play. These play circuits are highly sensitive to the modulatory influences of fear, aggression, and nutritional deprivation. Fear and irritability appear to inhibit play directly, making the absence of play a possible diagnostic indicator of fear and aggression. The researchers found that lesioning of the ventromedial hypothalamus (VMH) produces pronounced effects on an animal's disposition to play. Presumably such lesions disrupt play by lowering irritability thresholds in response to playful gestures and initiatives:

> When these VMH lesioned pups [rats] were paired with controls who initially responded with playful solicitation, the VMH lesioned animal seemed unable to reciprocate. Playful gestures provoked defensive biting, and the controls shied away from further interaction. It was as if the VMH pups were unable to correctly interpret the playful gestures. Such results suggest that continuance of vigorous play requires active inhibition of irritability. Thus, it might be hypothesized that the medial hypothalamus normally promotes play by inhibiting aggressive tendencies which may periodically emerge during rough-and-tumble activities. (478)

These findings suggest that the continuation of play depends on the relative absence of fear and irritability. Play itself appears to exercise a modulatory effect on both fear and aggression, perhaps with the help of various species-typical signals that modulate nervous arousal. However, the modulatory effects of play may be rapidly overshadowed by increasing levels of fear or anger. The inhibitory effects exerted by fear and anger over play are much stronger than the pacifying effects of play on fearful or aggressive arousal. Play and fear are motivationally antagonistic toward each other, but play is probably organized at a higher cortical level. Like other cortical functions (e.g., attention and impulse control), play's relation to limbic and autonomic arousal is asymmetrical—fear asserts a stronger influence over play than play asserts over fear.

Playful dogs are normally social extroverts exhibiting a strong willingness to initiate social contacts and to explore unfamiliar environments. Socially inhibited dogs, on the other hand, are usually introverts that are prone to be withdrawn, reserved, and suspicious when confronted with unfamiliar situations or social contacts. In cases where a very low fear threshold exists, introverted dogs may avoid all social contact outside of their immediate circle of familiar contacts. Such dogs are prone to form an intense compensatory attachment to the owner or other family members. They are prone to run away and hide if threatened, unless escape is blocked. If escape is prevented and the threat increased, such dogs may attack to get away. Finally, introverted dogs with low thresholds for aggression and fear (sharp/shy) are prone to exhibit fight-flight conflict behavior and may bite under stressful conditions. Under normal circumstances fear arousal regulates the expression of aggression through direct inhibition, but in some cases fear may actually facilitate the expression of aggression as an escape/avoidance response (see *Fear and Aggression* in Chapter 7). In the case of the dominance aggression, perhaps the behavioral threshold controlling aggression (fight) is reached before the threshold of inhibitory fear (freeze-flight) is reached.

REFERENCES

Aronson LP (1998). Systemic causes of aggression and their treatment. In N Dodman and L Shuster (Eds), *Psychopharmacology of Animal Behavior Disorders.* Malden, MA: Blackwell Science.

Askew HR (1996). *Treatment of Behavior Problems in Dogs and Cats: A Guide for the Small Animal Veterinarian.* Cambridge, MA: Blackwell Science.

Bandura A (1977). Self-efficacy: Toward a unifying theory of behavior change. *Psychol Rev,* 84:191–215.

Baum M (1970). Extinction of avoidance responding through response prevention (flooding). *Psychol Bull,* 74:276–284.

Beaver BV (1994). Owner complaints about canine behavior. *JAVMA,* 204:1953–1955.

Bolles RC (1970). Species-specific defense reactions and avoidance learning. *Psychol Rev,* 77:32–48.

Campbell WE (1986). The prevalence of behavior problems in American dogs. *Mod Vet Pract,* 67:28–31.

Catania AC (1998). *Learning,* 4th Ed. Englewood Cliffs, NJ: Prentice-Hall.

Denny RM (1971). Relaxation theory and experiments. In R Brush (Ed), *Aversive Conditioning and Learning,* 235–295. New York: Academic.

Denny MR (1983). Safety catch in behavior therapy: Comments on "Safety training: The elimination of avoidance-motivated aggression in dogs." *J Exp Psychol Gen,* 112:215–217.

Fox MW (1966). The development of learning and conditioned responses in the dog: Theoretical and practical implications. *Can J Comp Vet Sci,* 30:282–286.

Freedman DG, King JA, and Eliot O (1961). Critical period in the social development of dogs. *Science,* 133:1016–1017.

Gantt WH (1962). Factors involved in the development of pathological behavior: Schizokinesis and autokinesis. *Perspect Biol Med,* 5:473–482.

Gantt WH, Newton JE, Royer FL, and Stephens JH (1966). Effect of person. *Cond Reflex,* 1:146–160.

Glickman LT, Glickman NW, Schellengerg DB, et al. (2000). Incidence of and breed-related risk factors for gastric dilatation-volvulus in dogs. *JAVMA,* 216:40–45.

Hamilton E and Cairns H (1961). *The Collected Dialogues of Plato.* Princeton: Princeton University Press.

Heidegger M (1949). *Existence and Being,* RFC Hull and A Crick (Trans). Chicago: Henry Regnery.

Heidegger M (1977). *Basic Writings.* D Farrell-Krell (Ed). New York: Harper and Row.

Hothersall D and Tuber DS (1979). Fears in companion dogs: Characteristics and treatment. In JD Keehn, *Psychopathology in Animals: Research and Clinical Implications.* New York: Academic.

Lockwood R (1997). The abused dog: Recognizing and responding to its special training needs. Presented at the APDT Conference Program, Memphis, TN.

LoLordo VM and Droungas A (1989). Selective associations and adaptive specializations: Taste aversions and phobias. In SB Klein and RR Mowrer (Eds), *Contemporary Learning Theories: Instrumental Theory and the Impact of Biological Constraints on Learning,* 145–179. Hillsdale, NJ: Lawrence Erlbaum Associates.

Lore RK and Eisenberg FB (1986): Avoidance reactions of domestic dogs to unfamiliar male and female humans in a kennel setting. *Appl Anim Behav Sci,* 15:261–266.

Marks I (1987). *Fears, Phobias, and Ritual: Panic, Anxiety, and Their Disorders.* New York: Oxford University Press.

Menzies RG and Clarke CJ (1995). The etiology of phobias: A nonassociative account. *Clin Psychol Rev,* 15:23–48.

Mineka S (1979). The role of fear in theories of avoidance learning, flooding, and extinction. *Psychol Bull,* 86:985–1010.

Murphree OD (1973). Inheritance of human aversion and inactivity in two strains of pointer dogs. *Biol Psychiatry,* 7:23–29.

Panksepp J, Siviy S, and Normansell L (1984). The psychobiology of play: Theoretical and methodological perspectives. *Neurosci Behav Rev,* 8:465–492.

Pavlov IP (1927/1960). *Conditioned Reflexes: An Investigation of the Physiological Activity of the Cerebral Cortex,* GV Anrep (Trans). New York: Dover (reprint).

Pavlov IP (1928). *Lectures on Conditioned Reinforcement,* Vol 1, WH Gantt (Trans). New York: International.

Reese WG (1979). A dog model for human psychopathology *Am J Psychiatry,* 136:1168–1172.

Rescorla RA (1988). Pavlovian conditioning: It's not what you think it is. *Am Psychol,* 43:151–160.

Rescorla RA and LoLordo VM (1965). Inhibition of avoidance behavior. *J Comp Physiol Psychol,* 59:406–412.

Rosenblatt J (1983). Olfaction mediates developmental transition in the altricial newborn of selected species of mammals. *Dev Psychobiol,* 16:347–375.

Rotter JB (1966). Generalized expectancies for internal versus external control of reinforcement. *Psychol Monogr Gen Appl,* 80:1–28.

Scott JP and Fuller JL (1965). *Genetics and the Social Behavior of the Dog.* Chicago: University of Chicago Press.

Seligman MEP (1971). Phobias and preparedness. *Behav Ther,* 2:307–320.

Seligman MEP and Binik YM (1977). The safety signal hypothesis. In H Davis and HMB Hurwitz (Eds), *Operant-Pavlovian Interactions.* Hillsdale, NJ: Lawrence.

Seligman MEP and Johnston JC (1973). A cognitive theory of avoidance learning. In FJ McGuigan and DB Lumsden (Eds), *Contemporary Approaches to Conditioning and Learning.* Washington, DC: Winston-Wiley.

Seligman MEP, Maier SF, and Solomon RL (1971). Unpredictable and uncontrollable aversive events. In FR Brush (Ed), *Aversive Conditioning and Learning.* New York: Academic.

Shull-Selcer EA and Stagg W (1991). Advances in the understanding and treatment of noise phobias. *Vet Clin North Am Adv Companion Anim Behav,* 21:299–314.

Solomon RL and Corbit JD (1974). An opponent-process theory of motivation: I. Temporal dynamics of affect. *Psychol Rev,* 81:119–145.

Solomon RL and Wynne LC (1953). Traumatic avoidance learning: Acquisition in normal dogs. *Psychol Monogr (Gen Appl),* 67:1–19.

Solomon RL, Kamin LJ, and Wynne LC (1953). Traumatic avoidance learning: The outcomes of several extinction procedures with dogs. *J Abnorm Soc Psychol,* 43:291–302.

Voith VL and Borchelt PL (1996). Fears and Phobias in Companion Animals: Update. In VL Voith and PL Borchelt (Eds), *Readings in Companion Animal Behavior.* Trenton, NJ: Veterinary Learning Systems.

Voith VL, Goodloe L, Chapman B, and Marder A (1993). Comparison of dogs presented for behavior problems by source of dog. Presented at the AVMA Meeting, Minneapolis, MN.

Wells DL and Hepper PG (1998). Male and female dogs respond differently to men and women. *Appl Anim Behav Sci,* 61:341–349.

Wolpe J (1958). *Psychotherapy by Reciprocal Inhibition.* Stanford: Stanford University Press.

Wolpe J (1969). *The Practice of Behavior Therapy.* New York: Pergamon.

Wright JC (1983). The effects of differential rearing on exploratory behavior in puppies. *Appl Anim Ethol,* 10:27–34.

4

Attachment, Separation, and Related Problems

Genuine social contact requires distance, and not only in a metaphorical sense.

PAUL LEYHAUSEN, *"On the Natural History of Fear"* (1973)

PART 1: ATTACHMENT AND SEPARATION

ATTACHMENT AND SEPARATION DISTRESS

Social and place attachments owe their development to a puppy's strongly motivated desire to maintain close contact with its mother and to stay within the safe confines of a familiar home area or nesting site. The importance of social and place attachments for dogs can be readily and dramatically demonstrated by taking a puppy away from its mother and confining it to an unfamiliar place. Such isolation invariably elicits robust signs of heightened emotional distress, sustained vocalization, and vigorous efforts to regain contact with the mother and littermates (see *Social Attachment and Separation* in Volume 1, Chapter 3). These species-typical responses to separation are commonly observed by puppy owners and have been carefully studied in the laboratory (Scott et al., 1973).

Separation distress probably reflects an evolutionary adaptation to the dangers of being left alone, with distress reactions discouraging vulnerable puppies from wandering too far away from the safety of the lair. In addition to prompting her to locate puppies that have wandered too far away, separation-distress vocalizations (whining and yelping) may stimulate the mother to stay close by her young, at least until they are old enough to fend for themselves. Young animals that express this tendency are much less likely to fall victim to various natural calamities and, therefore, are more likely to reproduce successfully and perpetuate the genes mediating the trait. In testament to its evolutionary value, separation distress enjoys a significant evolutionary continuity among animals, with a wide variety of species exhibiting the tendency.

The enhanced contact and safety secured by distress calls not only increase a puppy's survivability, they also provide the emotional basis for the formation of lasting social relationships. Behaviorally speaking, separation distress functions as an *establishing operation* under the motivational influence of which distance-decreasing behavior is emitted by both the infant and the mother. In addition, as the result of relief from distress, distance-decreasing or contact-seeking behavior is strongly reinforced when contact between the mother and infant is restored. Animals that exhibit separation distress as young tend to maintain close social contact with one another as adults. From this perspective, adult attachment and bonding tendencies may be viewed as secondary elaborations built upon the distress-relief exchanges first occurring between the mother, the infant, and littermates.

Given such emotional exchange and dependency, it is natural to expect that some degree of lasting mutual attraction and affection should develop between the vulnerable infant, its mother, familiar conspecifics, and others providing comfort and care to the puppy. In fact, Peter Hepper (1994) demonstrated that offspring recognize the scent of their mother and the mother recognizes the scent of her offspring after 2 years of continuous separation starting at 8 to 12 weeks of age. William Carr and colleagues at Beaver College (Glenside, Pennsylvania) extended Hepper's research, showing that dogs recognize the scent of their mothers after 6 years and, possibly, as long as 10 years after separation. Interestingly, with respect to the durability of the social bond, they found that dogs could recognize the hand scent of the breeder for 4 years and possibly as long as 9 years after separation without any intervening contact (Appel et al., 1999). Essentially, these findings suggest that olfactory memory and social recognition are lifelong in dogs.

BOWLBY'S SOCIAL BOND THEORY

John Bowlby (1969, 1973) made many pioneering contributions to the study of attachment and separation-related behavior. Originally trained as a psychoanalyst, Bowlby had broad philosophical and scientific interests, including a combined appreciation of ethology and behaviorism. According to Bowlby's eclectic theory, separation distress is mediated by primitive, self-protective impulses to maintain close contact with the mother. He adopted a Darwinian perspective on separation distress, interpreting it as an ontogenetically adaptive response to imminent danger resulting from maternal separation and isolation.

Bowlby (1969) describes several developmental phases that infants undergo during the ontogeny of attachment. Phase 1 involves the display of bodily orientations and various signals, but the exchange lacks social specificity. Phase 2 also involves the display of bodily orientations and the exchange of signals but with evidence of a progressive preference being exhibited toward primary attachment objects. Phase 3 involves bodily orientation, signals, and locomotion in an effort to maintain proximity with the attachment object. The infant shows heightened arousal at times of separation and becomes more excited when reunited with the attachment object. During phase 3, the infant begins to use the attachment object as a security base for environmental exploration. Also, during this phase, the infant becomes more selective with regard to social contacts and may exhibit increased alarm and caution when approached by a stranger. Phase 4 involves the development of a more complex cognitive understanding of the attachment object as an independent entity or partner. With regard to human infants, at approximately 3 years of age, children may begin to appreciate their mother as having personal feelings and motives of her own, laying the foundation for a much more complex and empathetic relationship or what Bowlby calls a *partnership*.

Protest, Despair, and Detachment

Bowlby observed a regular sequence of events that infants go through when they are separated from an attachment object. These responses to separation include protest, despair, and detachment. The *protest* phase involves general arousal and behavioral activation, with loud vocalizations, disruptive behaviors, and searching activities aimed are regaining contact with the absent mother. Protest and increased general activity occur immediately after the mother departs and corresponds in many ways to the sorts of behavior associated with separation distress in dogs (Voith and Borchelt, 1985; Lund and Jorgensen, 1999). *Despair,* the depressive phase, is associated with depressed affect and mood, inactivity, and infrequent distress vocalizations; however, even though depressed, the infant still remains vigilant for the mother's return. Finally, the third phase, *detachment,* involves an apparent loss of interest in the mother when reunited with her. All of these various phases of separation distress appear to present in various forms in dogs, suggesting that dogs and humans share similar emotional substrates for mediating the expression of separation-elicited behavior. In addition to mediating both human and dog separation distress, these shared substrates probably provide the framework for humans and dogs to form lasting attachments with one another.

Attachment and Fear

According to Bowlby, the attachment object provides support and security to the infant for a wider exploration of the environment (Mineka and Suomi, 1978). With the security of the mother's protection nearby, an infant can more confidently venture away from the immediate nesting area and explore its surroundings, at least until it encounters a threatening situation. When frightened, immature animals tend to flee back to the security of their mother, thus simultaneously reducing fear while enhancing social attachment. In fearful situations where the attachment object is absent, an infant's sense of security may be undermined and its ability to modulate fearful arousal compromised. In the absence of the mother, thresholds for fear and separation distress may be significantly lowered, resulting in highly aversive and generalized fear and panic toward the environment (Harlow and Mears, 1979). As the result of traumatic experiences during separation, animals may learn to fear being left alone and exhibit signs of anticipatory anxiety at times when they expect to be separated. As a result, sensitized animals may develop an anxious or anaclitic attachment, with increased vigilance about their mother's whereabouts, as well as exhibiting increased efforts to maintain close proximity with her.

The concurrent arousal of fear and separation distress may account for many characteristic patterns of behavior exhibited by separation-reactive dogs. One hypothesis derived from Bowlby's account is that adult separation anxiety may be incubated out of early experiences in which intense fear is elicited without the presence of an attachment object to help modulate fearful arousal and restore emotional equilibrium. Such animals may develop a fear of separation, thereby amplifying separation distress while coactively lowering fear thresholds when left alone. Consequently, at separation both fear and separation distress interact in a synergistic and mutually escalating manner that results in the expression of fear-related separation behavior. According to this analysis, separation anxiety is a state of emotional arousal that combines separation distress with a fear of separation. Consistent with this interpretation, many dogs exhibiting phobias also exhibit secondary separation-anxiety problems. These observations suggest that separation-related problems have a complex etiology, with fear being a significant factor in some cases (especially in dogs with existing phobias), but certainly not all dogs exhibiting separation-related problems do so because of fear.

PSYCHOBIOLOGICAL ATTUNEMENT: THE BIOREGULATORY HYPOTHESIS

The withdrawal of an attachment object appears to exert numerous psychobiological effects, the sum of which produce disruptive emotional and physiological distress in a separated animal. Adopting this line of analysis, M. A. Hofer (1983) argues that attachment is mediated by the establishment of various maternal regulatory influences over biological processes and needs exhibited by the infant. When the attachment object is withdrawn, these modulatory influences are disrupted, and the young animal is caused to experience acute distress. According to the bioregulatory hypothesis, separation anxiety is the result of biological stress produced by the loss of maternal regulatory influences over physiological processes. Similarly, Tiffany Fields (1985) has proposed that various reciprocal interorganismic regulatory influences are instrumental in the formation of attachments occurring at various points in an animal's life cycle, including, but not limited to, the mother-infant relationship. She argues that separation distress is not due to a disruption of an hypothesized *attachment* bond between mother and infant, but rather distress results when the psychobiological synchrony or *attunement* between mutually attached organisms is disrupted by separation:

> Attachment might instead be viewed as a relationship that develops between two or more organisms as their behavioral and physiological systems become attuned to each other. Each partner provides meaningful stimulation for the other and has a modulating influence on the other's arousal level. The relationship facilitates an optimal growth state that is threatened by changes in the individuals or their relationship or by separation and the behavioral and physiological disorganization that ensue. Thus, attach-

ments are psychobiologically adaptive for the organization, equilibrium and growth of the organism. Because the organism's behavior repertoire, physiological makeup, and growth needs are an integrated multivariate complex that changes developmentally, multiple and different types of attachment are experienced across the life span. (15–16)

The psychobiological attunement hypothesis of attachment and separation distress is compelling. Dogs often exhibit their first acute episodes of adult separation anxiety following prolonged contact with the owner. Also, the disruptive events associated with separation are particularly common after long vacations or after an owner returns to work or school after a long stay at home. Theoretically, some dogs may undergo enhanced regulatory synchronization with the owner during these periods of prolonged contact. The sense of well-being achieved during these periods of prolonged contact is dramatically disrupted when a dog is separated from its owner, with the resultant evocation of separation-related disturbances and excesses.

OPPONENT-PROCESS THEORY AND SEPARATION DISTRESS

The opponent-process theory (Solomon and Corbit, 1974) may offer a useful construct for understanding certain etiological aspects of adverse separation reactivity in dogs (see *Practical Application of Opponent-process Theory* in Volume 1, Chapter 5). According to this theory, there exists a hypothetical neural system that regulates emotional arousal and prevents affective extremes from occurring as the result of attractive or aversive stimulation. This emotional regulatory function is believed to be performed by indirect and hedonically opposite *slave* emotions that shadow attractive and aversive stimulation. These underlying slave emotions serve to dampen affective extremes. For example, while being petted, a dog experiences a wide range of socially comforting emotions or *a-processes*. The opponent-process theory postulates that such feelings of well-being and comfort are shadowed by hedonically opposite affects (e.g., feelings of contact need) or *b-processes*. The antagonistic b-processes are of an opposite hedonic

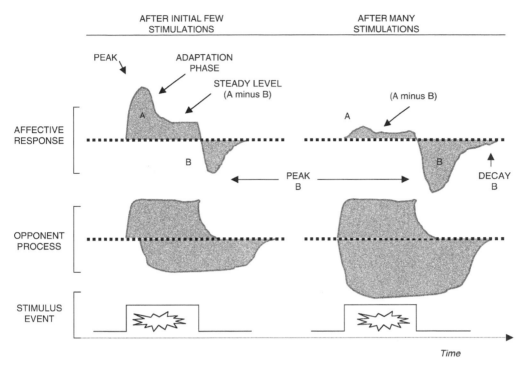

F IG. 4.1. Opponent B-processes restrain emotional responding elicited by affective stimulation. After repeated stimulation, A-process responding is significantly dampened. A similar pattern appears to occur in the case of separation anxiety, suggested by the progressively reduced magnitude of cyclic recurrence of distress during the day. See Fig. 4.2. After Solomon and Corbit (1974).

quality to the directly elicited emotion or a-processes (Figure 4.1); that is, if the eliciting a-processes are attractive, the opposing b-processes are aversive and vice versa. B-processes occur concurrently with a-processes, but the former become evident only after the eliciting stimulus is withdrawn. According to the opponent-process theory, the organism's hedonic state (general feelings of euphoria or dysphoria) at any given moment is determined by the interaction of a- and b-processes: If (a − b) > 0, the animal is in an A-state. On the other hand, if (a − b) < 0, the animal is in a B-state. Here, zero represents affective neutrality.

The latency, magnitude, and persistence of a- and b-processes gradually change as the result of repeated stimulation. Initially, a-processes are subject to robust arousal and decay rapidly after the eliciting stimulus is discontinued. On the other hand, antagonistic b-processes exhibit an initially sluggish onset and persist longer than a-processes when stimulation is withdrawn. However, after repeated stimulations (habituation), a-processes are weakened (slower latency and decreased magnitude), whereas underlying b-processes are gradually strengthened and become more persistent.

Theoretically, in terms of attachment phenomena, these differential effects of repeated a- and b-process stimulation would result in the gradual attenuation of affectional responses aroused by social contact, while at the same time progressively potentiating aversive emotions associated with the withdrawal of contact at separation. As the result of repeated separations and reunions, the psychophysiological effects associated with separation may become progressively more intrusive, while subsequent reunions may fail to satisfy fully a growing need for social comfort. Overall, the net result of these opponent dynamics is consistent with the development of an insecure or anxious attachment and increased separation distress when a dog is left alone.

Opponent Intensification of Separation Distress

Some experimental data support the opponent-process interpretation of attachment and separation distress. For example, Hoffman and Solomon (1974) reviewed several imprinting studies showing that repeated contacts with an imprinting object intensifies separation-elicited distress. In one of these experiments, ducklings that had been repeatedly exposed to alternating periods of contact followed by withdrawal of the imprinting object exhibited mounting signs of distress whenever the imprinting object was removed. After many repetitions of this pattern, the ducklings exhibited increased signs of distress even when the imprinting stimulus was presented, suggesting that a-processes aroused by the imprinting object were being concurrently overshadowed by ascending b-processes. It is noteworthy that the successive presentation and withdrawal of the imprinting stimulus produced corresponding attractive and aversive effects sufficient to modify instrumental behavior. Ducklings learned various voluntary responses based on the contingent presentation (reward) or withdrawal (punishment) of the imprinting stimulus. Ducklings can even be trained not to follow the imprinting stimulus, if doing so results in its removal. Also, Starr (1978) reported that the most intense and frequent distress vocalizations shown by ducklings were elicited either when the imprinting stimulus was presented and withdrawn repeatedly or when it was presented for long periods before being withdrawn. In addition, he found that the interval between repeated separation trials had a marked effect on the amount of distress vocalization emitted by the ducklings. Interestingly, 1-minute intervals between trials had the most pronounced effect on subsequent separation-distress vocalization, whereas 5-minute intervals produced proportionately less distress vocalization. These findings are consistent with an adjunctive analysis of separation anxiety (see below).

Opponent Processing and Imprinting

The opponent-process theory offers a viable theoretical model for understanding some aspects of canine separation-anxiety panic. Typically, separation reactivity rapidly mounts in magnitude and reaches a peak approximately 30 minutes after the owner leaves (Voith and Borchelt, 1985; Lund and Jorgensen, 1999). This rapid onset and intensification of separation reactivity is followed by a gradual adaptation period and a steady decline of distress over a variable length of time, ranging from minutes to hours, depending on the individual dog and the severity of its separation problem (Figure 4.2). This general pattern is consistent with the sluggish latency or slow buildup of b-processes and their tendency to decay slowly after the a-process stimulus is withdrawn. This picture is in contrast to the brief latency and vigorous buildup of intense greeting activity (via a-processes) when the owner returns. Another aspect of considerable interest regarding separation anxiety and opponent-process theory is the observation that, after repeated exposures to separation, many separation-reactive dogs fail to habituate (as might be expected) but instead continue to become increasingly distressed when left alone. It follows that the planned-departure method of repeatedly leaving and returning to a dog, if not properly performed, could inadvertently intensify separation distress rather than reduce it—an outcome that is fully consistent with predictions from the opponent-process theory.

Opponent Origins of Separation Depression

Opponent-process theory also provides a way for understanding some aspects of the depressive phase of separation distress. In response to chronic separation distress, some dogs appear to withdraw emotionally, become depressed, and exhibit signs of progressive detachment toward their owners' return home. These cumulative changes may be due to B-state dominance developing over time in response to repeated separation-reunion experiences. As a result of repeated separations,

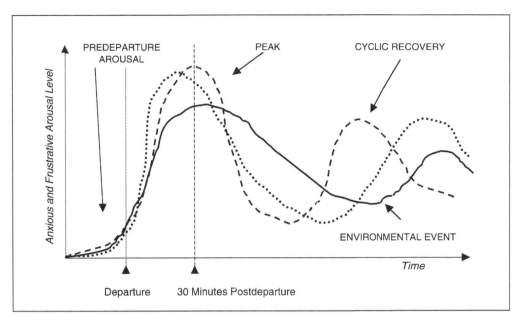

FIG. 4.2. Three hypothetical separation-reactive dogs exhibiting the general pattern of predeparture and postdeparture arousal, adaptation, and cyclic recovery. Note that anxiety and frustration levels follow a cyclic pattern of adaptation and recovery and often recovery after an environmental event (car passing by, dog barking, etc.). After Voith and Borchelt (1985) and Lund and Jorgensen (1999).

b-process feelings of loss may become sufficiently strong and persistent to overshadow a-process greeting excitement elicited by an owner's homecoming. The result is an appearance of detachment—what some owners may interpret as the dog being sullen or angry for leaving them alone. Detachment in such cases may reflect a situation in which a-process stimulation is dampened and offset by strong slave b-processes.

The duration of contact between an animal and an attachment object was a significant variable in some of the aforementioned experiments. Long periods of social contact produced more separation distress than did brief periods of contact. This finding parallels conditions often associated with episodes of separation distress in family dogs. Owners frequently report the occurrence of separation-related problems following long weekends or after holidays in which greater amounts of time are spent with their dog.

SUPERNORMAL ATTACHMENT HYPOTHESIS

Many experiments have shown that contact with a human handler has a pronounced ameliorative effect on separation distress in puppies and dogs. The presence of a person exercises a calming effect that is often greater than occurs in the presence of other dogs. Pettijohn and colleagues (1977) found that the presence of a human handler during periods of separation had a more pronounced effect on separation distress in puppies than did the presence of its mother or a littermate. Similar effects have been observed in adult dogs. For example, Tuber and colleagues (1996) reported that dogs restrained in a novel situation with a human companion had lower cortisol levels (a sensitive measure of biological stress) than did dogs restrained in a novel situation with a canine companion. Also, Gantt and colleagues (1966) observed that petting exerted a pronounced calmative effect on sympathetic arousal, reducing both heart and respiratory rates in separated dogs. In neurotic dogs, the effects of human presence and petting were often even more striking and robust than observed in normal dogs. Lynch (1970) reviewed the findings of various studies, comfirming that aversive arousal in dogs is significantly modulated by human petting. For most separation-anxious dogs, canine companionship does not provide ersatz comfort in the absence of human contact. Voith and Borchelt (1996) report that many separation dogs are highly distressed despite the availability of another dog during periods of separation. Also, videotapes of separation-distressed dogs left alone with nondistressed dogs show that they virtually ignore the presence of their nondistressed companions. Together these findings suggest that a human companion provides a strong modulatory effect over canine separation distress, apparently more so than the relief produced by the presence of conspecifics.

One way to interpret these findings is that humans represent a *supernormal* attachment object for dogs. According to Tinbergen (1951/1969), the supernormal stimulus is an artificial stimulus or situation that is more effective in evoking some species-typical behavior than is the natural stimulus situation. In short, the supernormal stimulus produces a response of stronger magnitude than does the natural one. It is interesting to speculate that the protective influence of human contact and petting against increased distress and aversive arousal associated with unfamiliar places and fear is due to such a supernormal influence. A supernormal attachment may help to explain the peculiar psychological dependency (anaclisis) that some dogs form toward their owners (and vice versa), inclining them to develop separation-related problems. Dogs rarely present with separation-distress or panic problems resulting from the loss of canine companions: although such loss is commonly associated with a variable degree of ennui or depression, it does not frequently rise to the level of producing separation distress or panic problems. Perhaps attachment with human companions creates a supernormal feeling of well-being and safety that is lost at separation, causing heightened levels of generalized distress and panic in predisposed dogs when left alone.

Many routine rearing practices may contribute to a supernormal attachment forming between owners and dogs. Normally, nearly every activity of significance is controlled by human caretakers, making dogs virtually dependent on the presence of human help to survive. In addition to contact comfort, dogs depend on human caretakers to provide food, exercise, play, and sundry other things. What may further magnify the human as an attachment object is a growing sense of helplessness on the dog's part. Helplessness is a natural cognitive, motivational, and behavioral outcome that develops under environmental conditions in which significant events occur independently of what a dog does or does not do. Supernormal attachment as a factor in separation distress has many obvious overlapping features with the attunement and bioregulatory hypothesis already discussed. The dog may also represent a supernormal attachment object for humans. This is a particularly appealing idea, given the behavioral and morphological changes in the direction of neoteny that have occurred to the dog over the course of its domestication. The infantlike appearance and dependency of dogs may stimulate intense attachment and parenting behavior in human caretakers (Figure 4.3).

NEOTENY AND DEPENDENCY

As a result of domestication, the dog has undergone a pervasive neotenic transformation, setting the foundation for enhanced dependency. Neotenization has emphasized immature behavioral tendencies and physical characteristics in the dog. Unlike the dog's natural progenitor, the wolf, most domestic dogs cannot hunt and provide for themselves. Neoteny and enhanced docility have resulted in dogs becoming permanently dependent on humans for the provision of many of their social and physical needs. These changes have encouraged behavioral solicitousness as a means for attracting attention and care. Dependency needs appear to be stronger in some dogs, especially in those inclined to develop separation problems. Lonely puppies or neotenic dogs may feel vulnerable and in

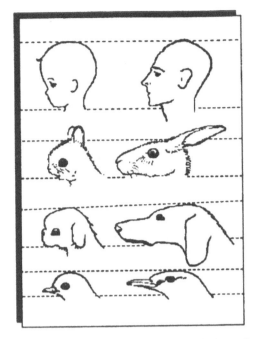

FIG. 4.3. In addition to babies, the morphology of the young of various species elicits attachment behavior, perhaps reflecting an innate releasing schema controlling attachment and parenting behavior. After Lorenz (1971).

danger when left alone—a natural reaction to separation for such dogs.

Under natural conditions, wolf pups are exposed to gradual doses of separation from group members. This exposure process is ontogenetically timed, so that a pup's increasing independence is correlated with the maturity of other physical and behavioral characteristics, ensuring readiness for greater autonomy. However, domestic dogs often grow up in an environment in which this natural learning and developmental process is impeded. They are sometimes kept in nearly constant contact with the owner and prevented from learning how to cope with the emotional demands of solitude. Instead of becoming progressively independent and secure when alone, they become overly attached, excessively dependent on the owner's presence and virtually helpless. Although physically mature, adult separation-reactive dogs may appear to be emotionally arrested at a very immature level of develop-

ment, responding to separation with puppy-like signs of distress and protest.

BIOLOGICAL STRESS AND SEPARATION DISTRESS

Separation distress evokes neuroendocrine activity involving the hypothalamic-pituitary-adrenocortical (HPA) system (see *Stress and Separation Anxiety* in Volume 1, Chapter 3). During stressful stimulation, corticotropin-releasing factor (CRF) is secreted by the hypothalamus and carried via the portal blood supply to the anterior pituitary gland, where it stimulates the release of adrenocorticotropic hormone (ACTH). ACTH, in turn, stimulates the adrenal cortex to secrete glucocorticoids, hormones that prepare and augment the body's ability to respond to physiological stress and to defend itself against danger. Rising glucocorticoid (e.g., cortisol) levels modulate hypothalamic CRF output directly and also indirectly via the combined influences it has on the amygdala (excitatory influence over hypothalamic CRF output) and the hippocampus (inhibitory influence over hypothalamic CRF output). The antagonistic effect of cortisol on the amygdala and hippocampus regulates the amount of CRF secreted by the hypothalamus and, ultimately, the peripheral release of cortisol by the adrenal cortex. Under conditions of chronic stress, the dynamic stasis modulating stress-hormone activity may undergo regulatory breakdown, along with various other destructive physiological and immunological impairments (Selye, 1976). The hippocampus, for example, as the result of excessive exposure to cortisol, may undergo degenerative changes that impede its ability to modulate emotional reactivity and associated neuroendocrine activities.

Stress-related hormonal changes have been found to occur as the result of separation in a number of animal species. For example, elevated cortisol output rapidly occurs and peaks within two hours after young monkeys are separated from their mothers, an effect that is reversed at reunion (Marks, 1987). In the case of dogs, Tuber and colleagues have (1996) identified a differential glucocorticoid (cortisol and corticosterone) response occurring under five conditions of separation: (1) alone in a novel environment, (2) together with a conspecific in a novel environment, (3) alone in a familiar environment, (4) together with a human in a novel environment, and (5) together with a conspecific in a familiar environment. As one might expect from the adverse additive effects of place unfamiliarity on separation distress, the researchers found that the highest levels of cortisol output occurred when the dogs were left alone in a novel situation. Conversely, the lowest levels of cortisol output occurred when the dogs were tested in their home kennel with a familiar conspecific. Interestingly, though, in light of the additive effects of an unfamiliar place on separation distress, they found that dogs tested in the novel situation in the company of a human companion exhibited significantly lower cortisol levels than measured when the dogs were restrained in a novel situation with a conspecific.

SEPARATION DISTRESS AND COACTIVE INFLUENCES

Fear and Anxiety

As already discussed, under some conditions fear of separation may significantly increase the magnitude of separation distress and lower fear thresholds. Despite the ostensive appearance of a potentiating effect of fear on separation distress, the relationship between the two emotional states is far from straightforward. A great deal of laboratory research supports the notion that separation distress per se is mediated by a relatively discrete motivational system that is functionally independent of fear but not without significant interaction with it (Panksepp, 1998). Davis and colleagues (1977) observed that among puppies separation distress was not increased by the startle of a loud noise. Although startle caused the puppies to carry their tails in a lower position, separation distress was not significantly altered by startling auditory stimulation. They concluded that "sound-induced fear and separation distress are separate and independent affective states" (203). Among chicks, separation-induced peeping is suppressed by a startling noise of a horn (120 dB) (Montevecchi et al., 1973)—the opposite effect of what one might expect to observe if fear motivationally augmented separation distress. Rather than potentiating separation-distress vocalization, fear appears to suppress separation-related distress behavior. Panksepp (1998) neatly summarizes the available data on the relationship between separation distress and fear:

> Thus, separation distress may promote activity in fear circuits, but behavioral data suggest that the converse does not occur. For instance, the presentation of fearful stimuli tends to reduce the frequency of separation calls, presumably because it would be maladaptive for young animals to reveal their locations when predators are nearby. (274)

The aforementioned separation-distress study reported by Tuber and colleagues (1996) provides data supportive of this general hypothesis. The researchers found that adult dogs exhibit different patterns of distress vocalization, depending on the familiarity of the test situation. Adult dogs, unlike puppies, tended to exhibit more distress vocalization when confined in a familiar situation than when they were confined in an unfamiliar situation. Among several adult beagles studied by Tuber's group, distress vocalizations were most strongly suppressed when the dogs were individually confined in an unfamiliar test situation. Apparently, in mature dogs the tendency to bark is more likely to occur under the *safety* of a familiar environment. When isolated in an unfamiliar environment, distress barking is inhibited, perhaps as the result of increased fear associated with novelty and unfamiliarity. Such inhibition would be adaptive under natural conditions, where, as Panksepp points out, distress vocalization might attract unwelcome attention in potentially dangerous and unfamiliar surroundings.

Panic

Again, although having some overlap and interaction at various levels of organization, separation distress and fear appear to belong to two separate neural systems in which distress-related behavior is subordinate to fear. Separation distress does not appear to depend on *anxiety* (in the sense of a foreboding or anticipatory fear of impending threat) but rather appears to operate under the influence of an independent social motivational system—one that exercises a pervasive influence on canine social development and behavior in its own right (Scott and Bronson, 1964; Panksepp, 1988a). Separation distress and fear of separation or separation *anxiety* are not the same thing. Further, although separation anxiety may not be strongly related to fear or *threat* anxiety per se, as will be discussed momentarily, it is strongly influenced by *need* anxiety and frustration.

In some ways, separation distress appears to be even more closely related to panic than anxiety. Among humans suffering panic attacks, many report having experienced separation anxiety as children (Torgersen, 1986). During panic attacks, "the victims feel as if their center of comfort and stability has been abruptly removed, leading to active solicitation of help and social support" (Panksepp, 1998:274). Adverse traumatic or chronic activation of separation-distress circuits may gradually result in lowered thresholds for panic triggered by the loss of significant attachment objects at separation. The linkage between separation distress and panic is further supported by pharmacological studies showing that both conditions are ameliorated by the tricyclic antidepressant imipramine. Anxiolytics (e.g., benzodiazepines) have little beneficial effect on panic attacks or separation distress, although in cases where a fear of separation or a need anxiety is evident, antianxiety medications appear to provide some measure of relief.

Another way of interpreting panic at separation is in terms of behavioral helplessness. Helplessness occurs when significant events are perceived as being both unpredictable and uncontrollable. In addition to anxiety, separation distress is also probably potentiated by high levels of frustration occurring at separation. Frustrative arousal occurs when a dog's control over its attachment object is somehow impeded. Whereas the anxiety component in separation distress is primarily under the control of classical conditioning, the frustrative component is more strongly influenced by instrumental learning mechanisms. Under conditions in which the behavior of the attachment object is perceived as being both unpredictable (classical input) and uncontrollable

(instrumental input), insolvable conflict may ensue at separation, resulting in behavioral helplessness (see *Conflict and Neurosis* in Volume 1, Chapter 9) and precipitous separation panic. Separation-panicked dogs often exhibit compulsive repetitive behaviors, suggesting that separation may evoke acute compulsive episodes in susceptible dogs.

Frustration

One need only consider the frustrative effects of unrequited love on attachment and proximity-seeking behavior among humans to appreciate the central role that frustration plays in the formation of social attachments. The more one becomes frustrated by some activity or goal, the harder it seems to let go, especially if the goal happens to be an intimate attachment object. Experimental evidence suggests that both frustration and discomfort may contribute to enhancing social attachment and dependency. Brodbeck (1954) performed an early experiment to compare a number of variables affecting the development of dependency in puppies, especially the relative effect of food on the development social dependency. To test his hypothesis, he built a feeding machine so that food could be delivered anonymously by a system of ropes and pulleys. Subsequently, one group of puppies was fed by machine and another group fed permissively by hand. Both groups appeared to exhibit approximately the same level of dependency during the testing phase of the experiment. He concluded that food per se did not facilitate social dependency. In a third group, puppies were fed by hand but deliberately frustrated before and while they took food from the experimenter's hand. Interestingly, he found that the frustrated, hand-fed group exhibited much stronger dependency behavior (proximity seeking) than either the permissively fed group or the machine-fed group. Similarly, Fisher (1955) found that puppies that were alternately exposed to both social indulgence and punishment exhibited a pronounced increase of dependency behavior (proximity seeking) in comparison to puppies that were indulged only with petting and play over the same period. These experiments by Brodbeck and Fisher demonstrate that frustration and discomfort (punitive interaction) may facilitate attachment and dependency behavior. Frustration, in particular, appears to exert a prominent motivational influence on the formation of excessive dependency between humans and dogs.

The most common response to a situation where some desirable goal is obstructed is for a dog to persist or try harder. Similarly, when a dog's efforts to gain contact with its owner are unsuccessful, frustration invigorates separation-distress reactions and prompts efforts to regain contact. Many unwanted behaviors associated with separation distress, such as incessant barking and destructiveness, appear to be motivated by frustrative arousal. As frustration mounts, associated behavior patterns become correspondingly stronger and more compulsive. The contributory effects of frustration on separation distress may be quite dramatic, resulting in generalized behavioral activation involving increased activity (pacing), exploration (searching cabinets and waste bins), destructiveness (scratching, biting, and chewing personal belongings and furnishings, woodwork, doorjambs, and carpets), and barking—all emitted under a high degree of aversive arousal. In a certain sense, the perception of many owners that their dogs are acting out of *anger* may not be too far off the mark [see Berkowitz (1990)]—a common assumption that has often been criticized and rejected as a misconception (Lindell, 1997). The barking of such dogs often has a complaining and demanding quality to it—it does not affect one like the vocalization of a fearful or anxious dog. Such barking impresses one as the vocalizations of a dog that is upset about not getting what it wants, rather than a plaintive expression of loneliness, anxiety, or fear. Affected dogs may persist in their barking at separation for long periods, appearing to expect that the owner will eventually give in to their noisy demands. In fact, these dogs are frequently very successful social manipulators, having learned that persistence in the face of nonreward and punishment frequently pays off. Modifying manipulative separation behavior and replacing it with more cooperative and obedient alternatives is an important aspect of treating such problems.

Many of the problem behaviors exhibited by separation-distressed dogs are highly ritualized, repetitive, and resistant to behavior modification. Although such dogs usually tire of their efforts and gradually give up, after a variable period of remission they may be alarmed by something happening outside and the pattern starts all over again (Askew, 1996; Lund and Jorgensen, 1999). The sound of a passerby, a barking dog, or the drone of a passing car may prompt additional frustrative effort. Since internal states associated with frustration have often been present when the dog was successful in the past, frustrative arousal may provide a source of conditioned reinforcement or continuous incentive to keep trying, thereby maintaining separation-related behavior over long periods. The evident benefits of obedience training for managing or preventing separation-related problems (Borchelt and Voith, 1982; Clark and Boyer, 1993; Jagoe and Serpell, 1996; Goodloe and Borchelt, 1998) may be, in part, the result of encouraging more constructive patterns of interaction in which frustration-related excesses are discouraged and more compliant and cooperative behavior is rewarded.

In addition to persistence, regressive behavior is a common coping response to excessive frustration. Finding that some behavior no longer works, a frustrated dog may resort to other previously effective behavior patterns, including some belonging to an earlier stage of development. A common example of this sort of coping behavior in humans is the temper tantrum—a regressive response to frustration that often persists into adulthood. Distressed dogs may, under the influence of chronic frustration at separation from their owners, turn to coping strategies that proved successful in puppyhood to gain social contact. A regressive interpretation of separation-related behavior emphasizes the invigorating influence of frustration, perhaps rising to a level in which separation distress directly evokes immature species-typical contact seeking or et-epimeletic (care-seeking) behavior patterns in adult dogs. Sustained distress vocalization (e.g., whining and yelping), loss of bladder or bowel control, and increased orality among such dogs may be interpreted along similar lines of analysis. Many separation-reactive dogs are strikingly immature, exhibiting a variety of regressive behavior patterns and needs, including excessive dependency and proximity-seeking behaviors. Frustrative perseveration and fixation, destructive (angry) acting out, and immaturity are commonly associated with dogs exhibiting separation-related problems.

Although frustration appears to be a strong motivational variable, many dogs distressed at separation also appear to be intensely worried or anxious about being left alone. Perhaps a coactive linkage between anxiety and frustration may occur in some cases of separation distress. Such motivational coactivity could produce powerful synergistic effects, perhaps leading to the more extreme and compulsive separation-panic symptoms observed in some dogs. Finally, some separation-distressed dogs may be anxious only to the extent that they fear that their efforts will not work (need anxiety), and that they will be left to endure more and more discomfort as their frustration grows and their efforts continue to fail. Panksepp (1998) has noted that the distress resulting from frustrative arousal may be more akin to *pain* than to fear, however. A dog may fear the pain of frustrative loss and, in that sense, become *anxious* about experiencing separations from its owner.

Boredom

Boredom has often been proposed as a significant cause of separation-related behavior problems (Hart and Hart, 1985; Niego et al., 1990). Turner (1997) suggests that boredom-related destructive behavior is often misdiagnosed as separation anxiety. He admonishes behavioral counselors to differentiate destructive behavior carefully due to separation anxiety from behavior caused by *boredom*. Unfortunately, he offers little edification as to what he precisely means by boredom or how it might result in stimulating destructive behavior. Although boredom is often mentioned as a possible cause of misbehavior, it is rarely described in operational terms or with the sort of precision required to assess its potential role in

separation-related destructiveness or other behavior problems described as being boredom related (e.g., compulsive disorders). Finally, surprisingly few scientific papers have been devoted to the study of boredom and its effects on animal behavior, but ethologists have emphasized the role of boredom in the development of abnormal behavior in zoo (Hediger, 1955/1968) and farm animals (Fraser, 1980). Other authors have questioned the role of boredom in the etiology of such problems and have rejected the boredom interpretation as usually "simplistic and wrong" (Overall, 1997:222).

As a motivational concept, boredom can be defined as an aversive or stressful state that occurs in the absence of optimal stimulation. How animals respond to boredom depends on many considerations, including temperament (see *Experimental Neurosis* in Volume 1, Chapter 9). Some dogs, especially energetic and outgoing ones (extroverts), may respond to boring circumstances by engaging in diversionary activity aimed at achieving a more favorable level of stimulation. In essence, boredom for such dogs is an aversive state or an *establishing operation* that prompts behavior aimed at finding a means to reduce it. In other dogs, who are more withdrawn and less active (introverts), boredom may be taken more in stride or precipitate depressive forms of separation distress.

A. F. Fraser (1980) emphasizes the role of stress in the development of abnormal behavior in animals, defining stress and its relation to boredom in the following way:

> An animal is said to be in a state of stress if it is required to make abnormal or extreme adjustments in its physiology or behavior in order to cope with adverse aspects of its environment and management. . . . A feature of this definition concerns the issue of environments involving 'boredom' or physical restraint. . . . It is widely accepted that animals in monotonous and restricting environments seek out opportunities for exercise and stimulation. Most veterinary ethologists now suggest that the restriction of movement, 'boredom', thwarting of drives, stressful stimuli and deficiencies of the environment may lead to abnormal stereotyped behaviour. (237–238)

In combination, boredom and loneliness may coalesce to form a highly potent and aversive motivational state, perhaps underlying the development of certain separation-related problems. Boredom may be a source of considerable stress for dogs receiving inadequate daily stimulation and exercise. Chronic compulsive licking, causing acral lick dermatitis, may be directly related to stress resulting from separation boredom. Such compulsive habits often present comorbidly with separation-distress problems. Repetitive self-licking might offer bored and lonely dogs a self-stimulatory outlet for the stresses and tensions produced by separation. Licking may also serve a self-medicating function. Clinical evidence suggests that the activity is maintained to some extent by the release of endogenous opioids (White, 1990).

Finally, boredom may interact coactively with frustration, especially in cases where boredom-related exploratory behavior or other efforts to escape the situation are thwarted. Finally, although boredom may be a contributing factor in the etiology of some separation problems, it is unlikely that boredom alone is a significant motivational factor in the precipitation of the classical symptoms of separation distress. Boredom takes time to build up and, consequently, one would expect it to exert its most pronounced effects on behavior after some significant period had elapsed following separation. Typically, however, separation-related arousal and distress usually begin before the owner departs and continues building up for many minutes thereafter before gradually leveling off and dissipating (Voith and Borchelt, 1985).

Compulsion

As already noted, a fear probably plays a relatively secondary role in the development of anxiety at separation. In addition to a premonitory apprehension about some potential threat at separation, another possible source of anxious arousal is anticipated loss or *need anxiety*, which is common among both dogs and humans in response to the anticipated loss of an attachment or appetitive object. In the case of an attachment object, need anxiety expresses itself as obsessive worry and vigilance about the whereabouts of a lost object of affection or comfort. The sense of loss and worry about the owner's whereabouts may trigger exaggerated exploratory activity and other behavior under the control of the seeking system [see Panksepp (1998)]. Under conditions of high conflict and stress, especially in cases where such efforts are intermittently successful to reduce distress (e.g., owner returns or dog obtains internal relief from the worry), adjunctive or displacement behaviors may emerge in a variety of forms (see *Adjunctive Behavior and Compulsions* in Chapter 5). Many of the behavior patterns exhibited by separation-reactive dogs at separation do, in fact, appear to take on a compulsive character. In the laboratory, under certain schedules of reinforcement, various adjunctive behavioral excesses are generated, including excessive drinking, wheel running, object shredding, self-licking, and even aggression—if an adequate target is available. Under such conditions, Panksepp (1998) notes, "Animals appear to vent the frustration of neuroemotional energy emerging from unfulfilled expectations on any available target" (161). Whereas threat anxiety refers to an apprehension resulting from an inadequately predicted threat, need anxiety results when a highly attractive stimulus is lost and its future return is inadequately predicted.

Separation-reactive dogs may be conflicted between a desire to remain in close social contact with their owners while being prevented from doing so by an intervening barrier. This barrier can be either physical or emotional, that is, the owners may be emotionally withdrawn or rejecting toward their dogs. The conflict involves two antagonistic pressures demanding two mutually exclusive and opposing responses. On the one hand, a dog is highly motivated to maintain intimate social contact with its owner, whereas, on the other, it is physically or psychologically prohibited from doing so. When left alone at separation, most dogs simply accept their state of affairs and slip into a stoic state, patiently waiting for their owner to return. Separation-reactive dogs, however, are unable to control or cope with their volatile feelings of loss and worry. The experience of separation loss triggers growing levels of anxious and frustrative arousal, causing them to worry over their owner's whereabouts and compelling them to act in compulsive ways to restore contact. The most common compulsive responses to separation anxiety are rituals involving distress vocalization, pacing, and checking for their owner's reappearance. In some dogs, such behavior can continue on for hours with only brief interruptions.

Fun

Some authors, most notably Ian Dunbar (1998), have popularized the rather misleading and problematic belief that destructiveness in the owner's absence is most often an expression of *separation fun* rather than separation distress or anxiety. According to Dunbar's thesis, predeparture arousal in such dogs is not necessarily the result of excessive stress or worry; on the contrary, such behavior is most often a sign of percolating excitement over the prospects of engaging in destructive play activities without interference or risk of punishment from the owner. Dunbar reasons that dogs simply cannot wait for their owners to leave the house so that they can go about their destructive rounds in safety. His solution to such behavior problems is to set up beer can booby traps and to provide such dogs with attractive rubber toys, thereby redirecting their destructive "fun" into more acceptable outlets.

Dunbar's thesis does not enjoy very much empirical support. Although a very small percentage of dogs may look forward to being left alone so that they can play in peace, personally I cannot recall any dogs exhibiting such pleasure about being isolated or any reports indicating that some dogs look forward to being left alone so that they can play by themselves. The phenomena may occur but must certainly be very rare. Undoubtedly, many dogs do engage in exploratory and playful activities that may result in the destruction of household items, and some of this behavior may increase during an owner's absence when it is not prevented (Voith and Borchelt, 1985); on the whole, however, when destructive behavior is motivated by play and exploration, it usually occurs regardless of the owner's presence or absence (McCrave, 1991;

Lindell, 1997). In fact, many destructive dogs exhibit little or no concern about their owner's displeasure at their destructive adventures and may even taunt the owner with a forbidden object in order to elicit a chase-and-catch routine. Nothing could be more *fun* for such dogs. However, with respect to the vast majority of separation-reactive dogs, separation is far from fun; on the contrary, it represents a significant source of psychological distress for them.

One can safely venture to assume that the vast majority of dogs that exhibit destructive behavior only at times when they are left alone probably do so as the result of separation distress. Providing such dogs with rubber toys stuffed with food, as recommended by Dunbar, will not hurt but will probably not provide much relief either, since appetite is typically suppressed in such dogs. Unfortunately, many owners, convinced that their separation-distressed dogs are simply having a good time at their expense, may not be so understanding, generous, or patient with their dog's "playful" excesses. Led to believe that their dogs are just having fun, and finding that they ignore the toys that they are given but instead continue to chew on pillows and woodwork, frustrated owners may elect out of desperation to take more drastic measures. Although Dunbar is careful to note the dangers of retroactive punishment, such owners, upon recognizing that the recommended method does not work, may resort to severe punishment at homecoming in an effort to take some of the fun out of their dog's destructive game.

PART 2: ONTOGENESIS OF SEPARATION DISTRESS

DEVELOPMENT OF ATTACHMENTS AND SEPARATION-RELATED DISTRESS

Many studies of separation distress indicate that both social and place attachments influence the level of distress expressed by isolated animals. Place attachments appear to precede and prepare developing puppies for the elaboration of social attachments. For example, a puppy's initial attachment to its mother is probably motivated more by place and physiological interests such as thermoregulation and nutrition than by social needs. In line with this idea, Scott (1980) proposes that the evolution of mammalian social attachment probably grew out of more primitive place attachment tendencies. Beginning at approximately 3 weeks of age (Scott and Fuller, 1965), with the emergence of maturing sensory, motor, and cognitive abilities, puppies turn progressively toward more organized and purposive social interaction with conspecifics. At about this time, a puppy begins to exhibit intense signs of distress when separated from its mother and littermates.

Social Comfort Seeking and Distress

The ontogenetic transition from primitive place attachments to social attachments may be mediated by the sense of smell. According to Rosenblatt (1983), early approach-withdrawal (A-W) reactions mediating vegetative functions like thermoregulation, feeding activities, and reflex elimination are ontogenetically elaborated into more mature seeking and avoidance patterns through the modality of smell. According to this theory, olfactory sensations that occur in association with tactile and thermal A-W reactions are classically conditioned, thereby becoming the basic positive and negative stimulus incentives governing seeking and avoidance behavior. Presumably, olfactory incentives also mediate lasting maternal attachments and social bonding between littermates. Evidence for the importance of olfaction in the development of social attachment and, probably, the evocation of separation distress comes from several kinship recognition studies (Hepper, 1986, 1994; Meckos-Rosenbaum et al., 1994). Additionally, it should be noted in this regard that separation-anxious dogs frequently seek out and "worry" personal belongings (e.g., socks, undergarments, and pillows) bearing a strong odor of their absent owner.

The owner's odor in such cases may elicit conditioned regulatory responses serving to maintain psychobiological attunement in the absence of the actual attachment object—learning that may be mediated by opioid activity (D'Amato and Pavone, 1993) and other neuropeptide systems (oxytocin and arginine vasopressin) involved in the formation of social memories (Panksepp, 1998). According to this hypothesis, an owner's scent may elicit conditioned opioid activity, thereby physiologically reducing separation-related distress and comfort-seeking behavior (see *Limbic Opioid Circuitry and the Mediation of Social Comfort and Distress* in Volume 1, Chapter 3). Low doses of morphine appear to reduce tail wagging and contact-seeking behavior in adolescent dogs, whereas the opioid antagonist naloxone increases such social behavior (Knowles et al., 1987). Interestingly, separation-reactive dogs often show signs of pruritus (itchiness), intermittently scratching themselves while excitedly greeting their owner. Halliwell (1992) suggests that this pruritic activity may be due to endorphin-released histamine activity:

> Opiates are well-known histamine-releasing agents, and so it was not surprising when it was shown that endorphins could also cause histamine release, both *in vitro* and *in vivo*. Histamine release is blocked by the opiate antagonist naloxone. It is possible that when dogs become pruritic while exhibiting signs of euphoria (e.g., upon the return of the owner), they may in fact be experiencing pruritus from histamine release rather than merely exhibiting a behavior quirk. (897)

This observation is consistent with the important role opioids play in the development of social attachment and distress. Perhaps, during excited greetings, dogs receive a high opioid dose followed by a sustained "drip" while in continuous contact with their owner, thereby facilitating a physiological *addiction* to attachment that results in withdrawal distress during periods of separation. In fact, dogs with separation distress present many of the same symptoms exhibited by human addicts suffering withdrawal from narcotics (Mauer and Vogel, 1967):

> When an addict misses his first shot, he senses mild withdrawal distress ("feels his habit coming on"), but this is probably more psychological than physiological, for fear plays a considerable role in the withdrawal syndrome. . . [after a passage of time] the addict becomes progressively nervous, restless and anxious, and close confinement tends to intensify these symptoms. . . he will begin to yawn fre-

quently. . . . [with more time] all the body fluids are released copiously; vomiting and diarrhea are acute; there is little appetite for food, and the addict is unable to sleep. (95–96)

A growing body of behavioral and neurobiological research has demonstrated that endogenous opioid activity plays a central role in the formation of social attachment (Panksepp, 1998) and imprinting (Hoffman, 1996). Among mammals, social attachment is also strongly influenced by the modulatory influences of oxytocin, prolactin, and arginine vasopressin. Oxytocin is a posterior pituitary hormone that is released by way of touch stimulation of the nipples, causing the contraction of smooth muscles in the mammary glands to pump milk. Oxytocin not only mediates maternal behavior but also appears to facilitate attraction of the young toward their mother. Panksepp notes that oxytocin exercises some significant agonist effects over opioid systems, sensitizing them to opiate substances and making them less responsive to the effects of opioid tolerance. Consequently, oxytocin may render a mother particularly responsive to attachment signals and help to sustain long-term nurturing bonds with her young. Like opiates, oxytocin and prolactin (a pituitary hormone that stimulates milk production) exert powerful inhibitory effects over separation distress. Finally, oxytocin (and arginine vasopressin) appears to facilitate the formation of lasting social memories, thereby complementing underlying neurophysiological attachment processes mediated by the neuropeptide.

Social Attachment versus Place Familiarity

Fredericson (1952) was first to perform controlled experiments to isolate the relative contribution of social attachment versus place familiarity in the expression of separation distress. He found that the most explosive separation reactions occur when a puppy is socially isolated in an unfamiliar place. According to his analysis, the goal of separation-distress vocalization is to restore a hypothesized state of perceptual homeostasis that is disrupted by the loss of social contact within a familiar

home setting. He proposes the following hypothesis concerning the relationship between social and environmental factors and the elicitation of separation distress:

A decrease in predictable social relationships and the absence of known environmental stimuli both elicit behavior patterns which are aimed at the immediate resumption of perceptual homeostasis. (477)

Ross and colleagues (1960) confirmed Fredericson's general observations. In their experiment, puppies ranging from 3 to 6 weeks of age were confined to a small triangular box located within the home pen. The authors observed that puppies exhibited the most frequent and strong distress vocalizations when they were restrained alone. When confined with a littermate, distress vocalization was significantly attenuated. In addition, they discovered an important fact that anticipated current therapies for managing separation-distress panic: puppies gradually learn to adapt to separation-distress-eliciting situations:

Over the period of 10 trials, the mean number of yelps for both the restrained alone and non-restrained-together groups showed a significant though gradual decrease. It is more likely that this decrease is due to adaptation to the situation and learning rather than to maturation. . . . The most likely explanation is that the puppy learns that it will be released after a short time, and hence becomes less disturbed emotionally. (4)

In addition to learning, ontogenetic changes also play an important role in the reduction of separation distress in developing puppies. Elliot and Scott (1961) found that separation-distress reactivity first appears with the onset of the socialization period at 3 weeks of age, peaks between weeks 6 and 7, and then rapidly declines over the next several weeks. Scott (1988) notes that distress reactions are extremely persistent in 3- to 4-week-old puppies:

Descriptively, puppies first show a response to separation from either a familiar site or from other animals when they are between three and four weeks of age by emitting continuous vocalizations at the rate of 100 or so per minute. These continue indefinitely unless alleviated, with occasional slowing down because of fatigue. During separation, puppies will not eat and sleep very little if at all. I have never tried to isolate puppies of this age for longer than twenty hours a day over five days. In this case, the puppies became so debilitated that I feared that they would die if the separation were continued. (33)

Separation-distress vocalizations by 6-week-old puppies are most frequent and intense during isolation in a strange situation (1400 vocalizations in 10 minutes) versus a familiar place (400 vocalizations in 10 minutes). Between weeks 12 and 16 (coinciding with the close of the socialization period), the amount of distress vocalization emitted continues to decline, providing evidence of increasing behavioral adaptation to the emotional distress aroused by isolation or, perhaps, reflecting the development of an underlying maturational process.

Cairns (1975) has also studied the effects of social isolation on puppies but has arrived at substantially different conclusions regarding the effects of isolation on behavior. He confirms that most isolated puppies exhibit pronounced signs of distress for several hours following separation from littermates but emphasizes that, by the end of 8 hours of isolation, they had recovered their composure and resumed normal activities like eating, chewing, grooming, and sleeping:

> Displacing the intense, high-arousal behaviors are actions of a normal, species-typical form. By the end of the second day, the shift to normative levels of eating and sleeping was virtually complete: the puppies had seemingly adapted to the companionless environment. . . . Recurrent introduction, and removal, at different intervals following the first separation indicated that the young had become accustomed to the absence of their companions. (7)

In conflict with earlier findings of Scott and coworkers (1973), Cairns found that long-term separation had little effect on appearance, weight, activity, or vigor; neither was there an observable increase in the susceptibility to disease. Many of Cairn's findings are at odds with previous assumptions and observations concerning the pathological effects of separation distress. He writes,

> Attention to the dramatic initial responses of the young to isolation—the first 10 minutes—

has preempted consideration of the more mundane settling down adaptation to the new living conditions. The course of dynamic changes in behavior seems not unlike that described by Canon (1929) in his account of the physiological responses to emergency situations. In brief, the change in social context serves to produce a state of heightened preparedness for action, with accompanying sympathetic arousal. The young become primed, in effect, to perform vigorous responses—flight or freezing, escape or crying, retreating or clinging—as these are determined by the circumstances and species-typical propensities. When these vigorous actions are ineffective or unnecessary, the arousal gives way to cyclic homeostatic process and the emergence of tonic levels of activity, including maintenance responses of eating and sleeping. Adaptation—both physiological and social—to the new circumstances occurs within a reasonably short period. (1975:9)

More recently, a study involving puppies separated from their mother at 6 and 12 weeks of age seem to side with Scott's findings regarding the deleterious effects of early and prolonged separation distress. The study found that 6-week-old puppies exhibited significant adverse effects as a result of early separation from their mother in terms of general health and weight gain, impairments that were not observed in older puppies kept with their mother until they were 12 weeks old (Slabbert and Rasa, 1993). Further, the authors noted that the untoward effects of separation from the mother at an early age were directly related to behavioral indicators of increased separation distress. The study appears to confirm Scott's findings that separation distress has serious psychosomatic implications for developing puppies. (Also, see *Social Attachment and Separation* in Volume 1, Chapter 2, for an additional discussion of the effects of attachment and separation on puppy behavior and development.)

The canine socialization process begins around week 3 after birth and continues through week 12 or so (Scott and Fuller, 1965). Throughout this period, as permitted by opportunity and circumstances, attachments are readily and concurrently formed with both conspecifics and humans. As already discussed, a very influential attachment object for a puppy during this time is its mother. Adoption is a process in which the human adult assumes the role of surrogate mother, and other family members (especially children) become substitute littermates. A significant outcome of secondary socialization is the perpetuation of a puppy's dependency into adolescent stages of development and, in many cases, persisting throughout its life. However, for puppies to develop a confident adult attitude with sufficient security and emotional stability to enable them to cope when they must be left alone, owners should follow the lead of canine mothers by gradually weaning the puppies, so that they acquire a healthy sense of self-security and independence.

ATTACHMENT AND LEARNING

The study of social affiliation has revealed that attachments are strengthened by a simple learning process, whereby "the puppy is punished for separation and rewarded for reunion" (Scott et al., 1973:10). Separation from significant sources of attachment elicits aversive arousal that prompts frantic efforts to restore contact with attachment objects. The restoration of contact evokes relief, enhanced well-being, and increased levels of attachment toward the group and place where reunion occurs. Proximity and contact-seeking behavior that results in reunion are negatively reinforced. In combination, separation distress followed by the comfort and relief associated with reunion reduces the likelihood that a puppy will lose contact with conspecifics or wander too far away from the nest site in the future—at least until it is developmentally ready to do so.

As a puppy develops and begins to explore the wider environment, the mother and nesting site provide a base of security for such excursions. If frightened during these exploratory jaunts, the puppy will quickly retreat to the safety of the mother and nest. An extreme form of this tendency can be observed in some dogs exhibiting intense fears or phobias. When scared, such dogs may frantically seek physical contact with their owners and press up against them (positive thigmotaxis) in an apparent effort to alleviate fear. Not only does such contact reduce fear, it may

also deepen the dog's attachment and dependency on the owner. As a result, fearful dogs may be more prone to develop separation-related problems involving anxiety and panic. Although not all dogs exhibiting separation problems are fearful, many do appear to have collateral fear-related problems.

The motivations underlying social and place attachments are epigenetically elaborated into various allelomimetic behavior patterns (packing) and territorial imperatives. Social attraction and affiliation fortify group cohesion and unity, thereby providing a foundation for complex social activity and cooperation:

> One of the most important motivational systems in dogs is allelomimetic behavior, seen also in schools of fish, flocks of birds, and herds of mammals. It is defined as doing what the other animals in the group do, with some degree of mutual imitation, and often results in a high degree of coordination. It is a major system of behavior in dogs, and *if one wishes to understand their psychology, the most important thing to remember is that dogs love company and suffer without it* [italics added]. Such company may be either canine or human, and in order to maintain it they must do what their companions are doing, i.e., express allelomimetic behavior. (Scott, 1980:136)

Dogs strive to maximize social contact and abhor separation from the group. This is a basic motivational principle of dog training and behavior modification. A dog's "desire to please" is really a desire to stay close and to avoid rejection.

In summary, the socialization process is driven (at least in part) by a dynamic interplay between an innate aversion toward separation and the relief experienced when contact with a familiar group and place is restored. These primitive separation dynamics are epigenetically elaborated into more complex social exchanges involving organized group activity that takes place within a familiar territorial space. The avoidance of separation, therefore, plays a prominent role in the development of a coherent and stable family-pack unit and the maintenance of a territory. This effect is significantly amplified when separation is associated with fear, as in the case of dogs having phobias.

Early Trauma and the Development of Behavior Problems

The etiology of adult canine separation distress is not fully understood. A commonly entertained, but unproven, account suggests that separation-elicited distress in adult dogs may be the result of early traumatic experiences or inadequate socialization. A significant body of literature indicates that a puppy's brain develops in response to sensory, cognitive, and emotional stimulation. During early sensitive periods when the brain is undergoing significant differentiation, stressor-activated neurotransmitters and hormones may permanently affect the organization of the puppy's brain (Fox, 1971) (see *Stress and Separation Anxiety* in Volume 1, Chapter 3). The available information on the relation between early trauma and adult separation distress is ambiguous and inconclusive, but some data do suggest that a significant linkage exists between certain early experiences and adult separation-related behavior problems. Serpell and Jagoe (1995) found that puppies that had suffered serious pediatric illnesses were more likely to exhibit separation-related barking problems as adult dogs. The authors speculate that increased attention and care shown toward the sick puppies may have predisposed them to develop separation problems later on in life. But, not only is excessive attention a potential source of problems, so is a lack of attention. Puppies left alone for 6 to 8 hours during the day exhibited an increased risk for developing separation-related destructiveness or excessive barking problems at maturity. Borchelt (1983) suggests that removing a puppy too early from its mother may predispose it to form excessively strong attachments with its owner. Similarly, he suggests that a failure to form satisfactory attachments until after 4 or 5 months of age may also result in overattachment and predispose the dog to separation-related problems.

Many young dogs appear to be highly resilient to the effects of traumatic punishment, as demonstrated by a series of controversial experiments performed by Fisher (1955). Fisher's study began with puppies at 3 weeks of age and continued until week 15.

One group, referred to as punished-indulged (P-I), was exposed to a daily round of intensive social contact involving affectionate petting and holding, followed by a half-hour of noncontingent punishment, consisting of very rough handling, switching, and shock. Puppies could escape punishment by fleeing from the experimenter and hiding behind a panel, but they were often chased there and punished more, essentially making the punishment inescapable. Also, these P-I puppies were individually exposed to severe social inhibitory training. At weeks 5, 6, 7, 9, 11, and 13, each P-I puppy was coaxed to come to the experimenter located at the far end of a runway, whereupon it received a strong shock.

Of relevance to separation-related problems, Fisher found that P-I puppies exhibited significantly higher dependency measures (proximity-seeking behavior toward the passive experimenter) than exhibited by another group of puppies (indulged) that had received only indulging and playful interaction during the same period. By week 12, P-I puppies spent nearly threefold as much time in close proximity with the experimenter than did indulged puppies. These findings suggest that puppies exposed to severe punishment in combination with rewards and social attention may form excessively dependent bonds with their owners. What is perhaps most surprising about Fisher's study was the finding that *all* P-I puppies rapidly recovered from overt signs of fear and timidity, with *no significant or lasting adverse side effects.* An even more striking observation was made involving a group of puppies that had been socially isolated throughout the 12-week period of the study (*punished-isolated*), except for a daily half-hour period of punishment that they received from the experimenter. According to Fisher, *nearly all* of the punished-isolated puppies also exhibited rapid recovery at the conclusion of the treatment phase of the study. Finally, puppies that had been isolated throughout the treatment phase, without any exposure to human contact, showed very pronounced and permanent social deficits in response to contact with humans and other dogs. Fisher summarizes his findings and conclusions:

The rapid recovery of all Punished-Indulged puppies and nearly all Punished-Isolated puppies was striking. Such rapid remission of symptoms provides evidence against the hypothesis that early trauma has extreme and persisting effects on later behavior. Since all early social and exploratory opportunity led to punishment for the Punished-Isolated group, the data would also seem to limit the application of the "critical period" hypothesis. Scott termed the third to tenth week of age as critical for development of social adjustment in the puppy and hypothesized that traumatic experiences occurring during this period should have the greatest effect on later behavior. Trauma and stress applied to the Punished groups during this entire period did not lead to an inability to make an adequate later social adjustment with both humans and other puppies. . . . The present study would suggest that very early trauma may not be chiefly responsible for abnormal social behavior in dogs. (79–80)

Etiology: Traumatic Loss and Other Adverse Separation Experiences

Dogs exposed to excessive or traumatic separation experiences early in life may fail to mature normally and instead develop regressive, puppylike reactions to being left alone. Normally, distress at separation attenuates as a puppy grows older, but in the case of separation-reactive dogs this normal pattern of progressive tolerance for the loss of social contact does not occur. Panksepp (1988b) speculates that many human psychiatric conditions may be traced to adverse exposure to separation distress in childhood. In particular, he notes that there is a positive correlation between frequent and intense childhood separation experiences and the development of panic disorders: "This suggests that intense early activation of separation-distress circuitry may sensitize the system for heightened activity of the system during adulthood" (61). The separation-distress substrate may be sensitized by the enhancement of perceptual mechanisms accessing the system or by trauma-induced "biochemical and neuronal proliferation of the circuit" itself (see *Limbic Opioid Circuitry and the Mediation of Social Comfort and Distress* in Volume 1, Chapter 3).

Adverse Rearing Practices That May Predispose Dogs to Develop Separation-related Problems

Normal puppies are prone to experience varying degrees of separation-related distress when left alone. Such distress is expressed in worried activities aimed at regaining contact with the absent attachment object. Under natural circumstances, separation-distress behavior is adaptive in the sense that it helps puppies to maintain contact with their mother and the nurturance, warmth, and protection that she provides. Naturally, such behavior has strong survival value for the biologically dependent and vulnerable puppies. In the domestic environment, however, separation-related behavior may become difficult to manage and possibly develop into more serious behavior problems in adult dogs.

As already noted, separation distress may suppress interest in food and water (psychogenic anorexia), and chronic distress may prevent puppies from thriving and growing properly. Like dominance aggression, separation anxiety is not easily resolved once it has established itself, and it behooves conscientious dog owners to take measures to prevent it from developing in the first place. Prevention is the key to managing separation distress (Voith, 1981). Consequently, training puppies to cope and respond appropriately to their owner's absence should be an integral part of early socialization activities.

Care should be taken to safeguard against traumatic handling or excessive isolation, especially during the first few days after the puppy enters the home. A sensitive and separation-reactive puppy may be strongly affected by these first impressions—experiences that may exert a pronounced and lasting influence on its subsequent social development. Unfavorable experiences, such as traumatic isolation or inappropriate punishment, are particularly problematic since they may elicit intense emotional arousal and distress at a particularly sensitive time. As already pointed, both punishment and isolation may increase social attachment levels and sow the seeds of unforeseen attachment and separation problems appearing later in life. Repeated noncontingent punishment and long bouts of isolation may be particularly problematic in this regard.

As the result of ill-advised rearing practices and abusive handling, a puppy's adaptation to domestic life may be disrupted and disorganized. Instead of finding conducive outlets for the orderly expression and satisfaction of its developmental needs, a puppy may be faced with overwhelmingly restrictive and desultory punitive demands aimed at suppressing its behavior rather than actualizing it. Meanwhile, the genetically timed opportunities for optimal adjustment inexorably pass by, leaving a permanent schism between the dog's biological potential and its actualization. In short, the domestic environment may consciously or unconsciously constrain, disrupt, or disorganize critical maturational processes during sensitive and influential periods of development. These early influences may exert lasting adverse effects on a dog's behavior and ability to adjust, possibly playing a functional role in the etiology of separation anxiety and other serious behavior problems.

As previously noted, a possible predisposing influence on separation distress is fear. Under the prompting of fearful arousal, a dog may seek the security of close proximity to its owner. If fearful arousal is reduced as the result of such contact, escape/avoidance behavior is negatively reinforced and attachment levels with the owner may be increased. Over time and repeated exposure to the fear-eliciting situation, the dog may develop an inordinate emotional dependency on its owner, expressing itself in a pronounced fear and unwillingness to be left alone. This effect may be even more pronounced in dogs affected by a negative cognitive set (learned helplessness), causing them to view the home situation as something outside of their control. From the perspective of the helpless dog, others may be perceived as the only reliable source of control and security. Consequently, such dogs may be more prone to form excessively dependent bonds with family members perceived to be in control of the situation. By attaching to such individuals, the dog may obtain a sense of heightened control and security by proxy. Along with other factors, such

considerations may affect the differentiation of attachment levels between the dog and various family members.

Although crate confinement can be useful for certain training purposes, it can also be easily abused by dog owners and become the source of considerable distress for dogs (Campbell, 1991). Excessive crate confinement represents a significant welfare and quality-of-life concern. Thousands of family dogs spend 10 to 18 hours or more every day confined to wire or plastic cages. Paradoxically, the daily tedium and loneliness of crate confinement may cause dogs to gradually acquire a dependency on such restraint, an outcome that their owners may wrongly interpret as a sign of positive adjustment to crate confinement. Such dogs may become bizarrely aroused with evident distress (pacing and panting) when they are let of their crates alone or when access to them is prevented. Consequently, when dogs that had been previously confined to a crate are permitted to move about the house, instead of relaxing and quietly enjoying their new liberty, they may instead become highly active and exploratory, perhaps becoming destructive or eliminate, even though they do not soil the crate. Likewise, after months of crate confinement at night in a kitchen or, worse yet, in a basement, access to the bedroom to sleep may result in restlessness and an inability to sleep. Some of these dogs may even rub against walls and furniture, seeming to seek the contact comfort of crate walls. These signs of distress and disorientation continue until the dog is put back into its crate, thereby confirming the owner's belief that the dog likes its crate. These effects may be related to what Fuller (1967) has described as "emergence-stress," a cognitive and perceptual overload resulting from the experience of novel and complex situations. Finally, although crate confinement may prevent some destructive behavior and elimination problems, its benefits may be offset by many untoward side effects associated with excessive isolation of the dog from family members and the home environment. Patronek and colleagues (1996) have reported that crate confinement represents a significant risk factor for relinquishment of the dog to an animal shelter, raising the possibility that excessive crate confinement may exercise an adverse influence on attachment levels and the performance of appropriate training activities. Instead of training the dog or treating a behavior problem, the owner may rely on the crate as a way to control the dog's behavior.

In summary, two significant and problematic influences converge on developing puppies that may incubate into serious separation-related problems appearing later in adulthood:

Learned helplessness: Having formed strong attachment bonds with its littermates, the mother, the breeder, and, perhaps, a family of children and other human caretakers, susceptible puppies may experience a traumatic loss of control (helplessness) as the result of being abruptly removed from one social situation and then abruptly thrust into an entirely different one. The sense of helplessness is further increased by excessive crate confinement, noncontingent punishment, and a general perception that significant events (both attractive and aversive) occur independently of what the puppy does.

Fear of separation: Social and place attachments are a dog's basis for security and contentment. During separation, thresholds for fear may be lowered, resulting in increased anxious arousal. With the loss of security that the owner represents, a dog's growing fear of *fear* may coalesce with mounting separation distress and result in heightened separation distress and panic. One would expect in cases where a history of traumatic attachment loss and helplessness exists that the separation-fear response would even be more dramatic because the dog believes that it cannot control it without the owner's help and comfort. Finally, where phobias (e.g., fear of thunder) exist, a dog may tend to form an abnormally strong dependency on its owner as a base of security and means for modulating fear and panic. In cases where a high degree of helplessness and phobia exist in the same dog, one would predict a high probability of severe separation-anxiety panic.

COMPARISON BETWEEN DOG AND WOLF EXPOSURE TO SOCIAL SEPARATION

Under natural conditions, wolf pups are left alone for extended periods as early as 3 to 4 weeks of age. At about this time, wolf pups first emerge from their den but will quickly flee back into its protection at any sign of danger. As a pup matures, it gradually moves away from the den and begins to explore the surroundings, often in the company of littermates or the protective supervision of a juvenile "sitter." Eventually the use of the den is abandoned altogether at approximately 10 to 12 weeks of age (Young and Goldman, 1944/1964; Zimen, 1981), requiring that the pup participate more actively in pack life. This period of development is associated with the further elaboration and refinement of emergent allelomimetic tendencies. Food is no longer brought to the pups, but now they are required to follow adults to distant kill sites that become "loafing spots" for a few days of eating and playing until a fresh kill is made somewhere else. This ontogenetic pattern is probably genetically timed, biologically preparing each behavioral step with the maturation of a physical and psychological substrate sufficient to support it. The transitions from the den to the wider surroundings (ultimately leading to the notion of territory) and from close attachments for the mother and littermates to other group members (ultimately leading to full integration within the pack) are gradually accomplished. It is a process of social and territorial integration, extending the primitive attachment impulse from the mother, littermates, and den to other attachment objects and places, thereby facilitating a more perfect adaptation of the wolf to its social group and environment in preparation for adult life.

Dog puppies are exposed to a very different pattern of socialization and environmental exposure than that just described. The usual clip of events is more composed of abrupt jumps and bumps rather than smooth integrative transitions. Essentially, puppies are taken from familiar and secure circumstances and thrust into an unfamiliar and insecure environment. This transition from the breeder to the home is often carried out without much being done to minimize the potential trauma resulting from the experience. For example, many puppies spend the first night isolated in a crate in a remote part of the house, where they may yelp and whine themselves to sleep. Some owners may even see fit to punish a noisy puppy severely before realizing that such treatment simply makes matters worse. These aversive events marking the puppy's introduction into the home may be conducive for the development of learned helplessness. [For an excellent review of the potential role of learned helplessness in the etiology of separation anxiety, see Mineka and Suomi (1978)]. Helplessness and dependency are inevitable outcomes in situations where excessive punishment and confinement are the primary means used to control puppy behavior.

Under the ideal conditions of a wolf pack, a gradual transition away from the mother and denning site takes place over several weeks, allowing wolf pups to form alternative relationships and place attachments with a minimum of disruptive stress. These lupine ontogenetic transitions are, metaphorically speaking, orchestrated in the form of an outward expanding spiral that gradually encompasses the total social and physical environment, thereby perfecting a wolf pup's behavioral adaptation. A wolf pup's individuation occurs under the influence of a highly conducive social milieu operating under an open sky, producing minimal amounts of emotional distress while maximizing opportunities to enhance its adaptation. In contrast, domestic dogs may be exposed to the most unfavorable and disorderly conditions that maximize emotional distress and severely limit adaptive opportunities. Finally, wolf pups gradually become independent with a strong sense of control over what occurs or does not occur to them. Puppies, on the other hand, become progressively dependent on their owners for everything. Their food, exercise, affection, and most other significant needs may occur independently of what they do or do not do, rendering them all the more helpless and dependent.

PART 3: SEPARATION-RELATED PROBLEMS

Long ago, Fowler Bucke (1903) collected a number of intriguing reports written by children about their family dog. Of particular interest was the way the children described separation distress. The sensitivity, simplicity, and objectivity of these childhood anecdotes give them lasting value:

> When I am away she will hunt for me every where, and whine if they show her any of my clothes.

> When all went out he would bark and cry.

> It never wanted to be left alone.

> When we left it alone it would go around the house crying looking out of the windows.

> Poor little thing was so homesick that he did not touch food for a day.

> He died because mamma, for whom he had so much love, was taken to the hospital for an operation.

> When my mother died he felt so homesick that he got sick and would not eat. We had to take him to the hospital. (1903:505)

These reports underscore the dog's perennial tendency to form strong bonds with people and to suffer when the attachment object is lost. Although the dog's devotion and faithfulness have been often praised throughout its long history with us (see *Dog Devotion: Legends* in Volume 1, Chapter 10), its distress at separation is not always welcome or the subject of celebration, especially when it is the cause of behavior problems. A fascinating psychiatric case study reported by the psychoanalyst Marcel Heiman (1956) contains a revealing reference to separation anxiety and the despair it sometimes causes for dog owners. A female patient under Heiman's care expressed dire concerns and worry about her dog's elimination problem—a problem that occurred only when she was away from home:

> I am concerned about Robin's "crapping" and "peeing". Maybe it is due to my leaving him and not giving him enough attention. Maybe

he feels we will never come back. I wonder about myself, coming home from school with nobody home. I was terrified that my mother and father would never come home. I would cry and cry. . . .

Later, she confided to Dr. Heiman,

My neighbors complain about the dog. He is howling and whining. I am buying a book, *How to Train Your Dog.* My neighbors are so unfriendly [weeps]. Do you have any suggestions? (573–574)

Unfortunately, Dr. Heiman was unable to provide her with the information and support she sought, leading her to break down with a mixture of angry accusations and tears.

WORRY AND GUILT: THE HUMAN DIMENSION OF SEPARATION DISTRESS

The comments expressed by Dr. Heiman's patient are common concerns among clients presenting dogs with separation-distress problems. Barking problems may result in nasty complaints from neighbors or even costly citations, destructiveness may cause thousands of dollars of damage to household property, and periodic house soiling causes untold frustration. But not only are owners likely to be highly distressed by the trouble and costs resulting from their dog's separation reactivity, they may experience numerous inconveniences as the direct result of attempting to manage their dog's separation problems. There is a tremendous amount of worry expended in response to separation problems, leading one to consider whether the term *separation anxiety* might not better be reserved to describe how the owners feel when they leave their problem dogs behind. The lives of such owners are often profoundly impacted by the problem, causing them to alter daily routines and limit outside interests in an effort to minimize their dog's exposure to separation distress. As a result, a complex mix of conflicted feelings, dilemmas, and resentment may daily stir a caldron of growing impatience and anger toward the dog. At one moment, owners may feel victimized and helpless, while, at the next, they may experience feelings of bitter resent-

ment and anger about their dog's misbehavior. This turmoil may cause them to respond irrationally or explosively toward their separation-distressed dogs, sometimes causing them to resort to harsh and futile retroactive punishment in an effort to solve the problem (see the discussion below). Such punishment does not do dogs any good and may actually make the problem much worse. When owners of separation-anxious dogs finally turn for help, they are often desperate and impatient for relief. Unfortunately, treating such problems is often time-consuming and difficult—unwelcome news to owners who are already at their wits' end or secretly considering the possibility of giving their dog up.

Separation anxiety is a quintessential cynopraxic problem. The central issues at stake involve modifying the social bond between owner and dog to enhance their relationship, while at the same time raising the dog's quality of life and its sense of well-being. Balancing these interests will naturally result in improved dog behavior, while restoring the owner's affection and attachment toward the dog. Many owners seek help in a state of exasperation and only after having tried what they believe to be everything. More often than not, it is clear that they have received bad or incomplete information. It is of utmost importance to gain the owners' confidence by offering them, first and foremost, sincere support and understanding (see *Cynopraxic Counseling* in Chapter 10). The next step is to assess the problem, develop a working hypothesis, and make various behavioral recommendations. These efforts should be realistic and matched as closely as possible to each owner's capabilities and circumstances.

BEHAVIORAL EXPRESSIONS OF SEPARATION DISTRESS

Dogs exhibit three general patterns of behavior in response to separation from their owners. By far the most common response is resignation and patient waiting for the owners to return home. It is truly amazing how well so many millions of dogs cope with the daily drudgery and emotional strain of loneliness and boredom (Figure 4.4). The next group

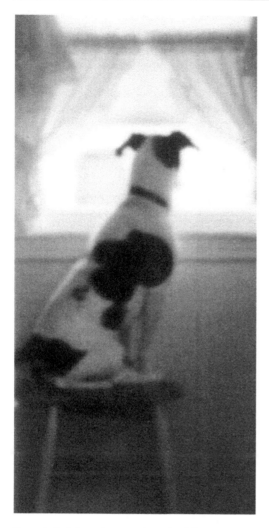

FIG. 4.4. Many dogs spend much of their time anxiously waiting for their owners to come home. (Photo courtesy of V. L. Voith.)

ing the chance of being detected by an enemy, thus making survival during long periods of separation more likely. Under adverse conditions, separation-depressed dogs may become progressively anxious and reactive. The third group, and the most commonly presented for training and behavior modification, exhibit signs of intense arousal, agitation, and behavioral activation (McCrave, 1991; Voith and Borchelt, 1996).

Some anaclitic or psychologically dependent dogs appear to *obsess* over their owners' whereabouts, following their *person* from room to room like a tireless shadow, whereas other dogs may exhibit more or less normal proximity-seeking behavior, at least until their owners prepare to leave the house. Dogs exhibiting separation distress often show signs of predeparture arousal and worry (e.g., restless, shaking, and whining) elicited by the owner's preparations to leave (Podberscek et al., 1999). Some dogs may engage in various efforts to forestall or prevent the owners' departure. For example, they may refuse to come or resist entering their crate or other areas used for confinement. In other cases, probably involving a strong element of frustrative arousal, dogs may threaten or even attack their owners in an effort to prevent them from leaving. Not only is increased arousal evident prior to leaving, separation-reactive dogs are also more likely to engage in intrusive and noisy greeting rituals, at which times they may repeatedly jump, run about, and bark, appearing to find it difficult to control their enthusiasm and *arrival elation* (Voith and Borchelt, 1996). Interestingly, many otherwise highly reactive and separation-anxious dogs may tolerate being left alone in a car without becoming overly distressed (Figure 4.5), but others may become reactive and potentially destructive to upholstery.

When separated from their owners, separation-reactive dogs may become highly agitated and exhibit various activities evidencing heightened distress or panic, such as becoming increasingly active and worried in appearance, pacing back and forth, looking out windows, and sniffing or scratching at doors. In addition, they may glance off countertops and furniture, all the while appearing to obsess over the whereabouts of their absent owners. After

encountered in large numbers includes those dogs who fall into a pronounced state of ennui or depression. These dogs appear to be held in a state of suspended animation. They do not move around much during their owners' absence and may refuse to eat or drink until they return home. They will sometimes howl or vent doleful and haunting moans—vocalizations expressing pronounced loneliness. Depression (reduced activity levels) in response to separation may serve an adaptive function by conserving energy and by reducing

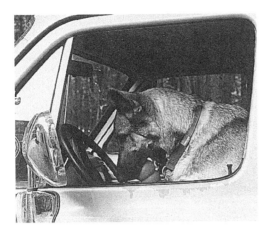

FIG. 4.5. Many dogs that cannot tolerate being left alone at home do well when left in a car. (Photo courtesy of V. L. Voith.)

a period of escalating activity, they may whine, followed by yelping and barking, and, finally, some may lapse into a panic of self-absorbed and persistent vocalization, pacing, and frustrative efforts to escape. These various attempts to restore contact may continue, off and on, for hours on end. Some separation-reactive dogs may pull pillows from sofas and chairs or target personal belongings like clothing, books, magazines, and television remote control devices—anything that might yield an ersatz connection with the absent attachment object. Separation-reactive dogs may lose bowel or bladder control—sometimes eliminating on furniture or beds. In fact, many house-soiling problems in adults dogs have been traced to separation anxiety. Of 105 cases of house soiling reported by Yeon and colleagues (1999), 39% of the dogs treated exhibited signs of separation anxiety. Another common sign of separation distress is evidence of excessive salivation at the base of the door or on the crate floor. Additionally, separation-reactive dogs may present symptoms of psychosomatic illness, including anorexia and diarrhea (Schmidt, 1968), with long-term separation distress possibly exerting deleterious stress-related effects on the animal's immune system (Coe et al., 1985; Ornitz, 1991; McMillan, 1999). Orphaned children have been reported to suffer various emotional and physical disturbances (even death) as the result

of long-term hospitalization, where they receive inadequate maternal care, contact, or stimulation [e.g., Spitz (1946)]. Dogs not exhibiting separation-anxiety distress may also exhibit some of these problems, so it is important to exclude other potential causes as part of the assessment process (Table 4.1).

ASSESSING SEPARATION-RELATED PROBLEMS

Separation distress is a common complaint presented to animal behavior consultants and trainers. Borchelt (1983) reported that from 1978 to 1981 he diagnosed 146 cases involving separation anxiety. This figure represented 39% of his caseload during that period. Other estimates have placed the incidence of separation-related problems at approximately 20% of the behavioral cases treated (McCrave, 1991). When presented with a behavior problem that only occurs in an owner's absence, separation distress, in one of its various forms, should always be considered as a possible cause. Most dogs experience some degree of distress when left alone, but a few experience very pronounced panic shortly after their owners leave the house, usually reaching a peak within 30 minutes or so after separation (Voith and Borchelt, 1985). As already noted, there appears to exist two general and opposing affective states associated with heightened separation distress. Some dogs become highly aroused, a state associated with panting, pacing, various distress vocalizations (including whining, barking, and howling), increased seeking and exploratory behavior, destructiveness, and loss of bowel and bladder control. As already noted, other dogs become depressed and simply lie down waiting forlornly for their owners to return home. Scott and colleagues (1973) early on recognized these two opposite tendencies resulting from separation distress and noted their respective roles in the development of behavior problems:

> That such a motivational system exists in the dog can be verified by any dog-owner who attempts to go away and leave his pet or to shut it up away from human beings and other dogs. Many animals in the latter situation become frantic, leaping at the door and gnawing on the woodwork. Or, if the dog belongs to an easily

TABLE 4.1. Separation-related Behavior Problems

Elimination	Destructiveness	Vocalization
Behavior Urination Defecation	*Behavior* Chewing Scratching Digging	*Behavior* Barking Whining Howling
Occurrence Owner absent Dog denied contact with owner	*Occurrence* Owner absent Dog denied contact with owner	*Occurrence* Owner absent Dog denied contact with owner
Significant signs Predeparture distress Exhibits pre- and postdeparture distress Elimination often occurs within first 30 to 60 minutes after departure Occurs with a high percentage of departures	*Significant signs* Destructiveness often directed toward personal belongings, doorjambs, and carpeting near doorways Exhibits pre- and postdeparture distress Destructiveness often occurs within first 30 to 60 minutes after departure Occurs in a high percentage of departures	*Significant signs* Vocalization may occur at various times during the day Exhibits pre- and postdeparture distress Vocalization often occurs immediately or within first 30 to 60 minutes after departure Occurs in a high percentage of departures
Differentiate Housetraining problems Fear-related elimination Excitement/submissive urination Urine marking	*Differentiate* Playful or exploratory destructiveness Destructiveness related to fear (e.g., thunder phobia) Related to external sources of stimulation (e.g., passing cat or dog) Hyperactivity	*Differentiate* Related to external sources of stimulation (e.g., presence of other dog, animals, passersby, deliveries) Vocalization occuring in response to fear-eliciting stimulation Occuring in reponse to other dogs barking Hyperactivity

inhibited breed, like the Shetland sheep dog we once owned as a pet, it may simply lie down in one spot and wait there until its owner returns, with a resigned lack of interest in anything around it. In common language, a dog's strongest and most continuous type of motivation is a desire for companionship, canine or human, and most of the dog behavior problems arise from deprivation of companionship. (11)

Although depressed dogs may be unhappy and discontented, they are not causing any problems and are only rarely presented for behavior therapy. A symptom shared by both groups is a loss of appetite or psychogenic anorexia. Some dogs appear to exhibit *bipolar* symptoms, alternately showing signs of both extremes, depending on circumstances.

Curiously, although the existence of separation distress in dogs has been recognized for many years, little systematic research has been done on the phenomenon until relatively recently. Albrecht (1953) appears to have been the first dog behavior counselor to clearly articulate a connection between excessive vocalization and destructive behavior with separation anxiety:

As silence settles over the empty house and the old scent of his master tells him that he is alone, he becomes apprehensive and begins restlessly pacing about, whining and sniffing in an attempt to catch a fresh scent or attract the attention of his master. Hearing nothing and finding no reassuring smell, his fear increases. Perhaps the telephone will ring or the doorbell. He always associates these familiar sounds with the answering voice or footsteps of his owner and so he sets up a frantic barking. But his master does not come and an ominous silence again reigns in the house. His barking becomes more hysterical and his restless pacing turns to frantic running about as he hunts for a means of escape. His frenzy increases, and he feverishly attacks any object within his reach and worries it until, if he is alone for a long enough time, he falls into an exhausted sleep with the evidence of his terror strewn around him. *Punishment is useless when his master eventually returns, for the dog's destructive panic is forgotten in his joy and relief at sight and scent of him.* (120, italics added)

Having diagnosed the problem, she then describes a procedure for reducing the separation-distressed dog's anxiety:

> To overcome this fear, you must teach your pet to have confidence that you will always come back to him. While you are at home, shut him in a room for a few minutes and go far enough away for him to be unable to hear you or scent you. After a short time open the door and fuss over him to let him know that you are as glad to see him as he is to see you. Repeat this several times a day for a few days, gradually increasing his period of solitude until he can be safely left alone for several hours. If you are always genuinely glad to see him when you return, he will not in any way connect his confinement with punishment or desertion; and in a week or so, unless he is an extremely shy and unstable animal, he will curl up and sleep knowing that you will com back to him. (120–121)

Albrecht's contribution is an important one, but, since then, several articles have appeared in the veterinary literature on the topic, confirming the efficacy of the general method and offering many additional insights and techniques for the management of canine separation distress. Unfortunately, however, besides the seminal clinical work reported by Hothersall and Tuber (1979) and its further develop-

ment and dissemination by Voith and Borchelt (Voith, 1980, 1981; Borchelt and Voith, 1982; Borchelt, 1983; Voith and Borchelt, 1985, 1996), little else of substance has been done to significantly broaden our understanding of the disorder and its treatment.

As already discussed, separation-related distress may be augmented by a number of motivational factors. Perhaps, as the result of early traumatic experiences or genetic predisposition, separation distress may coalesce with fear and gradually incubate into an adult global panic response at separation. Dogs exhibiting storm phobias and other fears elicited by stimuli likely to occur in the owner's absence may be susceptible to increased fear at separation. The development of separation-anxiety panic problems may be related to the presence of learned helplessness or excessive dependency on the owner for a sense of security. This sort of separation reactivity is clearly an anxiety-type disorder, but not all separation-related problems are due to a fear of separation and maladaptive panic. Many separation-reactive dogs do not appear to be motivated in the first place by a fear of separation but rather by frustration resulting from thwarted efforts to gain contact with the absent owner. Other dogs may simply have a low tolerance for boredom and an equally low threshold for boredom-related diversionary exploration and other activities aimed at obtaining optimal stimulation in the owner's absence. Such behavior is especially prevalent in breeds bred for high activity levels (e.g., sporting, working, and terrier breeds). Frustration and boredom have considerable overlap and motivational coactivity. Dogs that have a history of unresolved destructive behavior or have received excessive and ineffective interactive punishment as the result of stealing personal belongs or engaging in other oral excesses (e.g., mouthing or biting on hands and clothing) may resort to such behavior when agitated with separation distress. Clearly, frustrative-arousal and boredom-triggered activities play significant roles in the expression of separation-related behavior problems.

Diagnostically delineating separation-anxiety panic from separation frustration or separation boredom is not always easy. Some dogs may exhibit all four contributory elements: fear of separation, panic, frustrative arousal, and boredom. Others may exhibit a genuine fear of separation and an equally strong frustrative response to being left alone. Then there are those that are primarily motivated by frustration and that panic when they are unable to obtain contact. Active and helpless dogs (exposed to a pattern of retroactive punishment) may be particularly prone to separation-frustration panic problems, exhibiting frenetic and disorganized behavior (panic) when left alone. Even when a dog appears to exhibit clear signs of anxious arousal in response to its owner's preparations to leave, this behavior is not always positive proof of separation anxiety or fear. Askew (1996) has argued that in such cases *attention-getting behavior* routinely exhibited and reinforced prior to the owner's departure may be misconstrued as predeparture anxiety. Although fear certainly presents coactively with separation distress (e.g., the storm-phobic dog is prone to develop separation-anxiety panic problems), the role of fear in the development of separation-related problems is far from clear.

ETIOLOGIES, ETHOLOGY, AND RISK FACTORS

The predisposing and causal factors underlying separation-distress problems have not been fully worked out, but several prominent influences have been tentatively identified. Of first importance is the dog's proclivity to form strong and lasting attachments with humans and to remain dependent on human care throughout its life cycle.

Miscellaneous Causes and Risk Factors

Episodes of increased separation distress are often observed after an abrupt change of social or environmental circumstances (Borchelt and Voith, 1982). Many dogs exhibit their first episode of separation distress after being suddenly exposed to a period of separation following several weeks or months of near-constant contact with their owners. Frequently, dogs, that had been well adjusted to being left alone, are thrown into a crisis of separation distress after the family moves into a new home,

marking the onset of separation-related problems. Any abrupt change in daily routine and place may be more than predisposed dogs can handle. Some owners have noted heightened reactivity to separation in their dog after a lengthy period of boarding. Separation-reactive dogs are often highly sensitive and may present with various collateral fears and phobias, especially fears of loud noises and thunderstorms. In addition to fear and panic, frustration plays a significant motivational role in the expression of separation distress.

Although Wright and Nesselrote (1987) reported finding no significant difference between male and female dogs with respect to the incidence of separation-related problems, more recent studies have indicated that male dogs tend to present with separation problems more often than do female dogs (Podberscek et al., 1999; Takeuchi, 2000). Curiously, mixed-breed dogs appear to be significantly overrepresented in the canine population exhibiting separation-related problems. Statistical comparisons between purebred and mixed-breed dogs reveal that the most significant factor differentiating the two groups is their source: mixed-breed dogs are more frequently obtained from shelters than purebred dogs (McCrave, 1991). One explanation that has been proposed to explain the larger number of shelter dogs presenting with separation distress is that such dogs may be predisposed to develop such problems as the result of traumatic experiences associated with shelter relinquishment (Borchelt, 1983). Another possible explanation for the disproportionate representation of shelter dogs in this population is that owners of separation-anxious dogs may "dump" them on to the shelter system rather than treating the problem or having the dogs euthanized. In other words, the apparent higher incidence of separation-related problems in dogs acquired from a shelter may be due to the shelter system inadvertently recycling dogs with untreated separation anxiety (Van der Borg, 1991). Both of these explanations are probably at work, however. Relinquishment does involve some experience of traumatic loss for dogs, perhaps predisposing them to form an overly dependent attachment with the adopting owners. Further, dog owners may choose to relinquish mixed-breed dogs with separation-related behavior problems rather than seek costly behavior therapy and training or find new homes for their problem dogs. Finally, Mugford (1995) found that, among 220 dogs presenting separation-related problems, only 10% of the purebred dogs came directly from breeders, with the majority (55%) of them coming from "puppy mills" or similar places; unfortunately, he fails to define exactly what he means by a *puppy mill*. He speculates that early exposure to traumatic handling/transportation or inadequate sensory and social stimulation during a puppy's first 6 to 8 weeks of life may be involved in the development of adult separation-distress problems.

Unlike aggressive dogs, which are often destroyed, separation-distressed dogs usually escape euthanasia. For one thing, such dogs may be relinquished without mention of their separation problems, with owners making excuses for their dog's behavior like "not enough time" or "the dog needs more attention or space." The affectionate and outgoing enthusiasm of separation-reactive dogs may make them appealing to prospective owners, in comparison to less enthusiastic and retiring dogs competing for the attention of prospective adopters. Without treatment or training, separation-reactive dogs are recycled into new families, and the pattern is repeated until the dogs receive appropriate training or their luck finally runs out. Based on recent statistical studies, Tuber and colleagues (1999) estimate that 20% of the shelter population consists of dogs previously adopted and subsequently relinquished back into the shelter system, many as the direct result of behavior problems. In Europe (The Netherlands), the return rate has increased from 19% in 1983 to 50% in 1991 (Van der Borg et al., 1991).

Attachment, Proximity Seeking, and Family Size

Many dogs appear to develop separation problems as the result of forming excessively strong or exclusive bonds with one person. Clarifying the influence of owner attitudes and attachment levels on the development of separation distress is an important area of research. Surprisingly, in this regard, Voith and colleagues (1992) were unable to find a statistically significant relationship between anthropomorphic attitudes or spoiling activities and an increased occurrence of behavior problems. Further, Voith (1994) was unable to show a statistically significant difference between dogs diagnosed with separation anxiety and others not exhibiting the problem, in terms of whether they followed their owners about the house. Of these dogs (N = 100), 36 were diagnosed with separation anxiety, 64 were judged not to be exhibiting separation anxiety, and 3 presented ambiguous signs. Although the general tendency to follow the owner does not appear to be a reliable diagnostic indicator of separation anxiety, many separation-reactive dogs do exhibit pronounced proximity-seeking behavior toward their owners, especially at times immediately preceding owner departures.

Voith's findings question the importance of attachment levels as a predictor or causal factor in the etiology of separation anxiety. The literature on this issue is somewhat conflicted, however. Jagoe and Serpell (1996), for example, detected a significant relationship between sleeping in the owner's bedroom (a proximity measure) and an increased incidence of separation-related elimination problems, but emphasize that their data are inconclusive with respect to determining "whether the behavior problems are the consequences or the cause of the sleeping arrangement" (40). The strongest evidence to date questioning the role of attachment levels as a significant factor in the etiology of separation problems was reported by Goodloe and Borchelt (1998). Among 2018 dogs whose owners responded to a highly detailed questionnaire, the researchers found that measures of attachment, defined as efforts to maintain close proximity to the owner, showed no significant correlation with separation vocalization. They concluded that "panic at separation is not necessarily related to strong attachment. . . . Both humans and dogs can be strongly bonded to other individuals without experiencing anxiety or panic in their absence" (330). Nonetheless, many practitioners still believe that attachment levels play a significant role in the development of separation-related problems.

Although attachment per se may not always be a significant factor in the development of separation-distress problems, the quality of attachment, that is, the degree of dependency (anaclisis) versus secure attachment, may exert a significant influence (Clark and Boyer, 1993). Many separation-reactive dogs do, in fact, exhibit an exaggerated psychological dependency and anxious attachment toward their owners. They may appear insatiable for attention, exhibiting a constant desire for affection or need to maintain close physical contact, appearing uncomfortable unless they are in the owner's immediate proximity. They may engage in pestering antics or barking whenever their owners are distracted from them. Such behavior may occur when the owner diverts his or her attention away from the dog to use the phone. These demanding and persistent attention needs cause some owners to feel very uncomfortable and oppressed by it all. Some separation-anxious dogs will even refuse to eat unless the owner is nearby.

Despite the uncertainty and paucity of data regarding the influence of family size and structure on separation distress, there exists a general impression that separation anxiety presents most often in dogs living with a single owner or a couple. Recently, Topál and colleagues (1998) reported that dogs living in a large family situation tend to exhibit less separation distress when left alone than dogs living in smaller family groups. Perhaps, in larger family groups, with more people coming and going, dogs are exposed to separation in more safe and gradual ways. Also, large families may provide opportunities for multiple attachments to form, thereby preventing the development of an overly exclusive bond forming with one particular person, whose absence elicits separation distress. In regard to a possible connection between social group size and separation anxiety, Podberscek and colleagues (1999) reported that most of the separation anxious dogs in their study (N = 49) lived in homes with two adults and no children. Finally, the Ainsworth's (1972) strange-situation test used by Topál and colleagues provides an interesting nonintrusive means for evaluating some of the current con-flicting hypotheses concerning the role of attachment in the development of separation-related distress.

SEPARATION DISTRESS AND RETROACTIVE PUNISHMENT

Many owners presenting separation-distressed dogs for training believe that their dog's behavior is motivated by spitefulness or resentment at being left alone. In support of these beliefs, such owners may report various signs of guilt in their dog's demeanor, even before they discover the damage or mess made by the dog in their absence. The dog's appearance of *guilt in advance* is sufficient proof for them that the dog "knows" and is acting in a calculated manner (Vollmer, 1977). The first step in the counseling process is to convince them that their dog's behavior is better understood in terms of separation distress (anxiety, frustration, panic, or boredom) rather than vindictiveness. It is of utmost importance to explain in detail how such appearances of guilt probably result from a history of ineffectual punishment and that what they are observing is not guilt at all but rather apparent guilt or pseudoguilt (see *Misuse and Abuse of Punishment* in Volume 1, Chapter 8). It is also useful to point out that retroactive punishment may only worsen a dog's separation anxiety by enhancing its feelings of helplessness and, paradoxically, by increasing its attachment dependency toward the owner.

The owner may have trouble understanding and accepting the notion that dogs cannot causally connect punishment occurring in the presence of a *destroyed item* (e.g., the damaged sofa) with the *act of destroying it,* that is, behavior occurring at some in the past. But even the most resistant owner can be shown the dog's inherent limitations in this regard through thoughtful counseling. One method is to explore some of the differences in the way humans and dogs process, organize, and represent information. Appealing to the human's unique ability to think and symbolically represent experience through concepts and words provides a starting point from which to compare the dog's relative limitations with our own capabilities. It can be explained that humans can conceive of past events in terms of causal relations having deterministic effects on present events, largely as a result of our unique conceptual ability to symbolically represent and relate objects, events, and relations to one another. In addition, it should be emphasized that a dog's appearance of guilt is not an expression of remorse aimed at placating the owner about some past action but rather represents a fearful-submission display aimed at avoiding punishment in situations where it has occurred in the past, regardless of its association with the unwanted target behavior. This theory holds that pseudoguilt is maintained by a triad of conditioned associations involving the following elements (Borchelt and Voith, 1985):

- Evidence of a destroyed object or soiled area.
- The presence of the owner.
- A history of punishment under similar circumstances in the past.

Another scenario involves the possibility that separation distress itself becomes associated with belated punishment as an internal cue. According to this theory, a dog is destructive or eliminates only when it is under the influence of high levels of separation distress; that is, a dog may identify an increased probability of punishment with those occasions when it is particularly upset during separation, coincidentally those same times when destructiveness or elimination is most likely to occur in the owner's absence. This account could help to explain why some dogs appear to show guilt *before* the owner actually finds the evidence of misbehavior. The triad of associative elements in this case includes

- The dog feels distressed.
- The owner returns home.
- The dog has been punished in the past when it felt distressed.

Determining the various causes of pseudoguilt in dogs would provide valuable information. At this point, the debate concerning the causation of pseudoguilt revolves around little more than speculation and educated guesses. Unfortunately, these views have not been experimentally tested. Many anecdotal reports, however, are very supportive of a pseudoguilt interpretation. For example, it is not uncommon for an adult dog that is kept with a puppy during owner absences to exhibit guilt at homecomings, especially on those occasions when the puppy has been destructive or eliminates while the owner is gone.

AGING AND SEPARATION-RELATED PROBLEMS

A higher incidence of separation problems is observed in older dogs. Chapman and Voith (1990) found that half of 26 older dogs studied (mean age, 12.2 years; and range, 10 to 18 years) were diagnosed with separation anxiety. Milgram and colleagues (1993) studied the degenerative effects of aging on a dog's nervous system and behavior. Older dogs appear to undergo many of the same neurological and behavioral changes that are suffered by elderly people, including evidence of progressive cognitive dysfunction and degenerative brain disorders. In addition to performing basic research, members of Milgram's group have also evaluated the clinical and behavior effects of L-deprenyl (selegiline) on age-related symptoms presented by older dogs (Ruehl et al., 1995). They found that L-deprenyl appeared to enhance cognitive functioning in many of the geriatric dogs treated. As many as 62% of the dog population over 10 years of age may exhibit some sign of cognitive dysfunction (E. W. Kanara, 1998, Pfizer Animal Health Company). Collectively, these various neurological and behavioral changes are referred to as canine cognitive dysfunction syndrome (CCDS). According to K. A. Houpt (AVMA Press Release, 1996), increased susceptibility to separation anxiety and other emotional disturbances in older dogs are related to CCDS and other discomforts associated with aging. She has reported early successes using L-deprenyl in conjunction with behavior modification for the treatment of separation-related problems in older dogs.

REFERENCES

Ainsworth MC (1972). Attachment and dependency: A comparison. In JL Gewirtz (Ed), *Attachment and Dependency.* Washington, DC: VH Winston.

Albrecht RC (1953). *Living Your Dog's Life: How to Select, Care for and Train you Dog: A Method Based on Understanding Your Dog's Mind.* New York: Harper and Brothers.

Appel J, Arms N, Horner R, and Carr WJ (1999). Long-term olfactory memory in companion dogs. Presented at the Annual Meeting of the Animal Behavior Society, Bucknell University, Lewisburg, PA, June 27–30.

Askew HR (1996). *Treatment of Behavior Problems in Dogs and Cats: A Guide for the Small Animal Veterinarian.* Cambridge, MA: Blackwell Science.

AVMA Press Release (1996). Veterinarians uncover new treatments for separation anxiety in older dogs. http://www.avma.org/pubinfo/pi7a.html.

Berkowitz L (1990). On the formation and regulation of anger and aggression: A cognitive-neoassociative analysis. *Am Psychol,* 45:494–503.

Borchelt PL (1983). Separation-elicited behavior problems in dogs. In AH Katcher and AM Beck (Eds), *New Perspective on Our Lives with Companion Animals.* Philadelphia: University of Pennsylvania Press.

Borchelt PL and Voith VL (1982). Diagnosis and treatment of separation-related behavior problems in dogs. *Vet Clin North Am Small Anim Pract,* 12:625–635.

Borchelt PL and Voith VL (1985). Punishment. *Compend Continuing Educ Pract Vet,* 7:780–788.

Bowlby J (1969). *Attachment and Loss,* Vol 1: *Attachment.* New York: Basic.

Bowlby J (1973) *Attachment and Loss,* Vol 2: *Separation, Anxiety, and Anger.* New York: Basic.

Brodbeck AJ (1954). An exploratory study on the acquisition of dependency behavior in puppies. *Bull Ecol Soc Am,* 35:73.

Bucke WF (1903). Cyno-psychoses: Children's thoughts, reactions, and feelings toward pet dogs. *J Genet Psychol,* 10:459–513.

Cairns RB (1975). Beyond social attachment: The dynamics of interactional development. In T Alloway, P Pliner, and L Krames (Eds), *Advances in the Study of Communication and Affect,* Vol 3: *Attachment Behavior.* New York: Plenum.

Campbell WE (1991). "Learned helplessness," crate and forced training methods: Is this a factor when they succeed? *Pet Behav Newsl,* 93:3.

Chapman BL and Voith VL (1990). Behavioral problems in old dogs: 26 cases (1984–1987). *JAVMA,* 196:944–946.

Clark GI and Boyer WN (1993). The effects of dog obedience training and behavioural counselling upon the human-canine relationship. *Appl Anim Behav Sci,* 37:147–159.

Coe CL, Wiener SG, Rosenberg LT, and Levine S (1985). Endocrine and immune responses to separation and maternal loss in nonhuman primates. In M Reite and T Fields (Eds), *The Psychobiology of Attachment and Separation.* New York: Academic.

D'Amato FR and Pavone F (1993). Endogenous opioids: A proximate reward mechanism for kin recognition? *Behav Neural Biol,* 60:79–83.

Davis KL, Gurski JC, and Scott JP (1977). Interaction of separation distress with fear in infant dogs. *Dev Psychobiol,* 10:203–212.

Dunbar I (1998). *Dog Behavior: An Owner's Guide to a Happy, Healthy Pet.* Berkeley, CA: James and Kenneth.

Elliot O and Scott JP (1961). The development of emotional distress reactions to separation, in puppies. *J Genet Psychol,* 99:3–22.

Fields T (1985). Attachment as psychobiological attunement: Being on the same wavelength. In M Reite and T Fields (Eds), *The Psychobiology of Attachment and Separation.* New York: Academic.

Fisher AE (1955). The effects of early differential treatment on the social and exploratory behavior of puppies [Unpublished doctoral dissertation]. University Park: Pennsylvania State University.

Fox MW (1966). The development of learning and conditioned responses in the dog: Theoretical and practical implications. *Can J Comp Med Vet Sci,* 30:282–286.

Fox MW (1971). *Integrative Development of Brain and Behavior in the Dog.* Chicago: University of Chicago Press.

Fraser AF (1980). *Farm Animal Behavioural.* London: Bailliere Tindall.

Fredericson E (1952). Perceptual homeostasis and distress vocalization in puppies. *J Pers,* 20:472–478.

Fuller JL (1967). Experiential deprivation and later behavior. *Science,* 158:1645–1652.

Gantt WH, Newton JE, Royer FL, and Stephens JH (1966). Effect of person. *Cond Reflex,* 1:146–160.

Goodloe LP and Borchelt PL (1998). Companion dog temperament traits. *J Appl Anim Welfare Sci,* 1:303–338.

Halliwell REW (1992). Comparative aspects of food intolerance. *Vet Med,* Sep:893–899.

Harlow H F, Mears C (1979). *The Human Model: Primate Perspectives.* Washington, DC: VH Winston and Sons.

Hart BL and Hart LA (1985). Selecting pet dogs on the basis of cluster analysis of breed behavior profiles and gender. *JAVMA,* 186:1181–1185.

Hediger H (1955/1968). *The Psychology and Behavior of Animals in Zoos and Circuses,* G Sircom (Trans). New York: Dover (reprint).

Heiman M (1956). The relationship between man and dog. *Psychoanal Q,* 25:568–585.

Hepper PG (1986). Sibling recognition in the domestic dog. *Anim Behav,* 34:288–289.

Hepper PG (1994). Long-term retention of kinship recognition established during infancy in the domestic dog. *Behav Processes,* 33:3–15.

Hofer MA (1983). On the relationship between attachment and separation processes in infancy. In R Plutchik and H Kellerman (Eds), *Emotion: Theory, Research, and Experience,* Vol 2. New York: Academic.

Hoffman HS (1996). *Amorous Turkeys and Addicted Ducklings: A Search for the Causes of Social Attachment.* Boston: Authors Cooperative.

Hoffman HS and Solomon RL (1974). An opponent-process theory of motivations: III. Some affective dynamics in imprinting. *Learn Motiv,* 5:149–64.

Hothersall D and Tuber DS (1979). Fears in companion dogs: Characteristics and treatment. In JD Keehn (Ed), *Psychopathology in Animals: Research and Clinical Implications.* New York: Academic.

Jagoe JA and Serpell JA (1996). Owner characteristics and interactions and the prevalence of canine behaviour problems. *Appl Anim Behav Sci,* 47:31–42.

Knowles PA, Conner RL, and Panksepp J (1987). Opiate effects on social behavior of juvenile dogs as a function of social deprivation. *Pharmacol Biochem Behav,* 33:533–537.

Leyhausen P (1973). On the natural history of fear. In BA Tonkin (Trans), *Motivation of Human and Animal Behavior: A Ethological View.* New York: Van Nostrand Reinhold.

Lindell EM (1997). Diagnosis and treatment of destructive behavior in dogs. *Vet Clin North Am Prog Companion Anim Behav,* 27:533—547.

Lorenz K (1971). *Studies in Animal and Human Behavior,* Vol 1, R Martin (Trans). Cambridge: Harvard University Press.

Lund JD and Jorgensen MC (1999). Behaviour patterns and time course of activity in dogs with separation problems. *Appl Anim Behav Sci,* 63:219–236.

Lynch JJ (1970). Psychophysiology and development of social attachment. *J Nerv Ment Dis,* 151:231–244.

Marks IM (1987). *Fears, Phobias, and Rituals.* New York: Oxford University Press.

Mauer DW and Vogel MPH (1967). *Narcotics and Narcotic Addiction.* Springfield, IL: Charles C Thomas.

McCrave EA (1991). Diagnostic criteria for separation anxiety in the dog. *Vet Clin North Am Adv Companion Anim Behav,* 21:247–255.

McMillan FD (1999). Influence of mental states on somatic health in animals. *JAVMA,* 214:1221–1225.

Meckos-Rosenbaum V, Carr WJ, Goodwin JL, et al. (1994). Age-dependent responses to chemosensory cues mediating kin recognition in dogs (*Canis familiaris*). *Physiol Behav,* 55:495–499.

Milgram NW, Ivy GO, Head E, et al. (1993). The effect of L-deprenyl on behavior, cognitive function, and biogenic amines in the dog. *Neurochem Res,* 18:1211–1219.

Mineka S and Suomi SJ (1978). Social separation in monkeys. *Psychol Bull,* 85:1376–1400.

Montevecchi WA, Gallup GG, and Dunlap WP (1973). The peep vocalization in group reared chicks (*Gallus domesticus*): Its relation to fear. *Anim Behav,* 21:116–123.

Mugford RA (1995). Canine behavioural therapy. In J Serpell (ED), *The Domestic Dog: Its Evolution, Behaviour, and Interaction with People.* New York: Cambridge University Press.

Niego M, Sternberg S, and Zawistowsk S (1990). Applied comparative psychology and the care of companion animals: I. Coping with problem behaviors in canines. *Hum Innov Altern Anim Exp,* 4:162–164.

Ornitz EM (1991). Developmental aspects of neurophysiology. In M Lewis (Ed), *Child and Adolescent Psychiatry: A Comprehensive Textbook.* Baltimore: Williams and Wilkins.

Overall K (1997). *Clinical Behavioral Medicine for Small Animals.* St Louis: CV Mosby.

Panksepp J (1988a). Brain opioids and social affect. In P Borchelt, P Plimpton, AH Kutscher, et al. (Eds), *Animal Behavior and Thanatology.* New York: Foundation of Thanatology.

Panksepp J (1988b). Brain emotional circuits and psychopathologies. In M Clynes and J Panksepp (Eds), *Emotions and Psychopathology.* New York: Plenum.

Panksepp J (1998). *Affective Neuroscience: The Foundations of Human and Animal Emotions.* New York: Oxford University Press.

Patronek GJ, Glickman LT, Beck AM, et al. (1996). Special report: Risk factors for relinquishment of dogs to an animal shelter. *JAVMA,* 209:572–581.

Pettijohn TF, Wong, TW, Ebert PD, and Scott JP (1977). Alleviation of separation distress in 3 breeds of young dogs. *Dev Psychobiol,* 10:373–381.

Podberscek AL, Hsu Y, and Serpell JA (1999). Evaluation of clomipramine as an adjunct to behavioural therapy in the treatment of separation-related problems in dogs. *Vet Rec,* 145:365–369.

Rosenblatt J (1983). Olfaction mediates developmental transition in the altricial newborn of selected species of mammals. *Dev Psychobiol,* 16:347–375.

Ross S, Scott JP, Cherner M, and Denenberg V (1960). Effects of restraint and isolation on yelping in puppies. *Anim Behav,* 6:1–5.

Ruehl WW, Bruyette DS, DePaoli A, Cotman CW, et al. (1995). Canine cognitive dysfunction as a model for human age-related cognitive decline, dementia and Alzheimer's disease: Clinical presentation, cognitive testing, pathology and response to L-deprenyl therapy. *Prog Brain Res,* 106:217-25.

Schmidt JP (1968). Psychosomatics in veterinary medicine. In MW Fox (Ed), *Abnormal Behavior in Animals.* Philadelphia: WB Saunders.

Scott JP (1980). Nonverbal communication in the process of social attachment. In SA Corson, EO Carson, and JA Alexander (Eds), *Ethology and Nonverbal Communication in Mental Health.* New York: Pergamon.

Scott JP (1988). Emotional basis of the separation syndrome in dogs. In P Borchelt, P Plimpton, AH Kutscher, et al. (Eds), *Animal Behavior and Thanatology.* New York: Foundation of Thanatology.

Scott JP and Bronson FH (1964). Experimental exploration of the et-epimeletic or care-soliciting behavioral system. In PH Leiderman and D Shapiro (Eds), *Psychobiological Approaches to Social Behavior.* Stanford: Stanford University Press.

Scott JP and Fuller JL (1965). *Genetics and the Social Behavior of the Dog.* Chicago: University of Chicago Press.

Scott JP, Stewart JM, and DeGhett VJ (1973). Separation in infant dogs. In JP Scott and EC Senay (Eds), *Separation and Anxiety: Clinical and Research Aspects.* AAAS Symposium. Washington, DC: American Association for the Advancement of Science.

Selye H (1976). *The Stress of Life.* New York: McGraw-Hill.

Serpell J and Jagoe JA (1995). Early experience and the development of behaviour. In J Serpell (Ed), *The Domestic Dog: Its Evolution, Behaviour, and Interaction with People.* New York: Cambridge University Press.

Slabbert JM and Rasa OA (1993). The effect of early separation from the mother on pups in bonding to humans and pup health. *J S Afr Vet Assoc,* 64:4–8.

Solomon RL and Corbit JD (1974). An opponent-process theory of motivation: I. Temporal dynamics of affect. *Psychol Rev,* 81:119–145.

Spitz RA (1946). Anaclitic depression. *Psychoanal Study Child,* 2:313–342.

Starr MD (1978). An opponent-process theory of motivation: VI. Time and intensity variables in the development of separation-induced distress calling in ducklings. *J Exp Psychol Anim Behav Processes,* 4:338–355.

Takeuchi Y, Houpt KA, Scarlet JM (2000). Evaluation of treatments for separation anxiety in dogs. *JAVMA,* 217:342-345.

Tinbergen N (1951/1969). *The Study of Instinct.* Oxford: Oxford University Press (reprint).

Topál J, Miklósi A, Csányi V, et al. (1998). Attachment behavior in dogs (*Canis familiaris*): A new application of Ainsworth's (1969) strange situation test. *J Comp Psychol,* 112:219–229.

Torgersen S (1986). Childhood and family characteristics in panic and generalized anxiety disorders. *Am J Psychiatry,* 143:630–632.

Tuber DS, Hennessy MB, Sanders S, and Miller JA (1996). Behavioral and glucocorticoid responses of adult dogs (*Canis familiaris*) companionship and social separation. *J Comp Psychol,* 110:103–108.

Tuber DS, Miller DD, Caris KA, et al. (1999) Dogs in animal shelters: Problems, suggestions, and needed expertise. *Psychol Sci,* 10:379–386.

Turner DC (1997). Treating canine and feline behaviour problems and advising clients. *Appl Anim Behav Sci,* 52:199–204.

Van der Borg JAM, Netto WJ, and Planta DJU (1991). Behavioural testing of dogs in animal shelters to predict problem behaviour. *Appl Anim Behav Sci,* 32:237–251.

Voith VL (1980). Destructive behavior in the owner's absence. In BL Hart (Ed), *Canine Behavior.* Santa Barbara, CA: Veterinary Practice.

Voith VL (1981). Attachment between people and their pets: Behavior problems of pets that arise from the relationship between pets and people. In B Fogle (Ed), *Interrelations Between People and Pets.* Springfield, IL: Charles C Thomas.

Voith VL (1994). Profiles of dogs with separation anxiety and treatment approaches. Presented at the AVMA Meeting (July 10), San Francisco.

Voith VL and Borchelt PL (1985). Separation Anxiety in Dogs. *Compend Continuing Educ Pract Vet,* 7:42–53. [Also see update in Voith VL and Borchelt PL (1996). *Readings in Companion Animal Behavior.* Trenton, NJ: Veterinary Learning Systems.]

Voith VL and Borchelt PL (1996). Separation anxiety in dogs: Update. In VL Voith and PL Borchelt (Eds), *Readings in Companion Animal Behavior.* Trenton, NJ: Veterinary Learning Systems.

Voith VL, Wright JC, Danneman PJ, et al. (1992). Is there a relationship between canine behavior problems and spoiling activities, anthropomorphism, and obedience training? *Appl Anim Behav Sci,* 34:263–272.

Vollmer PJ (1977). Do mischievous dogs reveal their "guilt"? *Vet Med Small Anim Clin,* June:1002–1005.

Yeon SC, Erb HN, and Houpt KA (1999). A retrospective study of canine house soiling: Diagnosis and treatment. *J Am Anim Hosp Assoc,* 35:101–106.

Young SP and Goldman EA (1944/1964). *The Wolves of North America: Parts I and II.* New York: Dover (reprint).

White SD (1990). Naltrexone for treatment of acral lick dermatitis in dog. *J Am Vet Med Assoc,* 196:1073–1076.

Wright JC and Nesselrote MS (1987). Classification of behavior problems in dogs: Distributions of age, breed, sex and reproductive status. *Appl Anim Behav Sci,* 19:169–178.

Zimen E (1981). *The Wolf: His Place in the Natural World.* London: Souvenir.

5

Excessive Behavior

Persistence depends on inconsistent treatment of consistent behavior.

ABRAM AMSEL (1971)

PART 1: COMPULSIVE BEHAVIOR

Many compulsive and ritualized habits have been identified in dogs, including compulsive eating (hyperphagia), pica, excessive licking (directed toward the floor, furniture, and hands), rooting at food, digging, mounting, barking, pacing, fence running, and various aberrant aggressive displays. Some affected dogs suffer psychogenic dermatoses, compulsively licking lesions into their limbs and feet [acral lick dermatitis (ALD)]; others monotonously suck on their flanks [a habit most common among Doberman pinschers (Figure 5.1)]; and some appear mesmerized by phantom flies or may lunge and snap at flecks of light on a wall. Dogs taken too early from their mother are prone to develop compulsive, stereotypic habits involving blanket sucking and kneading—a compulsion frequently not appearing until after puberty. Finally, there is a tendency for certain breeds to present compulsive problems more often [e.g., bullterriers and German shepherds (whirling-tail chasing) and Labrador retrievers (ALD)], suggesting a probable genetic factor predisposing some dogs to develop such habits.

DEFINITIONS

Compulsive behavior disorders (CBDs) in domestic animals have received growing attention over the past several years. Some

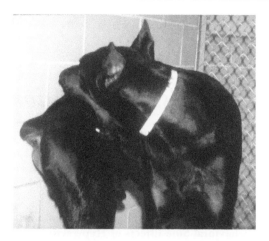

FIG. 5.1. Flank sucking is a compulsive behavior that is primarily exhibited by Doberman pinschers. (Photo courtesy of V. L. Voith.)

authors have unfortunately borrowed the psychiatric term *obsessive-compulsive disorder* (OCD) in describing the analogous conditions observed in dogs (Luescher et al., 1991; Overall, 1992a–c). This appropriation of terminology is apparently intended to emphasize the close similarity between human OCD and the stereotypic rituals and compulsive repetitive behavior exhibited by domestic animals. Rapoport and Ismond (1996) define *obsessions* in their *DSM-IV Training Guide for Diagnosis of Childhood Disorders* in the following way:

1. Recurrent and persistent thoughts, impulses, or images that are experienced, at some time during the disturbance, as intrusive and inappropriate and that cause marked anxiety or distress.
2. The thoughts, impulses, or images are not simply excessive worries about real-life problems.
3. The person attempts to ignore or suppress such thoughts, impulses, or images, or to neutralize them with some other thought or action.
4. The person recognizes that the obsessional thoughts, impulses, or images are a product of his or her own mind (not imposed from without in thought insertion). (230)

Although dogs may "obsess" like humans suffering with OCD, the possible role of obsession cannot be confirmed by direct report or quanti-

fied by any other scientific method currently available. Therefore, to refer to compulsive behavior exhibited by animals as obsessional is both excessively anthropomorphic and possibly misleading. Consequently, the term *compulsive behavior disorder* (Fox, 1963) is used in the following discussion to avoid such confusion.

Stereotypic rituals and compulsive repetitive behaviors are commonly seen in zoo and laboratory animals confined to spaces inadequate for their needs. Such animals can often be observed engaging in various *stereotypies,* including monotonous rhythmic pacing, rocking (chimpanzees), circling, excessive self-grooming, or various nonnutritive consummatory behaviors (e.g., pica). Since compulsive behaviors frequently occur in response to elevated arousal levels, especially as the result of frustration, it has been suggested that such behavior may serve a de-arousal function. In fact, several studies in humans and domestic animals have shown that compulsive repetitive behavior decreases heart rate (Seo et al., 1998). Some compulsive behaviors appear to involve aggressive behavior redirected toward the animal's body, often causing self-injury (Jones and Barraclough, 1978). Frustrative arousal is an establishing operation for aggressive behavior, supporting the notion that self-directed attacks may involve an aggressive motivation.

Compulsive repetitive behaviors are often referred to as stereotypies. Kuo (1967), however, has charged that strictly speaking stereotypic behaviors do not exist:

No animal responds twice to the same stimulation in exactly the same way. The pacing back and forth of a fox or a wolf in the zoo may appear to the onlooker to be stereotypical. But if one takes quantitative measurements of the pacing movements of the animal one will find that no two pacing movements cover the same ground, involve the same neuromusculature, consume the same amount of energy, and have the identical implicit gradients [that is, internal motivational organization]. (100)

It is important, therefore, to declare at the outset that when the term *stereotypy* is used here, it is employed in a less formal sense than suggested by Kuo and denotes a high degree of regularity, repetitiveness, and inflexibility.

The term *stereotypy* refers to a relatively invariant pattern of compulsive behavior, usually occurring under unnatural conditions, involving varying degrees of distress (e.g., conflict and frustration). *Stereotypies* usually consist of ordinary behaviors (e.g., appetitive, self-grooming, and locomotor activities) that occur out of context, in excess, or in an exaggerated form. The specific elements making up the *stereotypic* ritual consist of repetitive compulsive behaviors that intrude and interfere with normal activities or cause physical injury to the animal (e.g., automutilation). Finally, stereotypies have species-typical relevance and present similar forms in animals belonging to the same species. For example, crib biting (cribbing) is a common stereotypy observed among distressed horses. Affected animals engage in persistent and compulsive biting on wooden stalls and fence posts while simultaneously sucking in air. Dogs do not exhibit cribbing, but instead may lick sores into their carpus or mutilate their tail as the result of chasing it. Although stereotypies may serve a similar function in both species, the stereotypic forms expressed by the two species are different.

ETIOLOGY

The etiology of compulsive behavior in dogs is not fully understood; however, several prominent risk factors have been identified. Compulsive behaviors are most frequently reported in dogs that have been stressed by excessive confinement, exposed to sensory-motor deprivation (e.g., boredom and inadequate exercise), provided inadequate social attention and stimulation, or exposed to a conflict-dense environment. Stereotypic behavior patterns may develop as the result of neurobiological stressors; for example, hyperkinetic dogs under the influence of long-term amphetamine treatment may exhibit chomping behavior or spontaneous barking. Also, compulsive symptoms often appear in highly excitable or nervous dogs where no identifiable external precipitating causes or stressors can be identified, suggesting that a genetic predisposition may underlie the etiology of some compulsive behavior disorders. Once established, the frequency and range of contexts under which compulsive behavior occurs may increase and widen over time, making early diagnosis and treatment imperative (Hewson and Luescher, 1996).

Environmental Deprivation and Distress

Dogs may exhibit compulsive behavior when overly confined or deprived of adequate exercise, social contact, or sensory stimulation. Melzack and Scott (1957) reported the case of several 9-month-old Scottish terriers that had been exposed to 7 months of almost total sensory and social isolation (initiated at 4 weeks and terminated at 8 months of age). The dogs exposed to restricted rearing conditions exhibited a variety of motor deficits, increased excitability, and disorganized "wild, aimless" behavior. They also exhibited sharp differences in comparison to normally reared controls in terms of avoidance learning. When tested for nociceptive responsiveness, isolated dogs repeatedly approached the flame of a match even though they were burned by it again and again. Long-term restriction and social isolation have been implicated in the development of compulsive whirling and circling behavior by dogs (Fisher, 1955). Thompson and coworkers (1956) found that, among 11 Scottish terriers reared under restricted conditions, 8 developed the habit of whirling, together with intense vocalization, tail biting, and snarling—all lasting for up to 10 minutes at a time. Some breeds appear to be predisposed to develop the whirling compulsion. The English bullterrier, for example, is particularly prone to develop a serious whirling disorder with automutilation (Dodman et al., 1993; Blackshaw et al., 1994). Also, Hewson and Luescher (1996) note that German shepherds present relatively more often with the habit, but tail chasing and tail biting occur in a variety of breeds (Figure 5.2).

Vacuum Behavior

How is such behavior to be interpreted? Early ethologists proposed that such behavior might be viewed as a form of *vacuum behavior*. Vacuum behavior occurs under conditions of close confinement in which various drive pressures (including aggression) may gradually

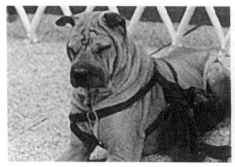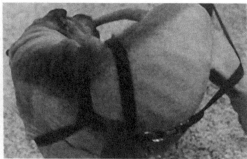

FIG. 5.2. This shar-pei appears to have difficulty staying awake, a sign that may reflect an underlying conflict or fear condition (Voith and Borchelt, 1996). When aroused, the dog turns and bites its tail. (Photos courtesy of V. L. Voith.)

build up and be triggered by objects and stimuli other than normal ones. Such behavior occurs especially in situations where normal outlets and opportunities for appropriate drive-reducing activity are not present. Vacuum behavior appears to spontaneously erupt out of frustrated internal drive tensions unable to find adequate expression otherwise. When vacuum behaviors are motivated by aggression, they frequently take the form of whirling topographies, with the aggression being directed at the animal's body (Lorenz, 1981). Whirling in dogs, therefore, may not be an entirely neutral motoric compulsion but an aggressive vacuum behavior directed at the animal's own body. This interpretation is consistent with the description of whirling given by Thompson et al. (1956) and others:

> Whirling can be described as follows: very rapid, jerky running in a tight circle; shrill, agonized yelping; barking and snarling; and tail snapping and tail biting. The syndrome may last from 1 to 10 minutes. It is usually heralded by certain characteristic signs. The dog suddenly becomes motionless, cocking its head up and back, as if looking at its own tail. It begins to growl viciously, and its eyes take on a glazed expression. These signs may continue for a minute or two, increasing in intensity until the full-blown fit occurs. (939)

Swedo (1989) proposes that compulsive behavior may be the result of a dysfunctional releaser and fixed-action pattern (FAP):

> Obsessive-compulsive rituals can be viewed as inappropriately released fixed-action patterns.

Our work with more than 200 children and adults has led us increasingly to view OCD in this fashion. For example, obsessive patients, who check and recheck that the coffee pot is unplugged, all seem to perform each checking pattern in an identical fashion. Their behavior is perfect in form, but after the first check, it is ineffectual and inappropriate. To follow an ethological model, one must of course, ask: what is the releasing stimulus in OCD? Is it internal (e.g., chemical) or external (e.g., environmental stress)? How does it effect the release of the ritualized fixed-action pattern? (273)

Given the relatively narrow range and specificity of compulsive behavior disorders, it makes sense to interpret them in terms of species-typical adaptations to persistent frustration or conflict. Under the stressful influence of adverse frustration or conflict, a *releaser* mechanism may become defective, causing predisposed dogs to inappropriately repeat the same rigid and perseverating loop of behaviors. Pathological compulsive behavior appears to operate independently of voluntary control and normal expectations. Like *instinctive* behavior, compulsive habits become progressively ritualized, stereotypic, and automatic—features consistent with an FAP interpretation.

Normal versus Abnormal Compulsions

Under extreme and adverse environmental conditions, it is reasonable to ponder whether such behavior is truly aberrant or simply an adaptive response to an aberrant environment, Mugford (1984) writes regarding this diagnostic dilemma concerning whirling behavior:

A heterogeneous species such as the dog, raised in a multitude of environments and social situations, presents even greater variability [than a laboratory mouse]. Thus, one generalizes about the behaviour of cats and dogs at one's peril, and the greater one's knowledge of the two species, the less appropriate seems the term "abnormal." For instance, "whirling" is a commonly occurring stereotype in kenneled dogs, but is unusual in free-roaming or home situations. If one examines the behavioural options available to a kenneled dog, one finds that restricted movement and reduced social contacts have made whirling a highly appropriate behaviour in this environment. It brings vestibular stimulation and attention from kennel staff, and in that setting is certainly not an abnormal behaviour. (134)

According to Fox (1974), many compulsive compensatory behaviors may be aimed at resolving internal conflict or other states of anxious arousal:

> If the environment does not provide varied stimulation, the subject may compensate by creating its own varied input by elaborating stereotyped motor acts or by directing specific activities toward inappropriate objects (such as copulating with its food bowl). The stereotyped motor acts (thumb-sucking, self-clutching, and rocking in primates) developed while in isolation may be performed when the subject is in a novel environment and may serve to reduce arousal or anxiety because they are familiar activities and may be comforting. (72–73)

Hewson and Luescher (1996) argue that most compulsive behaviors can be traced to conflict situations involving a high degree of frustrative arousal. Subsequently, the behavior may be "emancipated" from the original context and be expressed in other situations, when the dog is under the influence of increased excitement or stress. Obviously, drawing a definitive line is difficult when it comes to labels like "normal" and "abnormal."

DISPLACEMENT ACTIVITY

Classical ethologists interpreted and described compulsive repetitive behavior in terms of displacement activity. Displacement activity occurs when some course of action is thwarted (frustration) or when two opposing motivational tendencies are elicited at the same time (conflict). Under the influence of frustration or conflict, a substitute behavior may be emitted, often coming from a remote functional system and possessing little apparent motivational relevance for the conflict at hand. A classic example of such substitutive displacement behavior was observed by Tinbergen (1951/1969) in male sticklebacks. These fish are highly territorial and actively defend their nests from the invasion of conspecifics. However, if two male sticklebacks encounter each other on the boundary line between their respective territories, two antagonistic drives may be simultaneously induced. As a result, equally strong fight and flight drives are activated at the same time, resulting in approach-avoidance conflict. The resulting conflict is resolved when the two fish resort to digging behavior—a functionally remote species-typical displacement activity. While digging, sticklebacks point their heads downward and dig into the sand with their mouths as though making a nest. Interestingly, if male sticklebacks are forced to nest too closely together, "they will show nearly continuous displacement digging and the result is that their territories are littered with pits, or even become one huge pit" (117). According to Lorenz (1981), among animals, displacement activities are common everyday occurrences that are specific to particular conflicts and no others; that is, conflict situations among most animals and birds are highly stereotypic, producing only one displacement activity or "sparking over" action pattern.

Under conditions of behavioral or emotional conflict, requiring that a dog choose between two equally unacceptable courses of action, substitutive behaviors or *displacement activities* may help to restore balance and homeostasis within a behavioral system threatened by invasive anxiety or even (in the case of extreme conflict) functional collapse. Subsequently, the displacement activity may be activated whenever the animal is confronted with a difficult or insoluble conflict, providing a mechanism for safely killing time until a more adequate response can be found to resolve the situation. Since the substitute behavior results in the reduction (if only temporarily) of anxiety and the restoration of equilibrium, it may become highly reinforcing for animals to perform. This may help to explain why CBDs do not extinguish over time, as in the case of other behaviors occurring in the absence of reinforcement. Perhaps the substitute behavior is repeated again and again because it produces strongly gratifying and self-reinforcing effects.

The substitute response is often a behavioral non sequitur; that is, it does not follow from learned expectancies and predictions about the environment but rather represents a behavioral exception evoked under conditions of stress and conflict. The autonomous nature of the CBD gives it the appearance of being irrational, without purpose or apparent goal, and operating independently of normal constraints and inhibitions. Because the substitute behavior does not conform to the ordinary rules of learning, it may be refractory to modification. The substitute behavior is essentially an autonomous anomaly, presenting under the control of variables outside the scope of normal self-regulatory behavioral mechanisms. As a result of their exceptional character and origin, compulsions may exert a *superstitious* or obsessional fascination, further distinguishing them from ordinary behavior.

In fact, many compulsive behaviors appear to take the form of something like a superstition. Lorenz described in detail the behavior of one of his graylag geese that had developed a complex compulsion, apparently driven by anxiety reduction:

> At first, she always walked past the bottom of the staircase toward a window in the hallway before returning to the steps, which she then ascended to get into the room on the upper floor. Gradually she shortened this detour, but persisted in initially orienting towards the window, without, however, going all the way to it. Instead she turned at a 90 degree angle once she was parallel to the stairs. (Quoted in Swedo, 1989:282)

On one occasion, Lorenz forgot to let the goose in at the accustomed time. It was nearly dark outside, and she had become excited about the opportunity to get inside. As a result, instead of going through her typical ritual, she darted directly toward the stair steps and began to climb:

> Upon this something shattering happened: Arrived at the fifth step, she suddenly stopped, made a long neck, in geese a sign of fear, and spread her wings as for flight. Then she uttered a warning cry and very nearly took off. Now she hesitated a moment, turned around, ran hurriedly down the five steps and set forth resolutely, like someone on a very important mission, on her original path to the window and back. This time she mounted the steps according to her former custom from the left side. On the fifth step she stopped again, looked around, shook herself and performed a greeting display behavior regularly seen in graylags when anxious tension has given place to relief. I hardly believed my eyes. To me there is no doubt about the interpretation of this occurrence. The habit had become a custom which the goose could not break without being stricken by fear. (Quoted in Swedo, 1989:282)

This interesting anecdote is relevant to the way in which some common compulsive habits appear to develop in dogs.

Many ritualized habits develop around entryways and boundaries, often becoming extremely energetic and bizarre. For example, a common compulsion among dogs confined outdoors is fence running and fighting (see *Sources of Territorial Agitation: Fences and Chains* in Chapter 7). Sometimes, aggressive behavior is very dramatically increased under such conditions of confinement. Dogs with dog-fighting problems or exhibiting aggression toward strangers often exhibit intensely exaggerated displays while restrained on a leash or chain. In many cases, the aggressive behavior may seem vicious and virtually uncontrollable. Surprisingly, however, if such a dog happens to escape its owner's hold or confinement, the aggressive efforts may almost instantly fizzle out. On recognition that it is free, the previously uncontrollable dog may appear disoriented and confused about its intentions. This is definitely not always the case, though, with many dogs known to deliver particularly savage attacks after breaking free of a chain or slipping a leash. In general, any situation in which a dog is highly motivated to behave in some particular way but prevented from doing so by physical restraint or threat of punishment may increase the likelihood of compulsive behavior.

Adjunctive Behavior and Compulsions

Schedule-induced Excessive Behavior

Many experiments have been performed using intermittent reinforcement and observing confluent effects on behavior, especially exaggerations in drinking, pica, hyperactivity, and aggression (Falk and Kupfer, 1998). In the classic experiments performed by John Falk (1961), rats were trained to lever press on a variable schedule of reinforcement. A small pellet of food was presented on a variable-interval 1-minute schedule (i.e., the rats received reinforcement averaging 1 pellet per minute), so long as they lever pressed at least once between reinforcement opportunities. In addition, the rats were given free access to water. Falk noticed that the rats habitually drank after obtaining reinforcement, usually consuming around 0.5 ml before continuing to lever press. The cumulative result was the consumption of an extraordinary amount of water over the course of a typical 3-hour session. On average, rats drank 90 ml of water, a significant excess of consumption over the normal intake of 27 ml of water consumed by an average rat daily. In other words, the rats drank approximately 50% of their body weight in water during each training session. This phenomenon is referred to as *schedule-induced polydipsia.*

Additional experiments demonstrated that an important factor in the development of schedule-induced polydipsia is the duration of time between reinforcing events. Schedule-induced polydipsia is *time dependent,* with 2- to 3-minute intervals producing the largest magnitude of polydipsia. Shorter or longer intertrial intervals produce less polydipsia or result in normal water consumption. These findings suggest that the phenomenon is controlled by a *bitonic function:* "sessions with either short or long intervals between pellet consumption produce normal amounts of drinking, while intermediate values induce polydipsia" (Falk, 1981:317). Another important variable associated with the phenomenon is deprivation. Rats in Falk's studies were reduced to 80% of their free-feeding body weight. Rats of normal weight are significantly less affected by schedule-induced polydipsia, suggesting that *hunger tension* may influence the phenomenon.

Other forms of adjunctive behavior, including aggression and hyperactivity, have been associated with intermittent reinforcement. For example, a pigeon working on an intermittent schedule of reinforcement may turn and attack a nearby conspecific when the reinforcer is delivered. Although such frustration-related aggression is not uncommon, the magnitude of adjunctive attacks goes far beyond what is normally observed to occur under frustrative conditions (Campagnoni et al., 1986). Similar results have been observed in squirrel monkeys who were maintained on a variable-interval schedule. After receiving reinforcement, the monkey would aggressively grab and bite a rubber hose provided to receive such attacks. Increased activity has also been observed to occur as the result of intermittent reinforcement. For example, wheel running was significantly increased when rats were trained to work under a variable-interval 1-minute schedule of reinforcement.

Food is not the only reinforcer capable of generating schedule-induced excessive behavior. If a well-fed and watered rat is given intermittent access to an activity wheel, several adjunctive behaviors like rearing, licking, and position changes undergo an increase of emission. Studies of people under the influence of variable interval schedules have also shown increases in general activity levels, eating and drinking, and grooming activities. Finally, pica has been observed in animals stressed on brief-interval schedules, suggesting a possible role of schedule-induced motivations underlying the development of such behavior problems in dogs.

Schedule-induced Escape

An average pigeon is willing to work only so long as the schedule of reinforcement stays within certain limits. Rather than work on an exceedingly lean schedule of reinforcement, most animals will opt to press a second key wired to turn off (self-signaled time-out) the reinforcement contingency, even though the action postpones a possible opportunity for eventual reinforcement. This phenomenon is referred to as *schedule-induced escape.* Paradoxically, pigeons under the influence of food deprivation and weight loss tended to produce the most self-induced time-outs. This is counterintuitive to what one would expect from animals suffering from the effects of deprivation and hunger. An interesting example of schedule-induced escape behavior in dogs was reported by Luescher (1993b). The case involved a 2½-year-old German shepherd that, as a working police dog at an airport, searched planes for explosives. The dog was an enthusiastic and effective detector dog that routinely worked continuously for 1½-hour stretches. However, over the course of a year, his stamina and willingness to perform deteriorated until he was unable to work for periods exceeding 15 minutes at a time. After 15 minutes, he abruptly quit, appeared exhausted, and stood motionless looking at his handler. In addition, the dog developed over the same period a persistent collateral habit of whirling while in the police vehicle (perhaps a compulsion resulting from anticipatory conflict) and had become progressively aggressive toward pedestrians approaching it. The usual search of the plane took approximately 2½ hours, during which time the dog was provided one "successful" find of a dummy bomb, resulting in praise and tug with a toy. Luescher speculates that the schedule of intermittent reinforcement utilized was too lean; that is, the dog was required to search too long for a single reinforcement. He implicates the phenomenon of adjunctive escape as a possible explanation for the dog's behavior. The dog, rather than endure the aversive intermittent schedule, simply quit, even though it meant losing access to the eventual reinforcer:

> Although indicating was reinforced each time in the dog of this report, searching was reinforced as seldom as once in 2.5 hours. Hundreds of sniffing responses may have been performed over a period of up to 2.5 hours, before searching was reinforced by the smell of explosives. Thus, the ratio of nonreinforced to reinforced correct responses was large, and the dog would be assumed to perceive its work as increasingly stressful. . . Because the ride to the airport always preceded the work there, the

dog became classically conditioned to associate the ride in the truck with the stressful situation at the airport. The ride thus became a conditioned stimulus, in response to which the dog exhibited increased anxiety. (1539)

Displacement Activities and Compulsions

Falk (1977, 1981) views adjunctive behavior as natural response to equivocal circumstances in which decisive action is not possible. Such behavior may serve an important adaptive function by stabilizing conflict situations involving opposing motivational constraints. He argues that adjunctive behavior is commonly observed in nature when opposing motivational vectors are in equilibrium and *maximally equivocal* (Figure 5.3). These opposing motivations frequently involve defense of territory, feeding, sexual privileges, maternal protection of young, and self-preservation set against the possible need to withdrawal or flee from the situation:

> In terms of evolutionary processes, the adaptive function of adjunctive behavior is to delay commitment to either engaging a situation or escaping from it until one or the other vector becomes clearly ascendent. (Falk and Kupfer, 1998:341)

Among humans, various public rituals typically form around these important transitional cultural and social events (Falk, 1986). When opposing motivations are in approximate equilibrium, action is made uncertain. Under such circumstances, adjunctive behavior or displacement activity emerges in order to temporarily postpone decisive action, thereby preventing a potentially costly mistake. According to this theory, displacement activities stabilize the situation long enough for one of the opposing components to become ascendant and result in a stable resolution:

> The processes that produce displacement activities are precisely those responsible for adjunctive behavior. In both cases, an important activity is in progress or a crucial commodity is being acquired. These are usually territorial defense, courtship and mating sequences, and parental behavior in ethologic studies; scheduled access to food, water, activity, or money in investigations of adjunctive behavior. In one

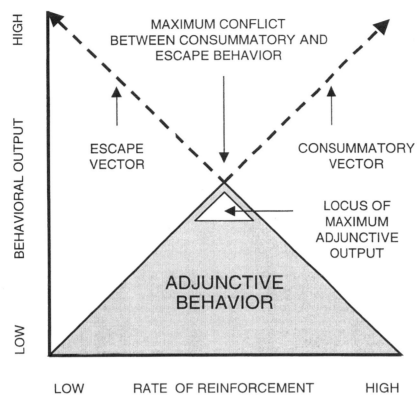

FIG. 5.3. Maximum adjunctive output occurs at the point of highest potential conflict between consummatory and escape vectors. After Falk (1981).

case the ongoing behavior is impeded by situational interruptions (intruders, inadequate releasing stimuli); in the other, by schedule constraints allowing only episodic access. The resulting behavior is described as incongruous or irrelevant in ethnologic observations and as persistent and excessive in adjunctive behavior investigations. I suggested that displacement activities have evolved because they serve an adaptive function: allowing stabilization of an unclear situation, with a nonprecipitous resolution of competing vectors. . . Adjunctive behavior, like displacement activities, is behavior that probably serves to block premature escape from nonoptimal situations. For example, a feeding environment providing a marginal amount of food induces a variety of adjunctive activities. In a natural environment, such behavior might function to delay abandonment of a feeding range or patch that, while marginal, is nevertheless adequate. (Falk, 1981:328–329)

There are several obvious implications of Falk's research for the understanding of compulsive behavior. In cases where biologically significant behavior is impeded by environmental constraints evoking opposing motivations of nearly equal strength, one would expect to observe the appearance of exaggerated adjunctive behavior. Adjunctive behavior functions to delay unnecessary retreat from anxious or frustrative arousal, perhaps allowing time for one or the other opposing motivational vectors to assume a definitively dominant influence over the conflict situation. Persistent and excessive adjunctive behavior (compulsive perseveration) results when neither side of a conflict assumes an ascendant role.

Schedule-induced paw grooming (licking) by rats has potential significance for understanding compulsive licking (ALD) in dogs. Lawler and Cohen (1992) observed that some rats operating under a fixed-time schedule of reinforcement (food was delivered every 2 minutes regardless of an animal's behavior) developed a habit of paw licking. The adjunctive grooming ritual occurred shortly after food was presented and lasted for approximately 30 seconds thereafter. Ordinarily, in rats, paw grooming is a brief initiating segment of a more elaborate grooming activity that includes nose wipes, ear wipes, and overall body grooming. In the case of persistent adjunctive paw grooming, there appears to be a stress-modulating function being performed under the condition of intermittent reinforcement. In the case of canine ALD, the initial increase in self-licking may begin as the result of a similar adjunctive or stress mechanism and then gradually come under the control of various other mechanisms (e.g., the endogenous opioid system), perhaps providing a source of intrinsic reinforcement maintaining the habit.

CONFLICT AND COACTIVE FACTORS

Compulsive behavior appears to be most commonly associated with situations where opposing motivational vectors (establishing operations) converge and require that the dog take one of two equally unacceptable courses of action. Given this definition of conflict, dogs are exposed to many conflictual situations in the course of their lives, but relatively few of them go on to develop compulsive habits that require professional intervention. In fact, most dogs appear to adjust to the adversity of conflict and frustration without developing any problems at all. Currently, it is not clear how compulsive disorders develop, but most behavioral theories incorporate some mix of influences, including adverse anxiety, frustration, learned helplessness, boredom, and attention seeking.

Anxiety and Frustration

Many compulsive behavior disorders appear to present under the influence of excessive frustrative arousal and stress (Hewson and Luescher, 1996). Anxiety, frustration, and other forms of stressful arousal have been fre-

quently implicated in the development of CBDs. These adverse emotional antecedents are frequently the result of conflict situations. Disruptive conflict, sufficient to disrupt purposive behavior, predictably occurs under circumstances in which dogs are strongly and equally motivated to behave in mutually incompatible ways at the same time. Presumably, under the influence of disruptive conflict, susceptible dogs are caught up in a psychologically intolerable state in which they are compelled to act but are unable to do so in a decisive way—a situation that cannot be merely escaped or ignored. Under such circumstances, a remote substitute behavior, irrelevant to both horns of the conflict, may be emitted and repeated as long as the conflict continues without resolution. This general theory has considerable appeal and is frequently referred to in the literature; however, it should be emphasized that the origin of many common compulsive behaviors cannot be readily traced to an identifiable precipitating conflict. In addition to conflict, many other environmental conditions may cause receptive dogs to exhibit compulsive behavior. Although the conflict theory may not explain the development of all compulsive behaviors, compulsions and other maladaptive behaviors have been produced and studied under laboratory conditions by inducing insolvable conflict.

Since the time of Shenger-Krestovnikova's famous experiments inducing neurosis in dogs (Pavlov, 1928/1967), many related experimental animal models have been used to investigate the etiology of neurotic behavior (see *Learning and Behavioral Disturbances* in Volume 1, Chapter 9). Several of these studies have stressed the importance of insolvable conflict in the development of neurotic compulsions. For example, Maier (1961) succeeded in producing a rigid behavioral fixation or stereotypy in rats by exposing them to an insolvable discrimination task. The rats in his experiment were unable to solve the "rigged" discrimination successfully and soon refused to jump, since doing so resulted in their bumping into locked discrimination cards and falling into a safety net below. The decision not to jump, however, was not a permanent solution, since the experimenter soon prodded them into action with a blast of air.

The result was the development of a position stereotypy or fixation. The rats chose one side or the other and persistently jumped in that direction even after the discrimination task had been restored to a solvable form. Maier speculated that the persistence of these abnormal behavioral fixations paralleled neurotic compulsive habits in human subjects.

A central feature of Maier's method for inducing neurosis is the imposition of a high degree of tension caused by avoidance-avoidance conflict. Such conflict is generated by placing an animal in an impasse between two equally undesirable alternatives. Avoidance-avoidance conflict is commonly observed in punitive situations where a dog is unable to abstain from some behavior or unwilling to perform a required behavior, but, nonetheless, is imposed upon to abstain or perform by threat of punishment. If this conflict situation is accompanied by the presence of poorly differentiated discriminative stimuli, then one is presented with a very similar scenario to the one described by Maier.

Another common configuration of conflict involves the evocation and collision of incompatible unconditioned responses, usually in the form of simultaneous approach and withdrawal behavior. The result is an approach-avoidance conflict. This form of conflict was studied by Masserman in his experiments with cats. Cats that were previously trained to expect food on approach to a hopper were exposed to an startling blast of air or shock as they began to eat. The unexpected aversive stimulation triggered a disorganizing expectancy reversal, causing the cats to exhibit a persistent pattern of phobic and compulsive behavior.

Workers in Pavlov's laboratory used a similar method to induce neurotic symptoms (Pavlov, 1928/1967, 1941). First, dogs were conditioned to expect the presentation of food following a certain number of metronome beats. Once the conditioned response was well established, an aversive stimulus was arbitrarily presented instead of the expected food. The approach-avoidance conflict generated by this expectancy reversal resulted in disturbances that Pavlov called *focal neuroses* or displacement stereotypies. Another procedure used in Pavlov's laboratory involved simultaneously eliciting potent incompatible emotional reactions (e.g., presenting food to a hungry dog together with shock). This arrangement caused a violent collision of incompatible expectations, precipitating internal approach-avoidance conflict and associated neurotic symptoms. Pavlov believed that approach-avoidance conflict was etiologically relevant to the development of OCDs in humans (Astrup, 1965). The disturbing effects of conflict led Pavlov (1941) to imagine what dogs might say, if they were able, about the causes of their various "neurotic" disturbances:

> One can conceive in all likelihood that, if these dogs which became ill could look back and tell what they had experienced on that occasion, they would not add a single thing to that which one would conjecture about their condition. All would declare that on every one of the occasions mentioned they were put through a difficult test, a hard situation. Some would report that they felt frequently unable to refrain from doing that which was forbidden and then they felt punished for doing it in one way or another, while others would say that they were totally, or just passively, unable to do what they usually had to do. (84)

Pavlov's observations emphasize that some dogs, especially overly excitable or inhibited ones, may respond adversely to aversive compulsion. Overly excitable dogs are less able to control impulses without extreme exertion and strain, whereas overly inhibited dogs may be unable to respond effectively under the pressure of punitive compulsion. Pavlov's observations also underscore the importance of providing dogs with adequate instrumental control over punitive events. When punishment occurs in an unpredictable or uncontrollable manner (i.e., independently of what a dog does or does not do), it may exert excessive or, potentially, pathological demands upon a dog's ability to adjust.

Negative Cognitive Set

Although conflict and stress appear to represent significant necessary conditions for the expression of compulsive behavior, as already noted, conflict alone does not provide an adequate explanation for the appearance of

CBDs. Identical exposure to conflict and stress may cause some dogs to develop a compulsive behavior problem, while leaving other dogs unaffected. A dog's ability to respond adaptively (or not) to conflict and stress is determined by various biological factors, the overall quality and cumulative effects of previous learning, and the animal's general ability to cope under adverse conditions. All three factors affect the manner in which dogs respond to conflict and stress. Dogs susceptible to CBDs may be more prone to exhibit compulsive behavior because they are unable to perform efficiently under stressful pressure. The cause of this impairment may be traced to an acquired cognitive deficit (see *Learned Helplessness* in Volume 1, Chapter 9). Some dogs exhibiting compulsive behavior may be affected by a pervasive belief or *negative cognitive set,* such that whatever they choose to do will be equally ineffectual and irrelevant to what actually occurs as a result of their action. The influence of a such an inimical efficacy expectancy may intrude most disruptively in emotionally stressful situations where a choice must be made between two highly emotional and opposing alternatives. As the result of a history of excessively unpredictable and uncontrollable learning events, vulnerable dogs may be predisposed to respond to stressful situations in more arbitrary and rigid ways. Under the stress of conflict, such dogs may be affected by a global pessimism or *learned helplessness,* inclining them to expect that all possible responses available to them will be equally useless and ineffectual. When exposed to heightened stress and conflict, predisposed dogs (unable to act functionally and voluntarily) may be compelled to adopt compulsive behavior as a stress-reducing strategy.

Boredom

Another factor putatively implicated in the development of compulsive behavior in animals is boredom (see *Boredom* in Chapter 4). Except in extreme cases of social isolation or excessive confinement, appealing to boredom as a primary cause of compulsive behavior is difficult to defend. Many dogs are exposed daily to incalculable boredom, but few of them develop compulsive habits. Boredom is common, but compulsive disorders are relatively rare. Further, if boredom were a primary cause of compulsive behavior, one would expect that supplemental activities, exercise, and social contact should reverse or attenuate observed symptoms. Although environmental enhancements aimed at optimizing stimulation for dogs may be helpful, once compulsive habits have formed the provision of environmental enrichment alone is rarely sufficient to modify the behavior.

Attention Seeking

Compulsive habits may be reinforced by social attention (both negative and positive) obtained by a dog from either its owner or other persons with whom it comes into regular contact. Many whirlers and tail chasers can be prompted to perform the behavior by waving a finger around above their heads. While the stimulus itself may elicit an unconditioned whirling response in some dogs, such behavior may have been learned as a result of deliberate or inadvertent training. Some rather bizarre habits have been identified as operating under the influence of attention-seeking motivations. Hart (1980), for example, has reported an *attention-getting* motivation underlying a wide array of compulsive behaviors and psychosomatic conditions:

> Attention-getting behavior almost defies categorization. The behavior may appear as a major disorder such as lameness, paralysis of the rear legs, shadow chasing or hunting for imaginary objects. The behavior may involve autonomic response such as diarrhea, vomiting or asthmalike reactions. Mutilation of a leg or tail, or seizurelike disorders, may also be attention-getting. (99)

Unfortunately, the way attention-seeking behavior is usually interpreted involves considerable anthropomorphic contamination, and the concept needs a scientific definition. In general, the significance of attention seeking is probably related to active-submission behavior, rather than a calculated effort by the dog to obtain enhanced social contact and recognition. The presence of affection and fear underlying active-submission behavior together with social frustration provides a potential locus of significant conflict, perhaps sufficient to support compulsive behavior (see *Adjunctive Generation of Hyperactivity*, below). Chronic conflict between the owner and dog involving affection and fear offers an alternative interpretation of attention-seeking behavior based on an adjunctive generator analysis—an approach that may be more useful than the usual social reinforcement theory. Active-submission behavior and associated excesses (e.g., jumping up, vocalizing, pawing, licking, and various other active-approach and contact excesses) are often the objects of considerable control efforts—efforts that aim to thwart or suppress their expression. Thwarting active-submission behaviors may simultaneously increase social conflict as well as introduce significant frustration, thereby possibly facilitating compulsive behavior in susceptible dogs.

The adjunctive conflict analysis offers an alternative way to understand how such diverse problems as those identified by Hart could operate under the influence of an *attention-getting* motivation. Figure 5.4 shows a Border collie that presented with a compulsion to retreat under a desk whenever the

owner picked up the telephone. Once there, the dog shadow chases, barks, and snaps at nonexistent objects. Although clearly suggesting an attention-seeking etiology (the behavior occurs primarily in the presence of one family member), oddly the owner expressed concern about the dog's lack of affectionate display and closeness. In addition, the dog is highly reactive, fearful of novelty, and intolerant of unfamiliar social situations. Besides the aforementioned compulsions, the dog exhibits several other variants that regularly occur under the influence of a variety of social triggers. Apparently, such behavior is emitted in the presence of adverse or stressful circumstances as a coping or holding pattern. The Border collie's compulsive behavior is probably due to a genetic susceptibility, fostered and incubated under the influence of active-submission conflicts and persistent frustration resulting from its failure to achieve more satisfying social relations.

COMPULSIVE BEHAVIOR PROBLEMS

Licking, Sucking, and Kneading

A common compulsive habit observed in dogs is sucking and kneading of blankets. This behavior is highly correlated with removing a puppy from the mother too early in its development. In many cases, the sucking-and-kneading compulsion does not appear until after puppies reach puberty, sometimes not until after 1 year of age. Dogs exhibiting this habit rhythmically suck and knead on a blanket as though quietly nursing on it. Owners note that it most often occurs when dogs appear slightly stressed by environmental events or are bored. In most cases, the habit is not self-injurious and is left untreated, partly because it gives such dogs so much apparent pleasure. The habit is best controlled through prevention. Puppies taken from the mother prior to normal weaning times should be fed by a method as similar to natural nursing activity as possible. Levy (1941) suggests that the sucking compulsion may be driven by frustration. He carried out an experiment in which puppies were given adequate milk to satisfy their nutritional needs but not enough time feeding to satisfy their sucking needs.

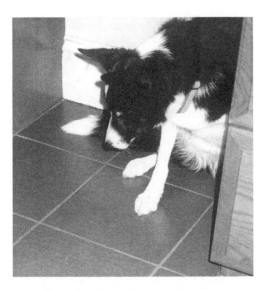

FIG. 5.4. This Border collie exhibits a variety of compulsive habits, especially lunging and snapping at shadows and at her reflections. Episodes are reliably elicited whenever the owner talks on the phone, at which time the dog runs under a desk and yelps, whines, barks, and lunges at shadows.

The control puppies, on the other hand, were given adequate milk to satisfy their hunger, as well as time to satisfy their sucking needs. In contrast to the satisfied group, the frustrated puppies exhibited increased sucking activity directed at nonnutritive objects (e.g., other puppies, their paws, and a variety of objects). In addition, as they matured, frustrated puppies engaged in excessive licking of their food plates.

Other compulsive oral habits commonly exhibited by dogs involve excessive licking directed toward the body, people, floor, or furniture. When dogs direct licking toward their extremities (usually the carpus or tarsus), this may cause physical effects ranging from minor alopecia (hair loss) and hyperplasia (thickening of the skin) to lick granulomas (Figure 5.5). Such problems usually involve both medical and behavioral causes and should be treated jointly by a veterinarian and a behavior counselor. Excessive self-directed licking is especially common among large breeds (e.g., Labrador retrievers, golden

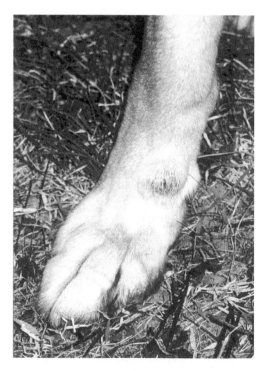

FIG. 5.5. This German shepherd exhibits a classic carpal granuloma resulting from compulsive licking.

retrievers, and Doberman pinschers). Licking directed toward furniture or flooring is usually less problematic, but occasionally dogs lick so much that they inflict minor abrasions and injuries to the lower jaw or lips.

Petra Mertens (1999) describes an unusual case involving a male 4-year-old miniature bullterrier. The dog, which the female owner characterized as being very oral and excessively interested in food, had developed a persistent habit of licking the arms and legs of her quadriplegic husband. One afternoon, the owner left the dog alone with her husband to find upon returning that the dog had erstwhile chewed off her husband's first toe and removed half of the second one. This rare example of allomutilation (from the Greek *allos* or "other") appears causally related to the dog's persistent tendency to lick the husband's skin, gradually resulting in gnawing, and, finding no inhibitory feedback limiting the extent of the oral behavior and its damage, resulted in the loss of the man's toes. This event underscores the importance of exercising caution when exposing persons who lack nociceptive sensitivity in their extremities to dogs with heightened oral interests. Dogs exposed to such individuals should be carefully supervised and receive inhibitory training to limit excessive licking behavior.

A key consideration in the treatment of compulsive behavior problems is the identification of social and environmental sources of stress and conflict. Excessive self-licking has been associated with socially conflicted situations, such as the introduction of a new animal (or person) into the household or separation-related distress. For some dogs, grooming and licking may be a way to cope with anxiety. Some compulsive licking habits appear to be under the influence of an attention- or comfort-seeking motivation. In such cases, licking may have been initially triggered by an actual traumatic event or injury, but, as the result of owner attention giving and comforting while licking, the licking behavior may have subsequently become a means to obtain attention from the owner. Finally, excessive crate confinement or neglect has been implicated in the development of grooming and licking excesses. For example, Hetts and colleagues found that isolated dogs tend to engage in more "bizzare movements" and distress vocalizations, and when confined to small cages they tend to exhibit more grooming activities (e.g., scratching, licking, and biting the skin). Finally, excessive licking is often associated with etiological factors other than psychogenic ones, including allergies, previous trauma, foreign bodies, infection, and arthritis (Veith, 1986). Such self-injurious licking habits often respond to medical treatment alone. Severe and refractory cases are sometimes treated with radiation therapy (Rivers et al., 1993). Once well established, ALD is rarely completely curable but is manageable through a variety of veterinary and behavioral interventions. In cases where psychogenic factors are also suspected to play a contributory role, systematic behavioral efforts should be introduced to prevent symptoms from reoccurring.

Locomotor Behavior

Many examples of locomotor compulsive behavior have been already discussed. The most common movement compulsions and stereotypies involve repetitive pacing, running fence lines, and other locomotor excesses. Under close confinement, dogs may develop persistent whirling habits. Other dogs may spend large amounts of time and energy unproductively pacing or charging up and down fence lines in a stereotypic manner or exhibit compulsions such as leaping up and down. Obviously, such dogs are motivated to move beyond the fence by the attraction of some external stimulation or desire to roam. The fence represents a conflict-laden barrier between what a dog would prefer to do and what it is constrained to do as the result of the surrounding fence, underscoring the role of frustration in the development of such problems. A compulsive factor appears to affect territorial aggression and fighting behavior occurring along fence lines (see *Variables Influencing Territorial Aggression* in Chapter 7). Similar conflict-generating conditions occur when dogs are restrained on leash. In this latter case, the dog is attracted by various impinging stimuli but prevented from acting on its impulses by the confinement of the leash. The result is compulsive investigatory and pulling behavior in spite of the dis-

comfort produced by the owner's frustrated yanking back. Dogs chained outdoors may develop compulsive digging or chewing habits, providing a substitute outlet for the frustration caused by such restraint. R. C. Hubrecht and colleagues (1992) found that dogs housed in small pens tend to develop stereotypic circling habits, behavior that is probably expressed as pacing when dogs are housed in larger pens. Finally, some forms of hyperactivity may be attributable to a compulsive etiology (see below).

Sympathy Lameness: Deceit or Compulsion?

When exposed to increased anxious arousal, dogs that have suffered injury to a limb or foot may display a pattern of limping or paw raising in the absence of actual injury or pain (Fox, 1962). The result is a compulsive reliance on the display of lameness in order to obtain *reward-sympathy* from the owner whenever the dog becomes distressed or anxious. Under conditions of emotional conflict, dogs may draw attention to themselves and gain relief by exhibiting *sympathy lameness*. To my knowledge, the first recorded case of sympathy lameness was reported by George Romanes (1888) in his interesting book *Animal Intelligence*. Romanes recounts the observations of a correspondent who had written to him about a peculiar behavior that gave credence (in his opinion) to the possibility that dogs can exhibit deceitfulness:

> He [a King Charles spaniel] showed the same deliberated design of deceiving on other occasions. Having hurt his foot he became lame for a time, during which he received more pity and attention than usual. For months after he had recovered, whenever he was harshly spoken to, he commenced hobbling about the room as if lame and suffering pain from his foot. He only gave up the practice when he gradually perceived that it was unsuccessful. (444)

Lorenz (1955) describes a similar case that he labeled a behavioral "swindle" (suggesting a similar interpretation to the one proposed by Romanes) involving feigned lameness exhibited by one of his dogs. The dog in question had suffered a severe strain with tendonitis that, consequently, required special attention and extended care. The dog recovered but apparently learned that limping produced sympathetic treatment from her owner. She subsequently developed a selective lameness whenever it was in her interest to do so:

> If I cycled from my quarters to the military hospital, where she might have to remain on guard by my bicycle for hours on end, she limped so pitifully that people in the road often reproached me. But if we took the direction of the army riding school, where a cross-country ride was likely to ensue, the pain had gone. The swindle was most transparent on Saturdays. In the morning, on the way to duty, the poor dog was so lame that she could scarcely hobble behind the bicycle, but in the afternoon, when we covered the thirteen miles to the Ketcher See at a good speed, she did not run behind the bicycle but raced ahead of it at a gallop, along the paths which she knew so well. And on Monday she limped again. (181)

From the foregoing anecdotes, it would appear that sympathy lameness is acquired as the result of increased attention given to a dog following a limb injury, with the dog learning to feign discomfort to get attention and affection from its owner (Hart and Hart, 1985), but another possible interpretation is that such behavior may stem from active-submission behavior and conflict (see above), resulting from increased petting and contact between the owner and dog following the injury. Whatever the case, sympathy lameness is a rather uncommon phenomenon, and before attributing an attention-seeking causation to the behavior, it should receive a careful veterinary evaluation. Differential diagnosis should exclude other more common and likely physical causes underlying signs of lameness. Limping should always be interpreted first in terms of a potential physical ailment and, only after such efforts fail to turn up a cause, should the possibility of sympathy lameness be seriously considered. If it is clear that the signs of lameness appear only under emotionally stressful situations, then *maybe* sympathy lameness is occurring rather than a strain, growth pains, or some other physical causation (e.g., Lyme disease).

Assessment and Evaluation

The first step in evaluating dogs with compulsive habits is to obtain relevant information, including a medical history. It is crucial for the consulting trainer to get a detailed picture of the dog's behavior, along with a thorough inventory of the various eliciting stimuli and contexts in which the behavior has occurred in the past, prevailing motivational conditions under which the behavior tends to occur, and the approximate frequency and duration of the behavior's occurrence. Additionally, the owner should be questioned with regard to previous methods used to control the dog's behavior, including both successful and unsuccessful ones. In severe cases involving acute onset, automutilation (self-injury), or seizure activity, the client should be referred to a veterinarian for a medical evaluation.

In many cases, finding a correlation between a compulsive behavior and a specific precipitating stimulus or environmental condition is not possible. In such dogs, a compulsive habit may be under the stimulus control of an internal cue and emitted to modulate a generalized state of frustration or anxious arousal. When such causes are suspected, steps should be taken to reduce adverse emotional arousal. Quality-of-life enhancements that often prove beneficial in reducing stress include increased daily exercise, play and training activities, and daily massage. In cases where a hunger tension is implicated, a dog's feeding can be adjusted by either increasing food intake or increasing the frequency of feedings. Some dogs are benefited by an ad libitum feeding schedule in which they are permitted to eat whenever they wish. Of course, not all dogs can be fed ad libitum without gaining weight, but many dogs can be fed in such a way without experiencing much, if any, significant weight gain. In those dogs where ad libitum feeding is inappropriate, the frequency of measured feedings can be increased during the day.

Compulsive behavior often occurs under the influence of excessive anxiety or frustration elicited by some external stimulus or situation. The most effective training method for managing CBDs involves a combination of graduated exposure, counterconditioning, and response-prevention procedures. For example, when the CBD is either precipitated or augmented by the presence of the owner or some other specific stimulus, it is often useful to gradually expose the dog to the eliciting stimulus while at the same time blocking the repetitive activity or by eliciting incompatible emotional responding (e.g., relaxation or appetence). In the case of intractable or refractory compulsions involving self-injury (e.g., ALD), aversive counterconditioning and punishment procedures may be effective (Eckstein and Hart, 1996). (Specific treatment recommendations for the control and management of CBDs is deferred for discussion in a forthcoming volume.)

PREVENTION

The etiology of compulsive behavior is only partially understood. Many dogs exhibiting locomotor compulsions exhibit general hyperactivity and impulse-control problems. Dogs with licking compulsions often exhibit anxious attachments toward their owners, may have suffered the loss of a significant other (animal or human), may be stressed by social competition or rivalry (perhaps involving the introduction of a new pet or baby), or may have undergone long-term neglect and social deprivation.

Compulsive behavior is commonly seen in dogs that exhibit signs of chronic stress, excitability, and insecurity. Such dogs can be provided with a sense of security and well-being by establishing strong leadership and making significant events predictable and controllable. Owners of such dogs should not neglect to establish definite boundaries and enforce them when necessary but should be careful to avoid highly charged emotional interaction triggering chronic fright-flight-fight conflicts. Other sensible precautions and suggestions include

1. Provide the dog with choices during stressful and conflict dense situations.
2. Interact with the dog in predictable, consistent ways, giving the dog a degree of control over what happens to it.
3. When discipline needs to be administered, make certain that appropriate alternative behaviors are prompted and reinforced.

4. Establish a daily regimen of obedience training based on positive reinforcement and play.
5. During training activities, emphasize clear communication and mutual understanding—not simply exercising one-sided control and dominance.
6. Make the dog feel secure in its social relationships by providing adequate daily affection and attention.

Finally, a dog's confidence is enhanced by providing it with structured training and socialization activities from an early age. Such treatment facilitates the development of behavioral optimism, causing the dog to believe that success is always possible, thus effectively immunizing it against acquired learning disabilities (negative cognitive set) and related compulsive habits.

PART 2: HYPERACTIVITY

HYPERACTIVITY VERSUS HYPERKINESIS

Excessively active dogs presenting with signs of impulse-control problems and other relevant symptoms (e.g., attention deficits, inability to calm down, persistent reactivity to restraint and confinement, aggressiveness, impaired learning abilities, and insensitivity to punishment) should be evaluated for hyperactivity and possible hyperkinesis syndrome. Dogs exhibiting hyperactivity (especially in those cases presenting with emotional instability, impulsivity, and aggressiveness) may be candidates for treatment with a central nervous system (CNS) stimulant (e.g., methylphenidate) and should be referred for a veterinary evaluation. Increased excitability and hyperactivity may be associated with various disease conditions (e.g., hyperthyroidism) that should be considered as part of a differential diagnosis performed by a veterinarian. In the discussion that follows, I have opted to use the term *hyperactivity* to designate the common form of excessive activity and attention deficits that occur in dogs without physiological concomitants. The term *hyperkinesis* is here reserved for those cases of hyperactivity and attention-impulse deficits that respond to stimulant medication.

SIGNS AND INCIDENCE

Impulse Control and Attention Deficits

Hyperactivity and attention deficits are frequently exhibited by puppies and adolescent dogs presented for behavioral training. These problems are widely distributed among dog breeds but are especially prevalent among hunting and working breeds—dogs selectively bred for enhanced environmental alertness, vigilance, and high activity levels. Affected dogs frequently exhibit an abnormally short attention span and impulsiveness. This attention impairment makes them unable to concentrate on any one thing or task for long before being distracted by something else. Some dogs appear as though everything encountered by them, no matter how trifling or insignificant, is treated with an equally active and fleeting interest. Hyperactive dogs are especially sensitive and reactive to novelty or the presence of unfamiliar persons or animals, often displaying a pronounced inability to habituate to such stimulation. Such dogs appear to be strongly influenced by a diffuse incentive or seeking mechanism that is activated by novelty, with resulting hyperarousal, exploratory and olfactory activity, and exploration-related problems (e.g., destructiveness). Consequently, such dogs may exhibit persistent restlessness and disorganized activity in search of rewarding stimulation. Frustrated owners often complain that their dog "can't sit still" or that it "gets into everything."

Reward, Inhibition, and Delay of Gratification

Another important behavioral manifestation exhibited by hyperactive dogs is their resistance to inhibitory training and physical control. Hyperactive dogs appear to be much less sensitive to aversive stimulation and punishment than are average dogs. Further, they often become even more excitable and unmanageable when efforts are made to constrain them forcefully. On the other hand, they are often very responsive to reward training, but rewards, if they are to work, must be given on a near-continuous basis in order to secure their wavering and easily distracted attention (Sagvolden et al., 1993). If reinforcement is scheduled intermittently or made contingent on the performance of a chain of intervening responses, hyperactive dogs may rapidly lose interest. The impulsive character of hyperactivity is reflected in the affected dog's inability to wait or to delay gratification. Although hyperactive dogs may attend and work well under conditions of continuous reinforcement, they exhibit clear deficits when it comes to situations requiring a long delay before reinforcement is delivered (e.g., a long sit-stay). This pattern is also evident among children with attention-deficit hyperactivity disorder (ADHD) who are easily distracted from deferred goals by the offer of more immediate but smaller rewards. To investigate the role of delay of reinforcement Sagvolden and colleagues (1992) performed a series of experiments with hyperactive rats. They confirmed the rat's preference for short-term reinforcers and the existence of deficits involving delay of reinforcement when compared to normal controls. In addition, they observed that CNS stimulants improved the effectiveness of delayed reinforcers for controlling repetitive operant tasks while simultaneously reducing the distractive strength of immediate reinforcers. These findings are consistent with the observed positive effects of CNS stimulants on impulse control and delay of gratification behavior in both hyperactive children and dogs.

Besides exhibiting a high degree of distractibility, impulsiveness, and various learning deficits, hyperactive dogs are impulsive and often emotionally unstable, possessing a low tolerance for frustration and sometimes exhibiting uncontrollable ragelike aggressive behavior. Parallel symptoms in child psychopathology have been identified and described (Hinshaw, 1994; Werry, 1994).

A biological factor certainly plays some role in the etiology of hyperactivity, but many social and environmental factors also contribute to its expression. Family dogs are especially vulnerable and prone to develop hyperactive behavior as the result of exposure to overly active and playful children. Additionally, hyperactive *play* may develop as an inadvertent result of ineffectual punishment. Although an owner may be quite sincere, the action taken is often attenuated as the result of affection for the dog or personal inhibitions about such interaction. A dog may misinterpret this self-restraint and *kindness* as an awkward human invitation to play rather than punishment. Active dogs play hard and, while playing, frequently exhibit subdued agonistic challenges and threats that may be ethologically analogous to the owner's ineffectual punitive efforts. Such play is often so intense that it may be confused with real aggression (Voith, 1980a,b).

ETIOLOGY

Social and Sensory Deprivation

Waller and Fuller (1961) found that puppies reared under conditions of semi-isolation exhibited excessive compensatory efforts to initiate social contact when permitted to do so. When the puppies were kept with littermates continuously, the number of social contacts was reduced by 75%. These observations suggest that dogs may possess a biological *need* for some relatively fixed amount of daily sensory stimulation, motor activity, and social contact. If these requirements are not met, then various compensatory and excessive efforts may be emitted by dogs to secure them. Clearly, there exists a great deal of individual variability from dog to dog with respect to their specific needs. Just as hypothalamic set points control many basic biological drives like hunger and thirst, it is reasonable to hypothesize that general arousal and activity may be controlled by a similar subcortical homeostatic mechanism (Fox, 1974). According to this theory, dogs are motivationally and behaviorally activated to secure stasis through compensatory and excessive behavior when environmental conditions prevent them from obtaining optimal stimulation or vital resources needed to sustain them.

Hyperactive dogs are often exposed to routine isolation due to their behavioral excesses. This points to another set of contributing factors underlying hyperactivity: inadequate social attention, insufficient or irregular exercise, and excessive confinement. Active dogs subjected to daily crate confinement tend to become increasingly hyperactive and solicitous of attention. When released from confinement, the demands made by such dogs are anything but welcome by family members, who may have all but entirely rejected them as a result of their behavioral excesses. The situation is a vicious circle, with excessive behavior resulting in further rejection and isolation, thereby generating more attention-seeking behavior and hyperactivity. Also, excessive or noncontingent (uncontrollable punishment) may contribute to the development of hyperactive attention-deficit symptoms. A result of such treatment is diffuse vigilance and disorganized responding, especially after startling stimulation or at times associated with a history of unpredictable and uncontrollable punishment.

Adjunctive Generation of Hyperactivity

Attention-seeking and active-submission behavior appear to play a significant role in both hyperactivity and compulsive behavior, perhaps stemming from strong adjunctive-generator influences localizing in affection-fear conflict. As previously discussed, Falk suggests that excessive behavior is likely to result under the influence of conflict-laden *marginal* intermittent reinforcement (see *Schedule-induced Excessive Behavior,* above). It should be noted that both rich and lean schedules of reinforcement are relatively immune to conflict and the adjunctive generation of excessive behavior. In the case of rich reinforcement schedules, conflict is avoided, since consummatory behavior is ascendant, whereas, in the case of lean schedules, conflict is avoided because escape behavior dominates, causing the animal withdraw from the situation. Under the influence of *marginal* intermittent reinforcement, a *conflict* may localize between a consummatory vector and an escape vector of equal strength. Compulsive habits or hyperactivity may result in cases in which marginal intermittent reinforcement occurs chronically. Attention-seeking behavior, for example, may succeed often enough to maintain a dog's effort but not enough to offset an opposing motivational vector to give up trying (escape)—an unlikely outcome, in any case, for a highly dependent and sociable dog.

Active-submission behavior (i.e., attention seeking) may itself become a compulsive activity in its own right. A conflict between affection and fear is embedded in submission behavior; that is, submissive dogs are simultaneously attracted to and repelled by the object of submission. *Affection keeps a dog in close contact with its owner, preventing the dog from resolving the conflict by running away, but fear prevents the dog from relaxing and fully enjoying the contact. As a result, contact comfort and reassurance may not satisfy a submissive dog, at least, not as long as it is engaged in active submission.* These observations may help to explain why some attention-seeking dogs are so insatiable, never seeming to get enough affection or contact comfort:

> Attention-getting behavior is found in the typical household situation in which the dog is already heavily indulged with love and petting. While it may seem illogical, dogs that are getting the most attention are those that will go to some effort to gain even more. It is probably impossible to satiate a dog with too much attention. Dogs that receive little attention from their owners have the least probability of acquiring this behavioral problem. (Hart and Hart, 1985:85)

Such dogs may engage in persistent licking, pawing, and other proximity-enhancing active-submission behaviors. This situation is very different from other drives, like thirst or hunger, that can be easily quieted by the consumption of food or water. For compulsive attention seekers, the consumption of social contact tends to generate more preparatory arousal (affection-fear conflict), resulting in more attention seeking but failing to quiet the escalating need for comfort and reassurance. Because of its motivational character, compulsive submission behavior is capable of generating high levels of anxiety. Because such dogs are often unsuccessful in their general social efforts, anxiety is joined by frustration to coactively increase activity levels and generate maladaptive and excessive behavior.

As a result, attention-seeking dogs may engage in a variety of adjunctive behaviors, such as destructiveness and hyperactivity. Treating such cases involves either (1) modifying generator conditions (alter the schedule of attention giving) or (2) directing the destructive or hyperactive behavior into more appropriate outlets. Although attention-seeking behavior may occur in close association with a variety of behavior problems, such behavior is probably not emitted as a means to obtain attention per se but as the adjunctive expression of marginal social reinforcement.

Neural and Physiological Substrates

During various classical conditioning studies involving the induction of stress by means of unavoidable aversive stimulation (shock), Corson and coworkers (1973) found that a small percentage of dogs were unable to relax while restrained in an experimental harness. Some of the dogs became so aroused and reactive that they attacked the harness and nearby equipment. These highly reactive dogs exhibited no signs of improvement over several training sessions. Hypothesizing that the symptoms were similar to those exhibited by hyperactive children, the researchers experimented with various CNS stimulants used to control hyperactivity in children. Children affected with ADHD respond *paradoxically* to CNS stimulants. Instead of causing them to become more active and excitable, as one might expect, the stimulants often cause them to become more calm and focused. They found that hyperkinetic dogs responded to amphetamines in a similar way, becoming less active, more focused, and even more affectionate.

Subsequent studies have confirmed many of Corson's original findings. Bareggi and coworkers (1979) have speculated that D-amphetamine enhances the activity of the neurotransmitters dopamine (DA) and norepinephrine (NE). At low doses, dopaminergic systems are activated whereas, at higher doses, both dopaminergic and noradrenergic systems are stimulated. Since high levels of amphetamine are required to generate the paradoxical effect, they reason that both catecholamine systems are probably involved. Recent studies with hyperactive rats and mice show that the differential response of animals to CSN stimulants is present in rodents. As a result, several new animal models of ADHD have been proposed. These models range from hyperactivity exhibited by "spontaneously hypertensive rats" to hyperactivity induced via chemical lesions of the rat brain. In one of these studies hyperactivity in rats was induced by destroying dopamine fibers with neurotoxins

(Kostrzewa et al., 1994). The lesioned rats responded in the typical manner to amphetamine treatment, thereby raising questions about the role of dopamine in the mediation of the paradoxical effects of CNS stimulants. These findings led the researchers to conclude that, in addition to dopaminergic activity, a serotonergic system is also involved:

> DA and 5-HT neurotransmission may mutually modulate spontaneous locomotor activity in rats and inhibit hyperactivity in humans. Either impaired ontogeny or injury of DA fibers, coupled with subsequent impaired ontogeny or injury of 5-HT fibers, may constitute the underlying basis of hyperactivity in ADHD. The effectiveness of amphetamine in controlling hyperactivity in ADHD is similarly thought to be due to the release of 5-HT, either directly or via action of released DA at 5-HT neurons. The implication is that 5-HT agonists, probably of the 5-HT$_{2C}$ class, could prove to useful in treating ADHD. Likewise, if amphetamine is not acting directly on 5-HT neurons, but via DA release, then direct-acting DA agonists could also become useful in treating ADHD. (165–166)

These findings support the *minimal brain dysfunction* theory of ADHD. Important neuroimaging studies of the frontal lobes and basal ganglia also suggest the possibility of an organic etiology underlying hyperkinesis and ADHD.

More recently, ADHD research has explored the possible role of defects in the DA reuptake mechanism, particularly involving DA-transporter molecules located on the plasma membrane of DA neurons. DA transporters mediate the reuptake and conservation of extracellular DA by absorbing and concentrating it within the cytoplasm for later use. Disturbances of transporter activity may cause a higher-than-normal concentration of DA to remain in extracellular fluids, thereby causing increased motor activity, stereotypies, impulsivity, and cognitive deficits. Research with *knockout* (KO) mice (mutants lacking the specific gene responsible for encoding the DA transporter) have revealed a number of interesting findings with respect to the differential roles of DA, hydroxytryptamine (5-HT or serotonin), and NE systems in the expression of hyperkinetic symptoms (Gainetdinov et al.,

1999). KO mice have five times as much DA concentrated in extracellular fluids than do normal mice. As a result, KO mice exhibit significantly higher levels of motor activity and show profoundly impaired cognitive abilities. Psychostimulants (e.g., dextroamphetamine and methylphenidate) were found to exert a significant attenuation of hyperkinetic symptoms in KO mice—effects that cannot be attributed to changes in DA-transporter activity. In addition to the aforementioned stimulant medications, the selective 5-HT reuptake inhibitor fluoxetine was found to attenuate hyperactivity significantly in KO mice but had no discernible effect on normal mice. Finally, the investigators selectively activated and inhibited NE transporters, thereby demonstrating that NE plays no significant role in the expression of hyperkinetic symptoms. In addition to the attenuating effects of fluoxetine, they found that treatment with 5-HT precursors [L-tryptophan and 5-hydroxytryptophan (5-HTP)] significantly reduced motor activity and stereotypic behavior in KO mice. Gainetdinov and colleagues conclude that the stimulants commonly used to treat ADHD probably produce therapeutic effects on downstream serotonin transporters rather than directly affecting DA receptors or transporters.

Kenneth Blum and colleagues (1997) at the University of Texas (San Antonio) have reported compelling evidence suggesting that ADHD, as well as a variety of other common impulse problems and conduct disorders (including aggressive behavior), may develop from an inability to obtain sufficient reward by engaging in everyday activities. This condition, referred to as *reward deficiency syndrome* (RDS), is believed to be a genetic aberration affecting dopamine reward pathways, in particular dopamine D2 receptors. In cooperation with several other neurotransmitters [e.g., serotonin, opioids, and γ-aminobutyric acid (GABA)], dopamine plays a central role in the mediation of reward and the experience of well-being. Blum's research group identified a gene variant (A1 allele) that appears to constrain the expression of D2 receptors on the dopamine neuron by 30%. They found that individuals possessing the A1 allele (especially those who are homozygous for it) are at a significantly greater risk of developing a variety of problem behaviors and appetites [see Singh et al. (1994)], including self-medication (addictions and excessive eating) and dysfunctional behavioral strategies (impulsive and compulsive tendencies), all apparently aimed at achieving improved reward satisfaction.

In the case of dogs, it might be likewise expected that failure to experience reward or well-being as the result of everyday social contact and activity may stimulate affected individuals to engage in impulsive-compulsive behavior and inappropriate appetitive gratification, such as increased attention seeking and pica. The inability of such dogs to achieve internal reward or satisfaction may prompt them to engage in excessive behavior (hyperactivity) seeking sufficient reward. Such a dysfunctional reward mechanism may help to explain why efforts to satisfy affected dogs with attention, exercise, and affection (or food) do not appear to reduce substantially their apparent need for such things. Dogs suffering from RDS may fail to experience social contact as a reward in a consummatory sense, but instead experience it as an incentive or prod to seek more attention or activity. Such dogs may never gain true satisfaction from social interaction because the neural substrates mediating the social reward cascade are not functioning at an optimal level. This is consistent with the observations of Sagvolden and coworkers (1993), who found that hyperactivity was reduced in genetically hyperkinetic rats when they received more frequent reinforcement.

The putative influences exerted by genes regulating the dopamine transporter system on ADHD as reported by Gainetdinov and coworkers seem to conflict with the receptor diminishment hypothesis of Blum and colleagues, suggesting that more research is necessary to uncover the neurobiological substrates controlling the expression of hyperkinesis and related impulsive and compulsive tendencies in dogs. Clearly, though, the dopamine limbic circuits appear to play a significant role in the development of excessive behavior. Interestingly, in this regard, Niimi and associates (1999) at Gifu University, Japan, have reported significant differences in genetic variants controlling the expression of dopamine D4 receptors in golden retrievers and Shibas. The D4 receptor is believed to be involved in

novelty seeking and other behavioral tendencies depending on the allele (short or long) expressed (Ebstein et al., 1996). In humans, the long allele is not only associated with novelty seeking, but also various personality dimensions, such as compulsiveness, excitability, quick temper, and fickleness, whereas the shorter allele is most often associated with reduced novelty seeking and an opposite set of personality characteristics (e.g., reflective, slow to anger, stoicism). Niimi's group found that the golden retriever was most likely to possess the short A allele (78.9%), whereas the long D allele was most common in the Shiba (46.7%). The D4 receptor is primarily found in the limbic system and expressed in neurons exerting direct effects upon cognition and emotional behavior. These findings support the view that the limbic dopamine system plays an instrumental role in the expression of canine behavioral traits.

Although the neural sites and pathways involved in the expression of hyperactivity (ADHD) are not definitively known, various neuroimaging studies suggest that the caudate nucleus and the striatum (basal ganglia) are involved to some extent (Hynd and Hooper, 1992). Both of these sites project to frontal lobe areas involved in the regulation of locomotor activity and impulse control. Studies with children exhibiting ADHD indicate that both the caudate nucleus and the striatum show low metabolic activity and blood flow— a condition that is ameliorated by the administration of methylphenidate and reversed as the drug wears off. Another distinguishing neuroanatomic feature of childhood ADHD is the finding that affected children do not exhibit the typical frontal lobe asymmetry (right > left) of normal children but instead tend to exhibit symmetrical (right = left) frontal lobe widths. Further, it has been found that hyperactive children have significantly narrower right frontal lobe widths than children not exhibiting ADHD (Hynd and Hooper, 1992).

Relevant studies were performed by Sechzer (1977) on split-brain kittens. The split-brain preparation involves surgically severing the corpus callosum (a large structure of interconnecting fibers communicating between the right and left hemispheres) and the striatal pathways connecting the right and left caudate nuclei. Split-brain kittens exhibited a constant, poorly focused hyperactivity not seen in normal kittens. At 6 months of age, kittens were injected with D-amphetamine and observed for behavioral changes. Striking reductions in general activity levels and distractibility were immediately seen, but hyperactive symptoms returned within 2 hours after the injection. At 1 year of age, normal and split-brain cats were compared in terms of their respective abilities to learn a simple discrimination task. As observed in hyperkinetic dogs, split-brain cats only very slowly habituated to the training environment, made frequent attempts to escape, and exhibited a high degree of distraction toward external noises. The results of discrimination training showed that split-brain cats were consistently slower than normal cats at learning the task. However, when split-brain cats were medicated with D-amphetamine, they learned the task slightly more rapidly than normal counterparts.

CNS-STIMULANT-RESPONSE TEST

Some authors have recommended a stringent diagnostic procedure for determining a dog's candidacy for stimulant therapy. The stimulant-response test is administered by challenging the dog with a dose of D-amphetamine and observing various physiological parameters (Luescher, 1993a). The dog's general activity level, demeanor, and various physiological parameters are observed. Hyperkinetic dogs respond to CNS stimulants paradoxically; that is, they calm down and become more focused. The stimulant-response test is performed by taking a baseline measurement of a dog's activity level, reaction to restraint (holding the dog in sit or down position), heart rate, and respiration rate, and (more rarely) salivary and urinary output are measured. Following an oral dosage of D-amphetamine, hyperkinetic dogs will tend to calm down, accept restraint more readily, and exhibit a generalized decrease in the aforementioned physiological measures (Voith, 1979). These effects usually take place within 2 hours—sometimes within 30 minutes after dosing a dog. Dogs that do not respond may

require a higher challenge dose. Voith (1980c) describes a method whereby the dose is increased by small amounts every 24 hours until the dog either becomes more active or begins to calm down. Dogs that respond by becoming more active and uncontrollable are not candidates for stimulant therapy. Although a real diagnostic entity, and perhaps underdiagnosed, true hyperkinetic syndrome probably does not occur at the frequency suggested by Campbell (1973, 1992), who claims that 75% of "hyperreactive" dogs given the stimulant-response test show positive results.

A study with hyperactive rats selected from a natural population offers an additional diagnostic dimension for evaluating hyperkinesis with attention deficits. Kohlert and Bloch (1993) observed that rats (not specifically bred for hyperactivity) frequently exhibited signs of hyperactivity similar to those presenting with ADHD. They found that a subpopulation of hyperkinetic rats can be easily isolated through a simple screening process involving three criteria: (1) presence of hyperactivity, (2) positive attenuation of activity levels in response to amphetamine, and (3) decreased ability to attend selectively to relevant stimuli during avoidance training. The study included an interesting test procedure for quantifying a subject's relative ability to attend selectively, that is, to pay attention to relevant cues while ignoring irrelevant ones. Disturbances of selective attention are frequently implicated in the diagnosis of hyperkinesis, but, unfortunately, objective criteria for its assessment have not been devised for dogs.

DIETARY FACTORS AND HYPERACTIVITY

Several studies have investigated the possible role of food additives and colorants in the development of ADHD in children. Most of this research has been unable to find a convincing causative link between ADHD and the various agents studied (Weiss, 1991). Likewise, among dogs, no scientific evidence exists to date supporting the popular belief that additives and colorants cause hyperactivity and other behavior problems. A study performed by Barcus and coworkers (1980) failed to show a causal linkage between FD&C red dye 40 or butylated hydroxyanisole (BHA)—substances suspected (but not proven) to play a role in the etiology of childhood ADHD—and hyperkinesis in Telomian hybrid dogs. Although the study failed show a direct linkage between red dye 40 and BHA in the development of hyperactivity, it should be noted that during a 28-day additive-free transition period all dogs exhibited a sharp decrease in hyperactive symptoms. Recent studies involving children have also discounted the role of excessive amounts of sugar and development of hyperactivity (Hynd and Hooper, 1992). However, studies with rats suggest that increased levels of dietary carbohydrates (including sugar) relative to decreasing protein intake results in the expression of higher activity levels (Spring, 1986).

Another potential source of hyperactivity in dogs is chronic lead poisoning. Two common sources of such poisoning are destructive chewing on linoleum or surfaces painted with lead-based paints. Silbergeld and Goldberg (1974) induced hyperkinetic symptoms in mice by exposing them to lead. The hyperkinetic symptoms were palliated with high doses of D-amphetamine. A large study performed by Thomson and colleagues (1989) found a positive correlation between lead blood levels and aggressive-hyperactive tendencies in children. Puppies exposed to lead should be tested and appropriately treated.

Inadequate nutrition may permanently affect general activity levels, especially when deprivation occurs early in life. Michaelson and coworkers (1977) found that hyperkinetic symptoms could be induced by manipulating dietary intake during a critical period for brain growth in mice. Mice were divided into two groups: group-I mice were raised in large litters in which 16 young were placed with a single mother (starved). Group-II mice were raised in small litters of 8 animals per nursing mother (controls). At 35 days of age, the two groups of mice were compared with regard to general activity levels and their response to D-amphetamine. Following a brief period of adaptation, starved rats exhibited a higher level of activity when compared with well-nourished controls. Upon administration of D-amphetamine, the starved rats became less active than the controls, a trajectory of

decreasing activity that continued to develop into the following hour after medication. Growth-retarded mice exhibited a strong paradoxical effect to D-amphetamine. These observations emphasize the importance of good nutrition during early growth periods in puppies. Breeders should be especially careful in their management of puppies belonging to large litters or those being nursed by a mother unable to produce sufficient nutrition through lactation alone. Further, the mother's dietary intake should be carefully evaluated and adjusted to meet the demands of nursing her litter.

TWO CASE HISTORIES

Jackson

A collateral discovery made by Corson and colleagues (1973) was the pronounced effectiveness of D-amphetamine for the control of aggressive behavior. A cocker spaniel-beagle mix named Jackson, described as being "incurably" vicious toward other dogs and people, responded dramatically to medication with D-amphetamine. Tranquilizers like chlorpromazine and meprobamate did not reduce the dog's aggressive behavior; however, an oral dose of D-amphetamine "within a period of 1 hr dramatically transformed the incorrigible, vicious, antisocial warrior into a peaceful, cooperative, lovable dog" (687). These effects lasted for up to 7 hours. An initially exciting aspect of CNS-stimulant therapy of hyperkinesis-related aggression was the finding that, after 6 weeks of drug and "psychosocial" therapy, the previously uncontrollable aggressive behavior largely disappeared and remained in remission even once the drug was withdrawn. Corson noted that no tolerance to the drug was observed during the treatment period. These early hopeful prospects have not been borne out by subsequent clinical experience, however.

Barney

In an anecdotal report, Jenny Drastura (1992) describes her personal experiences with a hyperkinetic male Lhasa apso named Barney that had developed a serious aggression problem. Even as a puppy, Barney exhibited incipient signs of a developing aggression problem. He resented being rolled onto his side and resisted various other forms of restraint and grooming. By the time he was 16 weeks of age, he began snapping during routine disciplinary interaction—discipline that involved verbal reprimands only. Barney proved recalcitrant to formal obedience training, biting his owners on three separate occasions while being trained. He was subsequently exposed to a more positive training process, employing food reinforcement and other rewarding activities in exchange for cooperation. Under the influence of such training, Barney proved much more compliant, but his aggressiveness continued to worsen. By the time he was 2 years old, it had become a serious behavior problem:

> Not only did he growl and snarl when challenged on his own turf, he was also beginning to go into a "ragelike" state any time he perceived that he was being threatened. In his rage state, he would withdraw into himself, growling and snarling, actually appearing to become smaller. His growling turned into screeching noises, his eyes appeared red as blood filled the blood vessels in his eyes and his gums turned white. Finally he reached a stage where he could not withdraw any further, and he attacked any object directly in front of him at about a 12 inch range. He appeared to have no peripheral vision. Oddly enough, this rage ended instantly if we yelled "cookie" or "cheese." His body relaxed and he immediately began jumping or dancing for whatever we had promised. It appeared that he had no idea what had just happened to him. (20)

As Barney's condition deteriorated, the owners contacted Victoria Voith for suggestions and guidance. Voith treated Barney with a combination of behavior modification and a panel of psychotropic drugs in an effort to control his ragelike aggressive symptoms. After a series of false starts and dead ends, it was found that Barney's aggressive symptoms were relieved by D-amphetamines. Barney was prescribed D-amphetamine to be taken twice a day. He responded to the medication by becoming more affectionate, more playful, and much less aggressive. The results were strikingly consistent with those described by Corson and coworkers in the case of Jackson.

Two significant divergences occurred between Corson's findings and the behavior of Barney regulated by D-amphetamine: (1) When Barney was taken off medication, his aggressive behavior returned. In Jackson's case, Corson observed a radically different therapeutic course. Instead of recovering after medication was discontinued, aggressive behavior remained quiescent. (2) Corson reported that dogs treated with D-amphetamine did not develop a tolerance to the drug. Barney did develop a tolerance to the drug (albeit after 3 years of treatment). He also exhibited a clear dependency on it. For instance, when he was periodically taken off the stimulant or when the drug simply wore off, he would become even more aggressive than he had been before treatment with the medication. Such heightened aggressiveness may have been the result of a combination of withdrawal symptoms and various neurological side effects of long-term D-amphetamine therapy. It should be noted that Barney exhibited other signs of neurological deterioration, including the development of various repetitive stereotypic behaviors (e.g., chomping with nothing in his mouth) and episodes of bizarre and inexplicable barking episodes.

COGNITIVE INTERPRETATIONS AND SPECULATION

Hyperactive dogs appear to be unable to modulate sensory input and to coordinate it with an integrated behavioral output. As the result of such cognitive impairment, a dog may attempt to keep pace and adjust to the changing environment by speeding up its behavior, increasing vigilance, or by intensifying its behavioral efforts to control fleeting events. Viewed from the perspective of a *minimal brain dysfunction,* the observed symptoms of hyperactivity are really the dog's best efforts to establish control over the slippery and transient stimulus events impinging on it.

Stimulus events reaching the attention of such dogs appear to compete for equal and undivided attention, suggesting a failure of cognitive functions dedicated to selectively collecting and processing sensory data and transforming it into information. Under normal conditions, a complex neural *gating* and comparator system serves to separate relevant from irrelevant sensory input, thus enabling dogs to match their behavior to changing circumstances. Sensory input is conditioned by at least three basic stimulus and contextual dimensions: (1) stimulus sequencing, (2) event boundaries and frames, and (3) figure/ground relationships. In the case of an inadequacy involving stimulus sequencing, dogs may not be able to sufficiently order events along a temporal dimension from which to derive causally meaningful relationships between them. In other cases, a dog may not be able to determine where one stimulus event begins and where another ends. In this case, the stimulus event is inadequately bounded and framed for cognitive representation and, therefore, insufficiently distinct to hold the dog's attention. Lastly, a dog may not be able to place stimulus events (although temporally well ordered and defined) into a spatial context in which they can be perceived as distinct and separate events set against a contextual backdrop. In this case, the event is obscured by competing and irrelevant background information. Of course, all of this is highly speculative but does provide a tentative framework for evaluating possible cognitive-perceptual impairments in hyperactive dogs.

An apparent exaggerated need for novelty and variety is a characteristic feature of many hyperactive dogs. They may be affected by an intolerance for boredom. In fact, some evidence suggests that hyperactive animals may actually be more intolerant of repetitive demands than are normal ones (Mook et al., 1993). Under experimental conditions where behavioral variability is rewarded, hyperactive rats may excel over normal controls. However, in situations requiring repeated performance of a similar response, hyperactive rats show clear signs of a disadvantage or learning deficit. On the positive side, these findings seem to imply that hyperactive animals are better adapted to situations requiring *creative* solutions. Perhaps an evolutionary pressure exists that alternately favors both general styles of learning, depending on changing demands placed on an animal by the environment. In times of change and crisis, a *creative* animal (greater behavior variability) would enjoy a distinct biological and adaptive advan-

tage over its more routine-oriented counterpart. These general findings suggest that hyperkinesis may serve a legitimate and important behavior-diversifying function. This line of reasoning leads to a novel appreciation of the biological and cultural significance of ADHD in children and hyperkinesis in dogs.

BEHAVIORAL SIDE EFFECTS OF HYPERACTIVITY

Many comorbid complications and long-term side effects frequently develop in the wake of hyperactivity. Affected dogs are often so behaviorally disorganized that normal developmental processes are adversely impacted. A striking characteristic of most hyperactive dogs is their immaturity. Because hyperactive dogs find it difficult to control their impulses, they are subjected to a high degree of frustration and other emotional tensions. It is interesting to note in this respect that hyperactivity is often most exaggerated during social encounters where such excesses result in a great deal of interactive punishment, disapproval, and rejection. An owner may also become progressively frustrated and respond by escalating punitive efforts or by relying on increasing amounts of isolation in order to manage a hyperactive dog's behavior. Since many attention-seeking behaviors are *active-submission* efforts, threats or physical punishment may serve only to stimulate even *more* of the unwanted behavior in a futile effort to appease the owner.

Not surprisingly, frustrative arousal is often associated with social excesses and hyperactivity. Dogs that are unable to achieve a satisfying social connection with their owners may, as a consequence, try even harder. Unfortunately, the dogs' efforts are rarely successful, and repeated failure may lead them to form corresponding negative expectancies about future efforts. In such cases, frustration is evoked by both obstructed access to the social goal, as well as a failure or deficiency of a dog's behavioral repertoire to achieve it. An expectation of failure may consequently evoke frustrative preparatory arousal whenever the dog is in the owner's presence. Consequently, the dog's moment-to-moment expectations of pending failure in social settings may stimulate a spiraling escalation of frustration and corresponding social excesses. The thwarted social intentions and motivations underlying unsuccessful social excesses provide a powerful locus for escalating frustration and anxious arousal in the form of attention seeking (i.e., excessive active-submission behavior). Problematic attention-seeking behavior may reflect persistent social frustration, resulting in disorganized and ineffectual social behavior, especially involving active submission. Attention-seeking dogs are not usually satisfied with getting social contact, and giving it to them may only evoke additional compulsive attention-seeking behavior, suggesting the presence of other motivational imperatives at work, besides the satisfaction of proximity or contact needs. Punishment in such cases appears to escalate attention-seeking efforts, underscoring the submissive character of such behavior—the punitive efforts simply serve to evoke more active-submission behavior. Punishment may be effective only if it results in passive submission. Interestingly, such dogs are often highly responsive to shaping procedures using positive reinforcement in combination with time-out, with brief isolation serving to calm them (see *Time-out and Social Excesses* in Volume 1, Chapter 8). The calming effects of brief time-outs away from the owner may work because the procedure removes (stimulus change) the operative cue (the owner) controlling frustrative submission behavior and restores contact only after the dog has calmed down (passive submission).

REFERENCES

Amsel A (1971). Frustration, persistence, and regression. In HD Kimmel (Ed), *Experimental Psychopathology: Recent Research and Theory.* New York: Academic.

Astrup C (1965). *Pavlovian Psychiatry: A New Synthesis.* Springfield, IL: Charles C Thomas.

Bareggi SR, Becker RE, Ginsburg BE, et al. (1979). Neurochemical investigation of an endogenous model of the "hyperkinetic syndrome" in a hybrid dog. *Life Sci,* 24:481–488.

Barcus R, Schwebel AI, and Corson SA (1980). An animal model of hyperactive-child syndrome suitable for the study of the effects of food additives. *Pavlovian J Biol Sci,* 15:183–187.

Blackshaw J, Sutton RH, and Boyhan MA (1994). Tail chasing or circling behavior in dogs. *Canine Pract,* 19:7–11.

Blum K, Cull JG, Braverman ER, et al. (1997). Reward deficiency syndrome: Neurobiological and genetic aspects. In K Blum and EP Noble (Eds), *Handbook of Psychiatric Genetics.* New York: CRC.

Campagnoni FR, Lawler CP, and Cohen PS (1986). Temporal patterns of reinforcer-induced general activity and attack in pigeons. *Physiol Behav,* 37:577–582.

Campbell WE (1973). Behavioral modification of hyperkinetic dogs. *Mod Vet Pract,* 54:49–52.

Campbell WE (1992). *Behavior Problems in Dogs.* Goleta, CA: American Veterinary Publications.

Corson SA, Corson EO'L, Kirilcuk B, et al. (1973). Differential effects of amphetamines on clinically relevant dog models of hyperkinesis and stereotypy: relevance to Huntington's chorea. In A Barbeau, TN Chase, and GW Paulson (Eds), *Advances in Neurology,* Vol 1. New York: Raven.

Dodman NH, Bronson R, and Gliatto J (1993). Tail chasing in a bull terrier. *JAVMA,* 202:758–760.

Drastura J (1992). Taming aggression with amphetamines: Drug therapy and obedience training help a Lhasa apso with temperament problems become more amenable. *Dog World,* Nov:18–25.

Eckstein RA and Hart BL (1996). Treatment of acral lick dermatitis by behavior modification using electronic stimulation. *J Am Anim Hosp Assoc,* 32:225–229.

Ebstein RP, Novick R, Umansky B, et al. (1996). Dopamine D4 receptor (D4DR) exon III polymorphism associated with the human personality trait of novelty seeking. *Nat Genet,* 12:78–80.

Falk JL (1961). Production of polydipsia in normal rates by an intermittent food schedule. *Science,* 133:195–196.

Falk JL (1977). The origins and functions of adjunctive behavior. *Anim Learn Behav,* 5:325–335.

Falk JL (1981). The environmental generation of excessive behavior. In SJ Mule (Ed), *Behavior in Excess: An Examination of the Volitional Disorders.* New York: Free Press.

Falk JL (1986). The formation and function of ritual behavior. In T Thompson and MD Zeiler (Eds), *Analysis and Integration of Behavioral Units.* Hillsdale, NJ: Lawrence Erlbaum Associates.

Falk JL and Kupfer AS (1998). Adjunctive behavior: Application to the analysis and treatment of behavior problems. In W O'Donohue (Ed), *Learning and Behavior Therapy.* Boston: Allyn and Bacon.

Fisher AE (1955). The effects of early differential treatment on the social and exploratory behavior of puppies [Unpublished doctoral dissertation]. University Park: Pennsylvania State University.

Fox MW (1962). Observations on paw raising and sympathy lameness in the dog. *Vet Rec,* 74:895–896.

Fox MW (1963). *Canine Behavior.* Springfield, IL: Charles C Thomas.

Fox MW (1974). *Concepts of Ethology: Animal and Human Behavior.* Minneapolis: University of Minnesota Press.

Gainetdinov RR, Wetsel RR, William C, and Jones SR (1999). Role of serotonin in the paradoxical calming effect of psychostimulants on hyperactivity. *Science,* 283:397–401.

Hart BL (1980). Attention-getting behavior. In BL Hart (Ed), *Canine Behavior (A Practitioner Monograph).* Santa Barbara, CA: Veterinary Practice.

Hart BL and Hart LA (1985). *Canine and Feline Behavioral Therapy.* Philadelphia: Lea and Febiger.

Hetts S, Clark DJ, Calpin JP, et al. (1992). Influence of housing conditions on beagle behaviour. *Appl Anim Behav Sci,* 34:137–155.

Hewson CJ and Luescher UA (1996). Compulsive Disorder in Dogs. In VL Voith and PL Borchelt (Eds), *Readings in Companion Animal Behavior.* Philadelphia: Veterinary Learning Systems.

Hinshaw SP (1994). *Attention Deficits and Hyperactivity in Children.* Thousand Oaks, CA: Sage.

Hubrecht RC, Serpell JA, and Poole TB (1992). Correlates of pen size and housing conditions on the behaviour of kennelled dogs. *Appl Anim Behav Sci,* 34:365–383.

Hynd GW and Hooper SR (1992). *Neurological Basis of Childhood Psychopathology.* Newbury Park, CA: Sage.

Jones IH and Barraclough BM (1978). Automutilation in animals and relevance to self-injury in man. *Acta Psychiatr Scand,* 58:40–47.

Kohlert JG and Bloch GJ (1993). A rat model for attention deficit-hyperactivity disorder. *Physiol Behav,* 53:1215–1218.

Kostrzewa RM, Ryszard B, Kalbfleisch JH, et al. (1994). Proposed animal model of animal attention deficit hyperactivity disorder. *Brain Res Bull,* 34:161–167.

Kuo ZY (1967). *The Dynamics of Behavior Development: An Epigenetic View.* New York: Random House.

Lawler C and Cohen PS (1992). Temporal patterns of schedule-induced drinking and pawgrooming in rats exposed to periodic food. *Anim Learn Behav,* 20:266–280.

Levy DM (1941). The hostile act. *Psychol Rev,* 48:356–361.

Lorenz K (1955). *Man Meets Dog.* Boston: Houghton Mifflin.

Lorenz K (1981). *The Foundations of Ethology: The Principal Ideas and Discoveries in Animal Behavior.* New York: Simon and Schuster.

Luescher UA (1993a). Hyperkinesis in dogs: Six case reports. *Can Vet J,* 34:368–370.

Luescher UA (1993b). Animal behavior case of the month. *JAVMA,* 11:1538–1539.

Luescher UA, McKeown DL, and Halip J (1991). Stereotypic or obsessive-compulsive disorders in dogs and cats. *Vet Clin North Am Adv Companion Anim Behav,* 21:207–224.

Maier, NRF (1961). *Frustration: The Study of Behavior Without a Goal.* Ann Arbor, MI: Univ of Michigan Press (Ann Arbor Paperbacks).

Masserman JH (1950). Experimental Neurosis. *Sci Am,* 182:38–43.

Michaelson IA, Bornschein RL, Loch RK, and Rafales LS (1977). Minimal brain dysfunction hyperkinesis: Significance of nutritional status in animal models of hyperactivity. In I Hanin and E Usdin (Eds), *Animal Models in Psychiatry and Neurology.* New York: Pergamon.

Melzack R and Scott TH (1957). The effects of early experience on the response to pain. *J Comp Physiol Psychol,* 50:155–160.

Mertens P (1999). Toe chewer. E-mail: Thursday, 18 November 1999, AVSAB-L@listserv.utk.edu.

Mook DM, Jeffrey J, and Neuringer A (1993). Spontaneously hypertensive rats (SHR) readily learn to vary but not repeat instrument responses. *Behav Neural Biol,* 59:126–135.

Mugford RA (1984). Methods used to describe the normal and abnormal behaviour of the dog and cat. In RS Anderson (Ed), *Nutrition and Behavior in Dogs and Cats.* New York: Pergamon.

Niimi Y, Inoue-Murayam M, Murayama Y, et al. (1999). Allelic variation of the D4 dopamine receptor polymorphic region in two dog breeds, golden retriever and Shiba. *J Vet Med Sci,* 61:1281–1286.

Overall K (1992a). Recognition, diagnosis, and management of obsessive-compulsive disorders (Part 1). *Canine Pract,* 17(2):40–44.

Overall K (1992b). Recognition, diagnosis, and management of obsessive-compulsive disorders (Part 2). *Canine Pract,* 17(3):25–27.

Overall K (1992c). Recognition, diagnosis, and management of obsessive-compulsive disorders (Part 3). *Canine Pract,* 17(4):39–43.

Pavlov IP (1928/1967). *Lectures on Conditioned Reinforcement,* Vol. 1, WH Gantt (Trans). New York: International.

Pavlov IP (1941). *Lectures on Conditioned Reinforcement*, Vol. 2: *Conditional Reflexes and Psychiatry*, WH Gantt (Trans). New York: International.

Rapoport JL and Ismond DR (1996). *DSM-IV Training Guide for Diagnosis of Childhood Disorders*. New York: Brunnel/Mazel.

Rivers B, Walter PA, and McKeever PJ (1993). Treatment of canine acral lick dermatitis with radiation therapy: 17 cases (1979–1991). *J Am Anim Hosp Assoc*, 29:541–544.

Romanes GJ (1888). *Animal Intelligence*. New York: D Appleton.

Sagvolden T, Metzger MA, Schiorbeck HK, et al. (1992). The spontaneously hypertensive rat (SHR) as an animal model of childhood hyperactivity (ADHD): Changed reactivity to reinforcers and to psychomotor stimulants. *Behav Neural Biol*, 58:103–112.

Sagvolden T, Metzger MA, and Sagvolden G (1993). Frequent reward eliminates differences in activity between hyperkinetic rats and controls. *Behav Neural Biol*, 59:225–229.

Sechzer JA (1977). The neonatal split-brain kitten: A laboratory analogue of minimal brain dysfunction. In JD Maser and MEP Seligman (Eds), *Psychopathology: Experimental Models*. San Francisco: WH Freeman.

Seo T, Sato S, Kosake K, Sakamoto N, et al. (1998). Tongue-playing and heart rate in calves. *Appl Anim Behav Sci*, 58:179–182.

Silbergeld EK and Goldberg AM (1974). Lead induced behavioral dysfunction: An animal model of hyperactivity. *Exp Neurol*, 42:146.

Singh NN, Ellis CR, Crews WD, and Singh YN (1994). Does diminished dopaminergic neurotransmission increase pica? *J Child Adolesc Psychopharmacol*, 4:93–99.

Spring B (1986). Effects of foods and nutrients on the behavior of normal individuals. In RJ Wurtman and JJ Wurtman (Eds), *Nutrition and the Brain*, 7:1-47.

Swedo SE (1989). Rituals and releasers: An ethological model of obsessive-compulsive disorder. In J Rapoport (Ed), *Obsessive-Compulsive Disorder in Childhood and Adolescence*. Washington, DC: American Psychiatric.

Thomson G, Raals GM, Hepburn WS, et al. (1989). Blood lead levels and children's behavior: Results from the Edinburg lead study. *J Child Psychol Psychiatry*, 30:728–732.

Thompson WR, Melzack R, and Scott TH (1956). "Whirling behavior" in dogs as related to early experience. *Science*, 123:939.

Tinbergen N (1951/1969). *The Study of Instinct*. Oxford: Oxford University Press (reprint).

Veith L (1986). Acral lick dermatitis in the dog. *Canine Pract*, 13:15–22.

Voith VL (1979). Behavioral problems. In EA Chandler, EA Evans, WB Singleton, et al. (Eds), *Canine Medicine and Therapeutics*. Oxford: Blackwell Scientific.

Voith VL (1980a). Play: a form of hyperactivity and aggression. *Mod Vet Pract*, 61:631–632.

Voith VL (1980b). Play behavior interpreted as aggression or hyperactivity: Case histories. *Mod Vet Pract*, 61:707–709.

Voith VL (1980c). Hyperactivity and hyperkinesis. *Mod Vet Pract*, 61:787—789

Voith VL and Borchelt PL (1996). Fears and phobias in companion animals: Update. In VL Voith and PL Borchelt (Eds), *Readings in Companion Animal Behavior*. Trenton, NJ: Veterinary Learning Systems.

Waller MB and Fuller JL (1961). Preliminary observations on early experience as related to social behavior. Am J *Orthopsychiatry*, 31:254–266.

Weiss G (1991). Attention deficit hyperactivity disorder. In M Lewis (Ed), *Child and Adolescent Psychiatry: A Comprehensive Textbook*. Baltimore: Williams and Wilkins.

Werry JS (1994). Pharmacotherapy of disruptive behavior disorders. In LL Greenhill (Ed), *Child and Adolescent Psychiatric Clinics of North America: Disruptive Disorders*. Philadelphia: WB Saunders.

6

Aggressive Behavior: Basic Concepts and Principles

But where danger is, grows
The saving power also.

FRIEDRICH HÖLDERLIN, *POEMS AND FRAGMENTS* (1966)

PART 1: INTRODUCTION

CHARACTERISTICS OF DOGS THAT BITE: AGE AND SEX

The etiology of aggressive behavior presents considerable variation from dog to dog. Aggressive behavior is most frequently exhibited by socially mature and intact male dogs (Reisner, 1997), but young puppies can have serious precocious aggression problems, as well. Mugford (1984) reported that among 50 English cocker spaniels the mean average age of dogs with dominance-related aggression was 7.4 months (range, 3 to 24 months). In another group of golden retrievers treated by

Mugford (1987), 24 with aggression problems averaged 2.9 years of age (range, 0.7 to 8.0 years). Of the 24 dogs treated by Mugford, 19 were males, two of which had been castrated. Beaver (1983) found that of 120 dogs with aggression problems (various diagnoses) the mean age was 3 years (range, 9 weeks to 11 years). She reported that 60.1% of the dogs were intact males (14% castrated), with 15.4% intact females (10.5% spayed). Wright (1985) found that the average age of dogs involved in severe attacks was 3 years (range, 0.67 to 10.5 years). All 16 dogs were males. These statistics suggest that considerable variation exists with respect to the time of onset associated with aggression problems. Although most dogs are presented for treatment at 1 to 3 years of age, incipient signs of a developing problem are frequently observed in young puppies, often prior to 4 months of age.

INCIDENCE AND TARGETS OF AGGRESSION

Although a number of studies indicate that dog bites against people represent a serious problem, perhaps even having reached epidemic proportions (Lockwood, 1996), the available statistics are incomplete and inadequate. A notable problem is the dog population sampled. Many of the statistics discussed below were obtained from urban populations that may be skewed by a disproportionate number of aggressive, guard-type dogs. Harris and colleagues (1974) note that urban dwellers frequently keep and socialize aggressive dogs to enhance home security in high-crime areas. Also, the number of social contacts in which bites might occur are probably substantially more numerous in the city than in the suburbs or the country. Consequently, it is difficult to draw any hard and fast generalizations, outside of those directly related to the particular populations sampled. In contrast, the statistical information concerning fatal dog attacks is considerably more reliable and complete. What is extraordinary about fatal attacks is the relative rarity of such incidents when considered in the context of the many millions of intimate contacts occurring between dogs and people every day. Statistically, a child's life is far safer in the presence

of its family dog than in the hands of human caretakers or parents.

Overall Situation: Total Number of Bites and Implications

The overall number of dog bites occurring in the United States is widely disputed among reporting authorities. These differences of opinion are attributable (in part) to statistical errors stemming from erroneous population estimates [see Mathews and Lattal (1994)], inconsistent definitions of what constitutes a dog bite, the absence of a consistent and reliable method for tallying dog-bite incidents, and widespread underreporting of dog-bite incidents. A task force on aggression, organized by the American Veterinary Medical Association (AVMA) (Golab, 1998), found that there is a need to standardize the ways in which dog bites are reported. The task force has suggested that standardized forms be produced for collecting information about the age of the bite victim, the circumstances of the incident, the extent of the injuries, and the signalment of the dog. In addition, the task force hopes to better define legal requirements for reporting dog bites and to develop better means for collecting and keeping dog-bite statistics. Unfortunately, the AVMA task force did not include a professional dog trainer—a significant oversight, since most owners with dog-aggression problems turn to such people for advice and guidance.

Despite the inherent limitations involved and the risk for erroneous generalizations, a careful study of relevant statistics is revealing and useful. According to the AVMA (1997), approximately 52.9 million dogs live in the United States. The AVMA figure is somewhat lower than the Pet Food Institute's (PFI) (1999) estimate of 57.6 million dogs, with approximately 37.6% of all American households keeping at least one dog. Calculating the number of dog bites is a much harder statistical task, with the current best guesses ranging from 2 to 5 million dog bites occurring each year. Pinckney and Kennedy (1982) estimated that approximately 2 million people are bitten each year in the United States, with a tenth of these victims requiring sutures, a third missing time away from school or work, and half receiving permanent scarring as the result of their injuries. Since many minor bites and bites delivered by familiar dogs are not reported, the actual number of dog bites is probably higher than this conservative estimate. In 1996, Sacks and colleagues (1996a) at the National Center for Injury Prevention and Control estimated that approximately 4.7 million people are bitten in America each year. Of these victims, 899,700 persons required medical attention. They estimate that children were 1.5 times more likely to be bitten, and over 3 times more likely to require medical treatment than adults. Besides the emotional and physical pain of dog attacks to the victims, dog bites represent a serious legal and monetary liability to dog owners. The Insurance Information Institute (1999) estimates that dog bites cost the public approximately 1 billion dollars per year in losses, with insurance companies paying out $250 million to resolve dog-bite claims in 1996. State Farm Insurance (1999) alone reported paying nearly $80 million in dog-related liability claims in 1997. According to State Farm Insurance, one in three homeowner claims involving personal injury pertain to a dog bite, with an average payout of $12,000 per bite incident.

Vital Characteristics: Age, Sex, Risk-taking Propensity, Location of Attacks, Time of Day/Season, and Bodily Target of Attack

Children are bitten at a disproportionate rate when compared to other population groups (Gershman et al., 1994). It should be noted in this regard, however, that children are also most commonly associated with homes that keep dogs as pets (Marx et al., 1988; Wells and Hepper, 1997). Approximately 1% of all children brought for emergency treatment are victims of dog bites (Brogan et al., 1995). Adams and Clark (1989) found that 38% of 105 dog owners interviewed reported that their dog had "nipped" at children or had bitten someone—62% of these bites were directed toward family members. The majority of dog bites are directed toward children 5 to 14 years of age (Riegger and Guntzelman, 1990).

Boys are bitten nearly twice as often as girls (Harris et al., 1974). Boys also receive the majority of severe bites (60% to 78%) (Wright, 1991). Sacks and coworkers (1989) found that, among 29 children between the ages of 5 and 9 who suffered a fatal dog attack, 23 (79.3%) of them were boys. The first clear sign of a sexual differentiation of victims is evident in the 1- to 4-year-old group, with 64.2% of the them being boys. A possible explanation for this difference may be due to the amount of time spent by boys versus girls interacting with dogs. Lehman (1928) performed a large statistical study involving 5000 respondents to determine how children spent their time playing. Children of various ages were asked to respond to a series of questions regarding their daily play activities. He found that boys tended to spend more time interacting with dogs than girls did, with both groups showing a steady decline in the amount of time spent playing with pets (both dogs and cats) as they matured. Another possible cause for the uneven distribution of dog bites between boys and girls may be attributable to a boy's greater inclination to engage in risk-taking behavior (Ginsburg and Miller, 1982).

Most bites occur during the summer months (peaking in June) and weekends. On the average day, they are most frequent from 1:00 to 9:00 PM, peaking between 3:00 and 7:00 PM (Harris et al., 1974). Wright (1990) has also reported seasonal and time-of-attack trends. Among 1724 dog bites reported in Dallas, the incidence of attacks peaked between March and May, with 34.6% of the bites occurring during those 3 months. The majority of dog bites (55.8%) took place from 2:00 to 8:00 PM, peaking between 5:00 and 6:00 in the late afternoon. Sacks and colleagues (1989) were unable to detect a similar seasonal trend in the case of fatal dog attacks. Fatal attacks involving pet dogs were actually more common in the winter, whereas stray-dog attacks occurred more often in the fall and least often in the summer.

The majority of bites involving young children are directed toward the face and head, with children under 4 years of age being bitten in the face, head, or neck 63% of the time (Chun et al., 1982; Podberscek et al., 1990). Beck and colleagues (1975) found that 35% of the bites involving children younger than 4 years of age were directed toward the face. In children between 5 and 9 years of age, this pattern shifts dramatically, with 84% of bites being directed toward the extremities or torso and 18.5% toward the face or neck (Beck et al., 1975). Among a population of children receiving severe injuries, 82% of the bites were directed toward the victim's head or neck.

Dog-bite reports analyzed by Wright (1991) indicate that 87.5% (range, 85.5% to 89.4%) of the dogs involved are owned, with attacks being directed toward family members in 10.5% (range, 5.9% to 15%) of the cases. These estimates probably underrepresent the actual number of persons bitten by their own dog. In a large study involving 3200 children between the ages of 4 and 18 surveyed, 45% had been bitten by a dog at some point in their life. About half of these children were bitten by a neighbor's dog, whereas nearly a third reported being bitten by the family dog (Jones and Beck, 1984).

EMOTIONAL TRAUMA OF DOG ATTACKS ON CHILDREN

Surprisingly, Jones and Beck found that the experience of being bitten had little effect on the person's later preference for the dog as a pet. This finding has significant implications for the study of cynophobia, since one would expect from the classical conditioning model of fear that a dog bite should have a lasting negative impact on a child's attitude toward dogs.

In fact, some recent and better-controlled research appears to indicate that there exists a significant independence between having experienced a dog bite as a child and the later development of cynophobia or fear of dogs. Two studies are of particular interest in this regard. First, DiNardo and coworkers (1988), utilizing heart-rate changes as a physiological measure of anxiety, were unable to detect a relationship between a previous dog bite and increased physiological arousal when people were tested in the presence of a friendly dog. Second, Doogan and Thomas (1992) found that most cynophobic adults report that their

fear of dogs began in childhood, but there is no clear correlation between the frequency of attacks in childhood and the subsequent development of fear toward dogs. The most important factor in the etiology of such fear is the amount of contact that a person had before the onset of fear. People having minimal contact with dogs as children are more prone to exhibit fearfulness as adults. The researchers suggest that prior "noneventful" exposure to dogs may impede the development of phobic reactions in response to dog bites and other sources of fear (e.g., inimical warnings about dogs):

> The role of conditioning events in producing fear of dogs must be considered as nonproven. If such conditioning events do play a causal role then it is only in conjunction with some other factor such as lack of prior uneventful exposure to dogs or in especially susceptible individuals. The present results from children suggest that information transmission may be more important in engendering fear of dogs than studies of adults might suggest. Although most fearful adults report that their fear of dogs began in childhood, it is clear that not all dog-fearful children grow up to become dog-fearful adults, which raises the question of why some children, but not others, eventually lose their fear of dogs. (393–394)

DOGS THAT KILL

Of particular concern for parents is the possibility of a fatal attack being directed toward an infant or toddler. Although such attacks occasionally occur, most serious attacks are directed toward older children, especially boys. Voith (1984) believes that the majority of fatal or serious attacks directed toward infants are probably instigated by aberrant predatory motivations rather than by sibling rivalry or other commonly cited motivations such as jealousy. Most fatal dog attacks are delivered by dogs known to the victim or the victim's family, with the majority of them being delivered by the family dog or a neighbor's dog. Most of the dogs involved had no prior history of aggressive behavior and attacked without known provocation by the victim (Pinckney and Kennedy, 1982).

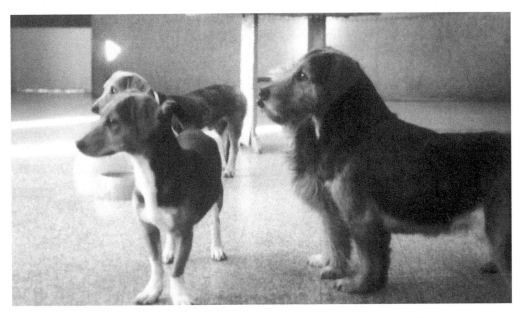

FIG. 6.1. These dogs do not fit the stereotypic profile of dogs that might be expected to kill, but they, together with two others not pictured, fatally injured an 81-year-old invalid woman. (Photo courtesy of V. L. Voith.)

It should be emphasized that fatal dog attacks on babies are extremely rare. From 1979 to 1988, the total number of infants (birth to 11 months old) killed as the result of a dog attack in the United States was 25. Children at the greatest risk for exposure to a fatal dog attack belong to the 1- to 4-year group, with 56 toddlers dying from dog attacks over that same period (Sacks et al., 1989). A more recent study by Sacks and coworkers (1996b), covering the years from 1989 to 1994, reported a total of 109 bite-related fatalities, with 57% of the deaths involving children under 10 years of age. Another age group at a higher risk is the elderly, with 18% of the fatal attacks involving persons over 70 years of age (Figure 6.1). The researchers found that 77% of the fatalities involved attacks occurring on the owner's property, with 18% of the dogs restrained and 59% of them unrestrained. Overall, the death rate involving fatal dog attacks has remained relatively constant over the past 16 years, with approximately 15 to 18 fatal dog attacks in the United States each year.

DOG ATTACKS VERSUS HUMAN FATAL ASSAULTS ON CHILDREN

Despite the tragic occurrence of dog attack fatalities, the average child is at a far greater risk of being seriously hurt or killed by a parent or relative than by the family dog. A recent report compiled by the U.S. Department of Health and Human Services (1999) found that 1196 children were killed in the United States as the result of maltreatment in 1997. An earlier government study placed that number closer to 2000; that is, approximately 5 children every day lose their lives to maltreatment and child abuse homicide (U.S. Advisory Board on Child Abuse and Neglect, 1995). Over 85% of the perpetrators are either parents (75%) or relatives (10%) of the victim. In addition to deaths, nearly 1 million children experience substantiated or indicated abuse and neglect annually. According to the USDHHS study, children 3 years of age or younger accounted for 77% of the reported fatalities. By way of comparison with dog attack fatalities, according to the aforementioned study performed by Sacks and colleagues (1996b), during the 5 years between 1989 and 1994, 45 children (from birth to 4 years of age) were killed by dogs. During a similar length of time, extrapolating from the foregoing statistics for 1997, among children 3 years or younger, an estimated 4605 were killed by humans. Given that approximately nine children of this age group are killed by dogs each year, these sobering statistics of child-abuse homicide reveal that it would take dogs over 100 years to kill as many children as are killed by their own parents, relatives, and other guardians on an annual basis. In other words, in any given year, children at greatest risk of abuse are 100 times more likely to be killed by a parent or relative than by the family dog.

Voith and Borchelt (1985) state the threat of serious dog attacks on children in a fair and balanced way:

> Few infants are severely injured by dogs, and the number of infants killed by dogs is very small, probably no more than 10 per year throughout the entire United States. In contrast, many thousands of infants in the U.S. are victims of automobile accidents, burns, drowning, choking, suffocation, and poisoning. It has also been estimated that each day in the U.S. one child under 10 years of age is killed in a handgun accident. Despite the small risk, there is still cause for concern about a dog's reaction to your infant and precautions are well worthwhile. (4)

When fatal or severe dog attacks occur, the situation is often exploited by "expert" media pundits who frequently fail to emphasize the statistical rarity of such anomalies, while pandering to the public's morbid interest in the gruesome details. Overall, the effect is to produce terror and media hysteria over a widespread threat that does not exist. Such incidents predictably spawn demands from dog-hating politicians and other busybodies for immediate action, including stronger animal control regulations and unfair legislation restricting dog breeding and ownership. Obviously, efforts must be made to educate the public about the risk of dog bites and how they can be prevented, but this can be accomplished without resorting to alarmist, unfair, and divisive breed-specific legislation punishing innocent dogs and owners for the actions of a few culpable and irresponsible offenders.

Despite the gloomy appearance of the foregoing statistics, most epidemiological studies have found that the majority of dog bites result in minor physical injury (Podberscek et al., 1990). In a major study by Parrish and colleagues (1959), 88% of the bite injuries treated were judged to be minor, with 2% producing no evidence of injury. This is not to say that serious attacks do not occur—they do and all too frequently—but the majority of dog bites are neither life-threatening nor disabling for the victim. Although dog bites result in relatively minor injuries, it is important that efforts be taken to prevent such attacks. These efforts should include appropriate education for both children and parents (Mathews and Lattal, 1994). Other key preventative measures include early training and socialization of dogs, responsible breeding and selection of dogs that are destined for homes with children, and early behavioral intervention when problems first appear. In addition, children should be taught how to interact more safely with dogs, and parents should become better informed about how to control their children around dogs.

BASIC CATEGORIES

Aggressive behavior is expressed in one of three general ways: threat, defense, or attack. The sort of aggression that a dog exhibits depends on its motivational state and the presence of significant triggers. Konorski (1967) divides aggressive behavior into two general types, depending on the behavioral traits of the organism and the environmental or motivational circumstances present at the moment of arousal (see *Preparatory and Consummatory Reflexes* in Volume 1, Chapter 6). He notes that the same trigger stimulus may elicit either fear or anger in the stimulated animal and consequently result in either defensive or offensive actions. For example, painful stimulation may evoke a massive fear-and-escape reaction in a solitary animal, whereas if the animal is in the presence of a companion, the same stimulation could result in an angry offensive attack (Ulrich and Azrin, 1962). Konorski also points out that the differential display of defensive or offensive behavior is strongly influenced by environmental circumstances, noting that an animal threatened on its own territory is more likely to become angry and engage in offensive aggression, whereas the same animal may show fear and react defensively if threatened while in an unfamiliar place. Fear- and anger-elicited attacks are forms of affective aggression, both involving the presence of a high degree of emotional arousal. As is discussed in greater detail below, affective aggression is distinguished from predatory or *quiet-attack* behavior.

Krushinskii (1960) argues that defensive behavior in dogs presents in two characteristic ways: passive and active defensive reactions. Passive defensive reactions take the form of fear and include all types of freeze and flight responses elicited, for example, by loud-unfamiliar sounds or the close presence of strangers. An active defensive reaction, or what Pavlov refers to as a "watch reflex," is expressed in two forms: (1) defensive barking without an effort to bite or (2) defensive behavior that includes an effort to bite. According to Krushinskii, the dog's active and passive defensive behaviors are the result of a combination of various *unitary reactions* that are coordinated to produce complex behavioral patterns having biological significance for the dog as a species. Unitary reactions are variably composed of both conditioned and unconditioned reflexes. However, unlike individual conditioned and unconditioned reflexes, whose pattern of expression is apparent from the beginning (stimulus) to end (response), the unitary reaction is only fully recognized during the final stages of its expression. Unitary reactions are functionally integrated and organized into species-typical behavior patterns and *epigenetic routines* in order to perform various social and biological functions efficiently by means of interacting with the environment. Consequently, although conditioned and unconditioned reflexes variably influence behavioral thresholds (e.g., fear and anger), the functional significance of defensive unitary reactions only become evident as they are organized into integrated species-typical patterns of active and passive defensive behavior.

In general, two broad categories of aggressive behavior exist, intraspecific and interspe-cific, depending on whether the aggression is directed toward conspecifics or toward other animals not belonging to the aggressor's species, respectively.

Intraspecific Aggression

Intraspecific aggression consists of both ritualized and overt forms of aggressive behavior directed toward conspecifics, that is, individuals belonging to the same species. Most intraspecific aggression is highly ritualized and serves some biologically significant function (e.g., social organization, population dispersion, or sexual selection). In general intraspecific aggression provides a countervailing and distance-increasing function over place and social attachment processes but without breaking down affiliative contact altogether. As such, ritualized intraspecific aggression imposes social order (e.g., the formation of a dominance hierarchy) and territorial limits on the interaction between individuals belonging to the same species. This ordering and distancing function of aggression is especially evident among familiar individuals belonging to the same social group. Whereas aggression directed toward conspecifics belonging to the same group is often highly ritualized and inhibited, aggression toward conspecific outsiders is usually not so well inhibited and may, as among wolves, result in an overt attack and the intruder's death if it cannot put up an adequate defense or escape by running away.

Interspecific Aggression

Interspecific aggression refers to aggressive behavior directed against another species and includes both offensive and defensive elements. Although intraspecific aggression is most often associated with competition between closely socialized animals belonging to the same species, interspecific aggression is most frequently associated with self-protective goals, as, for example, occur when a prey animal defends itself against the attack of a predator. The dog's relationship with humans is complex in this regard, with both competitive and self-protective aggression being exhibited under different situations. Many ritualized elements of intraspecific aggression are shown toward people with whom dogs are closely socialized. On the other hand, dogs may also exhibit defensive behavior aimed at self-protection and having nothing to do with the establishment of dominance and territory, as appears to be the case in most forms of intraspecific aggression. In the absence of adequate socialization, interspecific aggression predominantly consists of defensive behavior, lacking ritualization and inhibition, and performed with the intention of doing damage.

Many forms of aggression classified as dominance related (see Chapter 8) may be more defensive than offensive. For example, Line and Voith (1986) report that the majority of attacks by dogs diagnosed with dominance aggression occurred while the dogs were being disciplined. Some dogs may interpret human disciplinary actions (hitting, slapping, kicking) as physical threats and react aggressively in an effort to defend themselves. Predatory behavior is often viewed as a form of interspecific aggressive behavior, but, as will be discussed momentarily, predation is not influenced by the same motivational substrates mediating the expression of competitive and self-protective (affective) aggression. In fact, affective and predatory aggression appear to have evolved under independent pressures and are regulated by relatively distinct and segregated neural circuits and hormonal systems. In many ways, predation is more appropriately interpreted as a form of food-getting behavior motivated by hunger and mediated by the seeking system (Panksepp, 1998).

CLASSIFYING AGGRESSION: MOTIVATIONAL CONSIDERATIONS

Significant debate surrounds the question of how to organize and classify the dog's aggressive behavior into functionally discrete and logically coherent categories. Most trainers and counselors have adopted some variation of Moyer's classification system (Moyer, 1968, 1971; Hart, 1980; Borchelt and Voith, 1982; Borchelt, 1983; Beaver, 1983)—a system that has resulted in a great deal of confusion and misunderstanding (see below). Other authorities have argued with varying degrees of

cogency for a more simple classification system. O'Farrell (1986), for instance, has proposed a bipartite system, suggesting that canine aggression can be divided into two broad functional categories: dominance aggression and predatory behavior. This scheme places fear-elicited aggression under the same heading with dominance aggression: "'Fear-biting' is commonly distinguished from dominance aggression, possibly because it is felt to be understandable and excusable in a way that dominance aggression is not. It is, however, a variant of dominance aggression" (94). Although simplicity is often desirable, this arrangement is not very edifying or useful when one considers the numerous motivational assumptions it takes for granted and the equally numerous distinctions that it blurs for the sake of Ockham's razor. Further, the scheme stretches the concept of *dominance* in a way that further obscures its meaning and usefulness.

Since it is not clear how fear-related aggression might be used to enhance social status, O'Farrell's position would be made more appealing and defensible if she explicitly replaced the term *dominance* with the term *control related*. However, although such a revision would help to reduce some potential confusion in her scheme, the change would only open up another criticism. Reducing aggressive behavior to a control-related motivation still begs the question with respect to the special attributes of aggression that distinguish it from other control-related activities. Presumably, all voluntary behavior is control-related behavior, but not all voluntary behavior is aggressive, except, perhaps, in a philosophical sense. Furthermore, although many forms of aggression appear to be purposive and control related, some forms of aggression appear to occur as reflexive actions in response to specific triggers. Also, defining aggression as a control-related activity tends to obscure the unique motivational and situational factors differentiating aggression into varied species-typical forms—even predatory aggression logically collapses into a control-related category. Broadly speaking, both affective aggression and predatory behavior are control-related activities, but they are significantly different in terms of functional purpose, evolutionary history, and neurobiological origins [see *Neurobiology of Aggression (Hypothalamus)* in Volume 1, Chapter 3]. The most persuasive reason for adopting the concept of control-related aggression is that it conceptualizes offensive and defensive aggression in terms that are functionally compatible with the instrumental learning paradigm—learning concerned with establishing control over the environment. On the other hand, the underlying motivational factors (e.g., irritability, frustration, or fear) differentiating aggression into different forms represent the preparatory establishing operations facilitating the expression and potential reinforcement of control-related aggression. These emotional unitary reactions (conditioned and unconditioned reflexes) are under the influence of classical conditioning. In combination, instrumental control efforts and emotional unitary reactions converge on situations having species-typical significance for the dog, whereupon the specific intention of aggression is revealed (e.g., territory related, possession related, dominance related, or fear related).

Avoidance Learning and Aggression

Tortora (1983, 1984) has also suggested an alternative scheme for categorizing aggressive behavior. He interprets the development of aggression in terms of avoidance learning, arguing that what many dog behavior consultants refer to as dominance aggression is better understood as *avoidance-motivated aggression* (AMA). Social aggressors may not necessarily be dominant; instead, they may merely be incompetent and unable to respond appropriately under social pressure. Tortora argues that aggressive dogs appear to lack a repertoire of confident skills with which to cope and manage everyday challenges and stressors:

> The data suggest that the initial source of the aggressive avoidance response was one or more forms of elicited aggression such as species-typical aggressive reactions to pain, frustration, discomfort, territorial intrusion, or threats to dominance. Furthermore, it appears that these aggressive responses were exacerbated by trauma or punishment. Finally, the universal lack of behavioral control over these dogs implies that they had few operant alternatives to gain reinforcement by

compliance. From the case histories, it seems that these dogs were channeled down a path that allowed their initial innate aggressiveness to come under the control of the negatively reinforcing contingencies in the environment.

> The dogs in this study initially behaved as if they "expected" aversive events and that the only way to prevent these events was through aggression. The consequent reaction of the victim and the family, that is, withdrawal, turmoil, and belated punishment, confirmed the dog's "expectations" and reinforced the aggression. This positive feedback loop produced progressive escalation of the aggressive response, and the avoidance nature of the aggression presumably retarded or prevented its extinction. (1983:209)

The treatment program developed by Tortora is essentially a course of obedience training using various procedures, including remote shock, to enhance confidence and social competence. The operative assumption is that dogs exhibiting avoidance-motivated aggression need to learn systematically that they can *safely* control threatening or aversive events without resorting to aggression.

A strength of Tortora's functional analysis is that it rests on a strong body of supporting experimental research (Azrin et al., 1967; Hutchinson et al., 1971). In addition to being elicited by a variety of natural or learned triggers acquired through classical conditioning, aggressive behavior functions motivationally and behaviorally in a variety of ways, such as providing instrumental control over the physical and social environment. Animals can learn to avoid aversive stimulation by responding aggressively and may even learn and perform arbitrary instrumental responses to obtain an opportunity to attack a target provided as a reward (Azrin et al., 1965). The avoidance paradigm also offers an explanation for the persistence of some forms of aggressive behavior, since avoidance learning is marked by a strong tendency to persist over time and resist extinction (see *Fear and Conditioning* in Chapter 3).

Tortora does not reject the notion of elicited aggression (e.g., irritable, territorial, or dominance related), but stresses that the dog's repertoire of species-typical aggressive behavior and controlling natural triggers only represents part of the picture. Although aggression may be originally elicited by a *natural* trigger, it can subsequently come under the control of conditioned stimuli or *learned* triggers through avoidance learning. In fact, dominant-aggressive dogs frequently do exhibit behavior that appears to be influenced by avoidance learning. A common and often confusing characteristic of dominance aggression is the absence of an adequate trigger to explain the ferocity of the attack. In other words, the magnitude of dominance attacks is frequently far in excess to what one might expect to occur under the operative circumstances present at the time. Such attacks often appear to occur under minimal or no provocation at all. Low-threshold or unprovoked attacks may be explained along the lines of avoidance conditioning, whereby neutral stimuli present at the time of attack may become conditioned or learned triggers via association with unconditioned or natural triggers. As a result, these conditioned triggers may become capable of eliciting aggressive behavior in the absence of natural triggers. In other words, aggressors may learn to anticipate aversive arousal (frustrative, irritable, painful) by association with other stimuli present at the time when aversive arousal led to aggression. As a result, such stimuli may gradually become discriminative signals controlling avoidance-motivated aggression. According to this general account, most aggressive behavior is learned as a means to anticipate and avoid actual or perceived threats, especially threats occurring under circumstances where other means of control are unavailable or ineffectual. Bottom line, according the AMA hypothesis, *dominance* aggression toward human targets appears to be more about *defensive* control than *offensive* status-seeking efforts.

Many attack situations involving defensive aggression (that is, aggression influenced by a component of fear or avoidance) appear to present characteristics consistent with Tortora's AMA hypothesis; however, attacks motivated by anger do not appear to involve an underlying component of fear. The offensive aggressor may exhibit threatening postures and gestures (standing tall and stiff, ears up and turned forward, tail held erect, lips forming an agonistic pucker), behavioral signs indicating confident aggressive arousal—not preparatory fear. The offensive aggressor may learn that threats and attacks serve to secure or protect vital interests and resources. For example, a dog that has learned to threaten and displace its owner in the presence of food may learn through positive reinforcement (that is, the continued possession of food) that such behavior works. Determining whether the particular behavior is under the control of positive or negative reinforcement depends on whether the behavior functions to terminate or avoid stimulation or serves to obtain or perpetuate stimulation. When aggression occurs while the dog is sleeping, resting, or eating, the attack may be analyzed in terms of the perpetuation of these activities or resources, that is, understood by appealing to positive reinforcement. On the other hand, such attacks may also be analyzed in terms of negative reinforcement, especially if the behavior is primarily motivated to terminate the presence of a threat, a source of irritation, or frustration. In general, the determination of whether aggression is defensive (avoidance motivated) or offensive depends on the presence of behavioral signs at the time of attack. However, distinguishing between these two forms of aggression on the basis of postural signs of fear may become progressively difficult in the case of the experienced avoidance-motivated aggressors, who may not exhibit any signs of overt fear, especially as they become progressively confident and sure about the likelihood of success. In general, though, whether defensive or offensive, aggressive behavior aims at establishing control over some intruding target. The notions of positive and negative reinforcement may actually obfuscate the vital concern; that is, aggression is reinforced by the control it succeeds to establish, regardless of the motivational substrate operative at the moment of attack (see *A Brief Critique of Traditional Learning Theory* in Volume 1, Chapter 7). According to this perspective, punishment occurs when the aggressive threat or attack fails to avoid or terminate an aversive-thwarting situation or when it fails to obtain or perpetuate some gratifying activity or resource. These considerations are of vital importance for the effective control and management of aggressive behavior.

Social Dominance and Aggression

One of the most well-studied areas in ethology is aggression, especially aggression exhibited with the apparent purpose of establishing or defending social status or rank (Scott, 1992). The most widely adopted conceptualization of dominance aggression incorporates several interactive components, including an ethological dominance concept, species-typical signalization (gestures and postures signaling agonistic intent and rank—dominance and submission), early socialization, and learning. Dogs and humans both socially organize themselves by rank order (often involving very complex alignments) within a dominance hierarchy. Such organization is accomplished by various means, including the utilization of species-typical gestures and body postures employed to advertise and ritually defend the individual's status against challenges presented by others belonging to the same group. Sometimes, communication breaks down as the result of a misunderstanding or an outright power struggle, giving rise to conflicts and challenges that may escalate into overt attacks and fighting. The role of social dominance in the expression of aggression is examined in detail in *Social Dominance and Aggression* in Chapter 8.

Fear and Aggression

Normally, fear significantly inhibits aggressive behavior and causes the animal to freeze or flee—if it can. A fearful dog usually makes frantic efforts to escape when it feels threatened or is attacked. It is only under circumstances in which escape or appeasement is thwarted that a fearful dog may resort to aggression. First and foremost, the goal of fearful behavior is to escape or control threatening stimulation, with counterthreats and aggression emitted as a last resort. Fear aggression is always a defensive strategy and is most likely to occur when other means of escape or avoidance are thwarted. However, in cases in which fear aggression succeeds, the defensive threat or attack may undergo reinforcement and, under similar circumstances in the future, the behavior may be triggered by conditioned stimuli associated with the original

eliciting situation. As already discussed, the result is the development avoidance-motivated aggression—behavior that may closely parallel dominance aggression but remains essentially defensive rather than offensive. Fear aggressors can be distinguished from dominance aggressors by the exhibition of defensive postures indicative of fear (e.g., ears back, tail tucked under the body, nervous snarling, and showing of teeth) and approach-avoidance conflict. In addition, the fear aggressor may engage in barking (a possible repetitive conflict behavior) and other signs of fearful arousal (licking movements) and agitation that occur when it is exposed to eliciting stimuli, such as a doorbell, the approach of a stranger, noisy children, skaters and other similar stimulation, or the approach of other dogs. Typically, the fear aggressor is most likely to threaten or bite when it is suddenly approached by a fear-eliciting person or dog, where escape is preempted (Borchelt, 1983). Once fear aggression has graduated into avoidance aggression, many of the telltale signs of fear may be replaced with increased confidence and reduced latency and occur under minimal provocation.

Fear-related or defensive aggression stands opposite to dominance-related or offensive aggression on the agonistic continuum. Whereas dominance aggression occurs most often in situations involving competitive conflict between conspecifics, stimulated by the coactive influences of frustration, irritability, and anger, defensive aggression is most often directed toward another group member or species, under the influence of acute threat, fear, or anxiety. The tendency to bite out of fear is most commonly seen among shy or nervous dogs that have learned to rely on biting as means of self-defense. Paradoxically, fear-related aggression and dominance aggression sometimes present together in the same dog. The term *bipolar aggression* is a good descriptive term for this condition, since opposing ends of the agonistic continuum appear to be alternately involved, depending on the situation.

Since fear-related aggression depends on the presence of fear for its expression, an important initial step in the counseling process is to make an exhaustive inventory of the evoking stimuli and situations where aggression has occurred in the past. Detailed information should be gathered concerning the location, magnitude, and type (superficial, puncture, laceration, etc.) of the bites involved. Further, the originating causes of fear and aggression should be fleshed out and clarified. This is not always practical or possible, but an effort should be attempted in every case since the results are often very useful in terms of accurately describing the problem, prognosticating the likely outcome and benefit of training, and helping owners to understand their dog's problem. Fear-related aggression appears to be strongly influenced by predisposing genetic factors. Thorne (1944), for example, found that a single "fear-biting" Basset hound had a tremendous influence on a large group of descendants in terms of their relative fearfulness and reactivity. Of 59 dogs related to this highly reproductive female, 43 (73%) were shy and unfriendly. In addition to genetic predisposition, most etiological profiles show significant causality in terms of early socialization and exposure deficits or the contribution of learning. It is not uncommon to find cases involving all three factors. Voith and Borchelt (1996) suggest that excessive punitive interaction with puppies during house training may play a significant predisposing role in the development of fear-related aggression problems in adult dogs.

Distinguishing the effects of learning from other potential causes of fear is assisted by obtaining a behavioral history and performing a detailed evaluation. Dogs that are affected by a genetic predisposition are distinguished by a chronic, lifelong, and generalized fearfulness. They often suffer heightened or extreme sensitivity to sensory input and overreact in situations involving novel stimuli (neophobia), strangers, or unfamiliar animals. Differentiating cases exhibiting a genetic predisposition from those involving a socialization deficit is not always easy, since undersocialized dogs frequently exhibit similar signs and tendencies as genetically affected individuals. Temperament information about a dog's sire and dam could be helpful in making such determinations. Puppies isolated until week 14, or in cases where they come into the home at an unusually late date from an

unknown situation, should be suspected prima facie as suffering a socialization problem. A lack of proper socialization and inadequate or traumatic environmental exposure occurring early in development are commonly associated with adult dogs' reactive fear toward strangers (xenophobia), fear of children (pedophobia), or fear of outdoors and new places (agoraphobia). In cases where fearfulness is the result of learning (e.g., startle, trauma, or abuse), a dog's reactions are usually limited to a more specific range of eliciting stimuli and situations. Of the three aforementioned etiologies, fearfulness stemming from past learning events is usually the most responsive to remedial training, with problems involving a genetic predisposition being the most difficult to work through in my experience. Fear biting suspected of being predominantly under the control of an underlying genetic causation should be carefully assessed and the owner informed of the limited benefits to be expected from behavior modification before proceeding. Although such dogs *may* respond to behavioral intervention, the goals of training should be discussed in terms of amelioration and management—not cure.

Obviously, reducing fearfulness is central to effective behavioral control and modification of fear-related aggression. Several methods have been employed for this purpose with varying degrees of success. The most beneficial techniques involve some combination of graded interactive exposure, counterconditioning, relaxation training, modeling, and response prevention. The most important consideration recommending the use of such procedures is that they help to facilitate the disconfirmation of a dog's adverse expectations of social contact while at the same time encouraging a more affirmative set of expectancies and interactive behaviors.

Cognition and Aggression

Dogs appear to form various prediction-control expectancies about future events based on the accumulation of information extracted from past experiences (see *Prediction-Control Expectancies and Adaptation* in Volume 1, Chapter 7). In general, these expectancies help to promote a more secure existence by coordinating a dog's behavior relative to the most probable, although not yet actual (certain), circumstances. Prediction-control expectancies are continually undergoing appraisal and modification in order to most accurately fit or *adapt* a dog's behavior to the environment. These expectancies are influenced by emotional concomitants of success (elation) or failure (disappointment). In cases in which a high degree of correspondence exists between what a dog expects to occur and what actually occurs, effects of well-being and confidence prevail; whereas, under opposite circumstances in which their is little correspondence between what the dog expects to occur and what actually occurs, effects of depression and helplessness may ensue. Expectancies are adjusted in accordance with the occurrence of satisfying or distressful emotional concomitants resulting from the confirmation or disconfirmation of expectant arousal or action. For example, when a prediction expectancy is disconfirmed or proves inadequate, then *anxiety* ensues. On the other hand, when a control expectancy is disconfirmed or proves inadequate, then *frustration* ensues. These emotional concomitants of expectancy disconfirmation promote adaptive optimization through the activation of increased sensory vigilance and behavioral invigoration. Adaptive change is mediated through learning, and learning is guided by the affects of anxiety and frustration, resulting from the disconfirmation of prediction-control expectancies. Theoretically, when prediction-control expectancies are fully matched and coordinated with the environment, utopic adaptation is achieved, and further learning is unnecessary and does not occur. Under ordinary circumstances, anxiety and frustration promote learning and adaptive optimization of environmental resources. However, under conditions in which the environment is both highly unpredictable and uncontrollable, then pathological disorganization (learned helplessness) and behavioral disorder (impulsive-compulsive behavior) are prone to follow. In other words, a small amount of anxiety and frustration promotes adaptive success, whereas high levels of anxiety and frustration disturb learning and disrupt behavioral adaptation.

Preparatory arousal, attention, intention, and functional behavior are guided by prediction-control expectancies. Under ordinary circumstances, dogs select courses of action based on cognitive expectancies, unless the particular expectancy has been disconfirmed or the environment provides inadequate information with which to form adequate prediction-control expectancies. Under such circumstances, dogs may depend more on direct sensory information, until a more adequate expectancy is formed. This shift from expectancies to reliance on sensory information may be highly disruptive and stressful. In addition to resorting to sensory information, dogs may also be more inclined to rely on instinctive or species-typical impulses to secure the environment. Under highly threatening social situations which violate a dog's prediction-control expectancies (e.g., *trust*), increased sensory vigilance and behavioral invigoration may facilitate intense aggressive arousal and significantly lower thresholds for aggressive behavior. Unfortunately, as a result, the dog may modify prediction-control expectancies so that, under similar circumstances in the future, it may learn to preemptively prepare and respond aggressively under minimal stimulation and continue doing so until the operative expectancy is disconfirmed.

Although prediction-control expectancies may accurately reflect reality, under the influence of adverse learning dogs may form faulty expectations that may not adequately represent actual circumstances. This risk is particularly problematical in the case of escape and avoidance learning, in which case the avoidance response may preemptively interfere with a dog learning that the response is no longer necessary to control the anticipated threat (see *A Cognitive Theory of Avoidance Learning* in Volume 1, Chapter 8). For avoidance to discontinue, the operative prediction-control expectancy guiding the behavior must be first disconfirmed (e.g., via graduated interactive exposure and response prevention) and replaced with an alternative expectancy more adequately fitted to the actual situation. In addition to forming specific expectancies, dogs also appear to appraise and interpret events in very subtle ways that predispose them to preferentially engage in certain behaviors rather than others. Cognitive appraisal assists dogs in modulating their moment-to-moment arousal levels as well as finely regulating appropriate actions to achieve a more subtle behavioral adaptation to the environment. These interpretive cognitive functions are especially evident in the case of complex social circumstances requiring a high degree of communication and cooperation, such as play. In the case of play, aggressive elements and sequences are interpreted in terms of the play partner's intention and various play metasignals confirming that the interaction is *just play*. Interpretive appraisal of the social intention of others provides the basis of communication. The mutual communication of intent determines whether competitive or cooperative behavior will ensue between interactants. Communication of intent may not only predict aggressive or affiliative action, it may also define the most likely outcome of the encounter. A highly motivated dog (e.g., starving) may show a very strong intent to defend a bowl of food, sufficient to cause a less hungry potential competitor to withdraw—even though under other circumstances the competitor may be dominant and the aggressor submissive. The way a dog interprets the intention of interaction strongly influences how it will respond to it. Petting or hugging coming from one person may be welcomed and reciprocated with expressions of shared affection, whereas the same actions coming from another person may be interpreted as a threat and, perhaps, evoke an aggressive response. Such interpretations of intent are strongly influenced by the quality of attachment and communication between the human and the dog. Interpretive appraisal of social intention under the influence of high levels of affection, familiarity, and trust appears to promote strong and durable inhibitory effects over aggression between closely bonded interactants.

Another important cognitive influence over aggressive behavior is cost-benefit assessment and risk taking. Engaging in aggressive conflict brings with it considerable risk. Cost-benefit assessment appears to play a significant role in the case of offensive aggression, where the goal is to achieve some benefit or resource. In the case of a starving dog, the risk of injury that may result from fighting is offset by the benefit of eating. In situations where the potential cost of behaving aggressively (loss or injury) exceeds what might be conceivably gained by the action, a dog is more likely to steer away from initiating an aggressive conflict. Aggression is most likely to occur in motivationally significant situations, where the risks of aggression are minimal (costs) and the potential benefits are substantial. Finally, dominant dogs appear to be more inclined to engage in risk-taking behavior, whereas submissive dogs may be more conservative and careful regarding risky behavior. A predisposition to take risks may be a genetically expressed trait that is more characteristic of dominant individuals than submissive ones. Submissive individuals may be genetically prone to avoid risk taking, unless the perception of risk is motivationally offset by a pressing biological need or threat and the potential benefit of success is sufficiently enticing.

A potential factor altering risk assessment abilities is stress. Quatermain and colleagues (1996) have found that stressed mice more rapidly engage in risk-taking behavior than unstressed controls. In the case of dogs, stress may lower thresholds for aggressive risk taking, causing otherwise submissive and compliant dogs to become periodically more irritable and aggressive. Stress appears to impair normal attention and memory functions (Mendl, 1999) and cortical impulse control over subcortical activity (Arnsten, 1998), potentially lowering behavioral thresholds for aggression or liberating species-typical offensive and defensive behavior in response to wrongly interpreted social signals. The systematic reduction of stress is an important aspect of effective behavior therapy. Such treatment efforts may facilitate risk-assessment normalization and improve other cognitive functions involved in the modulation of aggressive arousal and the regulatory control of aggressive behavior. A neural site of particular interest in this regard is the amygdala (see *Limbic System* in Volume 1, Chapter 3), which appears to serve a central role in social communication by mediating direct eye contact, by interpreting socially significant facial expressions, and by assessing the interactants emotional disposition and intent (Allman and Brothers, 1994). Under the dysfunctional influence of excessive stress, the intent of social signals may be distorted and misinterpreted, causing a dog to respond with inappropriate fear or aggression. The amygdala may play a particularly prominent role in the case of dominance-related aggression (Fonberg, 1988).

A NOMENCLATURE OF AGGRESSIVE BEHAVIOR

Functionally speaking, aggressive behavior, not stemming from idiopathic or pathological causes, can be viewed as an adaptive effort to establish control over some vital resource or situation that cannot be effectively controlled through other means. A variety of motivational and functional factors are presumed to influence the expression of aggressive behavior in dogs (Table 6.1). Obviously, these types of aggression exhibit a great deal of functional overlap. Although useful as a descriptive inventory, the list fails to provide a consistent functional framework for analyzing aggressive behavior. Instead, like other similar lists in the dog behavior literature, it brings together various forms of aggression under the discordant rubric of species-typical elicitors, physiological causes, and functional purposes. As a classification system, such discordance precludes productive analysis and the extraction of general principles.

Moyer (1968) has devised a classification system that is based primarily on stimuli or situational conditions that regularly evoke aggression (Table 6.2). Moyer's inventory of stimulus situations evocative of aggression ends up including general physiological and psychological influences as part of the evocative situation. The inclusion of instrumental learning is particularly confusing and discordant in the framework of the system's stated purpose. Instrumental learning may certainly influence a dog's propensity to bite, but such learning is not part of the evoking situation, at least not in the same sense, for example, as an intruder is part of a situation that evokes

territorial aggression. Instrumental learning does not logically belong to the list, especially if other forms of learning such as classical conditioning are excluded as situational influences—an exclusion that makes very little sense, given the inclusion of instrumental learning. But, most importantly, Moyer's taxonomy chiefly fails because it does not properly emphasize the very active and purposive character of aggressive behavior. Aggression is not just passively evoked by an adequate stimulus situation or physiological state. On the contrary, most often, aggressive behavior is guided by an intention to actively control or change the environment somehow, especially those parts of the environment that otherwise resist control or *bite* back.

Moyer's decision to include instrumental learning in his list of evocative situations underscores the vital role that learning plays in the acquisition and expression of aggressive behavior. Aggression is not merely a passive response to circumstances—it is more often an active and purposive effort aimed at obtaining various ends through the assertion of threats or attack. As such, aggression can be adequately understood and controlled only by recognizing that it is motivated and emitted under the influence of both emotional (reflexive) and purposive (instrumental) components. Functional aggressive behavior depends on the presence of significant setting events (broad contextual and motivational variables), transient emotional *establishing operations* (e.g., frustration, irritability, and anxiety), and an evocative target or situation toward which the threat or attack is directed. *The goal of aggression is control.* In effect, Moyer's taxonomy is an incomplete list of setting events, establishing operations, and targets under whose influence aggression is most likely to occur and *potentially result in reinforcement*—that is, result in enhanced control over the environment.

Although some forms of environmental stimulation may at times elicit *reflexive* attack (rage), such behavior is rather rare in comparison to the incidence of functionally integrated and purposive aggression. Aggression is often aimed at controlling the behavioral trajectory of another whose interests or

TABLE 6.1. Descriptive and functional characteristics of aggression

Behavior	Etiological factors	Description-function
Avoidance-motivated: Often socially insecure and incompetent.	Fear Anxiety Control Learning Socialization	Occurs in situations where the dog has learned that aggression successfully postpones or avoids an aversive stimulus or situation.
Control (dominance)-related: Dogs often lack appropriate boundaries and social inhibitions. Often limited to family members. Occurs around defended areas (e.g., bed, doorways, furniture) or items. Most often observed in male dogs.	Frustration Anxiety Learning Hormonal Genetics Socialization	Aggressive behavior occurring under a variety of situations involving competition and control. Dominance aggression generates social distance and establishes hiearchical stratification or status between socially familar competitors.
Dysfunctional: Explosive behavior may be related to PTSD (see *Low threshold*).	Frustration Anxiety Helplessness Learning Socialization	Occurring under inappropriate stimulus conditions and vastly exaggerated (disproportionate) within the context. Frequently, observed in cases involving dominance aggression.
Fear related: Attacks associated with postural signs of fear (e.g., lowered posture, tail down, ears back).	Fear Anxiety Helplessness Genetics Learning Socialization	Occurs only as a last resort when escape from an intensely fearful situation is not otherwise possible. Fear-related aggression is employed to escape but not to otherwise control or change the situation.
Idiopathic: May involve epilepsy.	Neurologicial Pathology Genetics	Aggression occurring as the result of unknown causes (see Pathophysiological).
Instrumental: Most forms of aggression are affected by learning.	Pain Anxiety Fear Frustration	Aggression enhanced or acquired through classical or instrumental learning but not specific to any single stimulus situation.
Intermale/interfemale: Aggression between females is most often seen among dogs sharing the same residence. Appears with sexual and social maturity.	Fear Dominance Hormonal Genetics Learning Socialization	Provoked by the close proximity of conspecifics of the same sex. Occasionally, dogs will fight with members of the opposite sex, but this is much less common.

TABLE 6.1. Descriptive and functional characteristics of aggression—*Continued*

Behavior	Etiological factors	Description-function
Irritable: Results from painful stimulation associated with injury, various grooming and veterinary procedures.	Pain Fear Frustration Pathology Genetics	Associated with situations involving cumulative stress: crowding, frustration, punishment, pain, and deprivation. Includes threats, biting, and scratching to escape painful stimulation.
Low threshold: Aggressive behavior occurring with little or no apparent provocation or warning. Commonly associated with dominance aggression and so-called springer rage syndrome.	Frustration Anxiety Neurological Helplessness Learning Socialization	A form of dysfunctional agression occurring in cases where normal inhibtions and central control over aggressive behavior is compromised—sometimes referred to as episodic dyscontrol syndrome.
Maternal: May be directed toward inanimate objects when pseudopregnancy is present.	Hormonal Genetics	Occurs when the nesting area or young are approached. Most often directed toward strangers.
Pathophysiological: If should be considered especially in the cases of aggressive behavior with an acute onset and presenting under poorly defined triggers.	Hormonal Genetics Pathology	Results from various underlying physical causes from hypothyroidism (Reinhard, 1978; Dodd, 1992; Dodman and Mertens, 1995) to various neurological disorders (neurogenic) such as epilepsy (Holliday et al., 1970). The role of hypothyroidism in aggressive behavior remains controversial (Polsky, 1993).
Playful: May be directed toward the owner as a nuisance. Excessive mouthing and biting on hands and clothing.	Competition Learning Socialization	Noninjurious aggressive displays during playful encounters, including stalking, pouncing, bumping, gentle biting, and pawing.

(*continued*)

TABLE 6.1. Descriptive and functional characteristics of aggression—*Continued*

Behavior	Etiological factors	Description-function
Possessive: Although commonly associated with dominance-related aggression, it may also occur independently. Appears in puppyhood and thoughout the life cycle.	Frustration Anxiety Learning Socialization	A form of aggression provoked by competition over a possession like a toy or food item.
Predatory: Distinguished from other forms of aggression by the absensce of affective arousal.	Learning Genetics Socialization	Attack released by the presence of prey animals or preylike stimulation. Most often triggered by fleeing movement.
Protective:	Fear Anxiety Learning Genetics Training	Agression emitted in the context of a socially significant other that would not likely occur otherwise.
Redirected: Commonly observed when an owner attempts to break up a dog fight.	Fear Frustration Anxiety Socialization Pain	Threat or attack that occurs when agression is blocked toward a preferred target and directed instead toward a more immediately available one.
Territorial defense:	Fear Anxiety Control Learning Training	Aggression that is directed toward a target intruding on an established territory.
Trained:	Frustration Anxiety Control Learning Play	Aggressive behavior that has been systematically agitated and brought under the control of specific releasing and inhibitory cues (e.g., protection-dog training).
Xenopic: See *Fear-related aggression*.	Fear Anxiety Genetics Learning Socialization	Agression that is directed toward strangers regardless of situation or territorial priority.

Table 6.2. Moyer's taxonomy of aggressive behavior

Predatory: evoked by a prey animal.

Intermale: evoked by the presence of a strange male conspecific.

Fear induced: preceded by efforts to escape a threatening situation.

Irritable: evoked by pain, frustration, deprivation, and other stressors and directed toward either animate or inanimate targets.

Territorial: evoked by an intruder entering an established territory.

Maternal: evoked by an intruder perceived as a threat by a mother to her young.

Sex related: evoked by the same behavior that elicits sexual behavior.

Instrumental: enhancement of any of the above through learning.

intentions conflict or collide with the aggressor's interests or intentions (see *Control-seeking Vector Analysis of Territory* in Chapter 7). Control-related aggression denotes any threat or attack aimed at controlling another animal or person, especially in response to social challenges and conflicts or intrusive threats on territory. Finally, control-related aggression is typically employed under adverse conditions (involving heightened frustration, anxiety, or irritability) to control social prerogatives, biological imperatives, or territorial space (any area defended by the dog). Dogs exhibiting aggressive behavior typically do so to secure or defend some vital resource or place against unwanted intrusion or to counter a perceived or actual threat asserted by a rival.

PREDATORY BEHAVIOR

Moyer's inclusion of predatory attack as a form of aggression alongside fear-induced or irritable attack is questionable and potentially misleading. As previously mentioned, predatory behavior might best be treated under some independent category such as "killing for food." This seems appropriate, since predatory behavior is not primarily motivated by affective arousal (anger). In addition, predatory aggression or *quiet attack* typically occurs without signs of sympathetic arousal. In contrast, affective attack is distinguished by the presence of strong sympathetic arousal and

anger. Predatory behavior appears to belong to a distinct behavioral and neurological system operating independently of affective aggression, perhaps involving the appetitive seeking system (Panksepp, 1998). An interesting neurobiological finding in this regard is the observation that the neurotransmitter norepinephrine inhibits predatory aggression while facilitating affective aggression like fighting (Siegel and Edinger, 1981). These findings (and many others like them) support the assumption that predatory aggression and affective aggression are mediated by very different biological and behavioral systems (see *Neurobiology of Aggression* [*Hypothalamus*] in Volume 1, Chapter 3). Although predation belongs to an independent motivational system, predatory behavior may be influenced by coactive anxious and frustrative influences that may ultimately lead to the expression of *affective aggression,* a possibility emphasized by Panksepp:

> Of course, this does not mean that the whole predatory attack sequence or any other real-life emotional pattern ever remains under the control of a single emotional system. A predator surely experiences irritability or frustration if the prey struggles so vigorously that it seems liable to escape. Thus, in real life, there are sudden shifts in emotions depending upon the success or failure of specific behavioral acts, as well as in the changing cognitive expectations and appraisals of each situation. (193)

None of the foregoing should be construed to imply that predatory aggression is innocuous or in any sense less dangerous than other forms of canine aggression. Predatory motivations have been implicated in several cases involving vicious maulings and deaths of humans by dog packs (Borchelt et al., 1983). In one of these cases, a large pack of eight dogs, with a known history of predatory behavior, attacked and killed a 14-year-old boy who was riding a motorcycle. Reportedly, the pack had been observed earlier attacking a deer that they had brought down but that managed to escape. This incident occurred approximately 1 hour prior to the attack on the boy. In another incident, a pack of dogs attacked an 11-year-old boy who survived severe injuries to report hearing the dogs "baying, as if chasing something" approximately 15 minutes before the attack. In both cases, there appears to have been a frustrated or redirected predatory motivation involved in the attacks, suggesting that some forms of "predation" are motivated by more than simple hunger and nonaffective neural circuitry. Another case involved a pack of several dogs that was kept by an elderly couple in rural Indiana (Figure 6.2). The dogs, which were permitted to run free, attacked a 10-year-old girl riding her bicycle near the couple's property. In an effort to escape the attack, the child ran into a nearby wooded area, where she was later found dead. The child received numerous wounds and parts of her flesh had been torn away and apparently eaten by the dogs (Borchelt et al., 1983). Winkler (1977) reviews the case histories of 11 fatal dog attacks and cites "threatening behavior or territorial invasion" as the most common causes, without mentioning the possible role of predation or a history of predatory behavior in the dogs involved. Although not mentioned specifically, several of the cases he describes are not entirely inconsistent with a predatory interpretation. Incidentally, of the nine cases where the sex of the dog was known, males accounted for seven of the attacks, with the remaining incidents involving a female and a male and female pair. These data suggest that male dogs may be at a significantly greater risk of delivering a fatal attack than are female dogs.

GENETICS AND AGGRESSION

There appears to exist a strong heritable factor affecting the predisposition of dogs to behave aggressively. Numerous studies have identified a genetic influence affecting animal behavior in the opposing directions of increased fearful behavior, on the one hand, and increased aggression, on the other (see *Genetic Predisposition and Temperament* in Volume 1, Chapter 5). In general, domestication has exerted selective

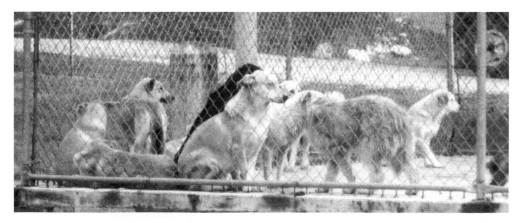

FIG. 6.2. Under the influence of packing behavior, large groups of dogs can represent a serious predatory threat. These dogs were involved in a fatal attack on a young girl who was riding her bicycle near their home property. (Photo courtesy of V. L. Voith.)

pressure toward behavioral thresholds conducive to reduced fear and aggression, thereby making dogs more socially responsive and tamable by humans (Price, 1999). Although the general trend has been toward a reduction of fear and aggression, significant variations of excitability exist between breeds and individuals within these different breeds. With respect to aggression, some dog breeds appear, on the whole, to be more aggressive and reactive than others to emotionally provocative stimulation. Scott and Fuller (1965), for example, found clear differences in the aggressive behavior of different breeds emerging at an early age. Of the five breeds observed and tested, they found wirehaired fox terriers to be the most aggressive, basenjis and shelties somewhat less aggressive, and beagles and cocker spaniels much less aggressive. Hart and Hart (1985b) analyzed the cumulative opinions of 48 veterinarians and 48 obedience judges with respect to the ranking of 56 breeds according to 13 behavioral traits. They found that the surveyed professionals shared significant uniformity in their assessment of various traits, enabling the authors to perform a cluster analysis for the various breeds represented in terms of such things as their relative aggressiveness, trainability, and reactivity. Their results show some conformity with Scott and Fuller's earlier findings. For example, the fox terrier is included in the cluster characterized by "very high aggression, high reactivity, medium trainability," whereas beagles and cocker spaniels are included together under the cluster "high reactivity, low trainability, medium aggression." Although such statistical studies as the above represent a good starting point, the results are difficult to generalize because they are limited to personal opinions about behavior—not objective assessments. Even the opinions of professionals are subject to considerable individual and cultural bias. In other words, the study tells us more about how veterinarians and obedience judges feel about the behavior of various breeds than it tells us about the actual behavior of the breeds specified. To make the results reliable with respect to dog breeds, they must be validated by comparison with more objective assessment tests and experimental observations of breed differences, such as provided by Scott and Fuller's work.

A putative heritable factor in the expression of dominance-related aggression has been identified in the English springer spaniel (ESS). As the result of a random national survey of ESS owners, Reisner (1997) found what appears to be a significant breed disposition toward developing dominance-related aggression. She reported that 26% of the ESS had bitten someone, with 65% of those persons bitten being family members or people with whom the dog was familiar. In addition, 48% of the dogs had growled at, snapped at, or bitten family members in a dominance-related context. Finally, the tendency to exhibit dominance aggression was associated with dogs coming from one particular kennel, suggesting the possibility of a popular sire effect. The influence of breed predisposition is apparent in some epidemiological studies of reported dog bites (Wright, 1991). Although mixed breeds are most often implicated in biting incidents, representing between 41.1% and 47.4% of bites reported, some specific purebred dogs appear to represent a greater risk than others. For example, Gershman and colleagues reported that German shepherds and chow chows were most likely to bite nonhousehold members, victims who were often children. It should be emphasized, however, that interpreting breed-related bite statistics is fraught with difficulties (Lockwood, 1995), not the least of which is breed identification. Many dogs may be misidentified and lumped together under a particular breed. Also, as Wright points out, statistical bite rates relative to breed must be carefully weighted against the numbers of a particular breed living in the geographical area from which the sample is derived—a requirement that is not usually satisfied by statistical analyses comparing dog bite rates by breed.

HORMONES AND AGGRESSIVE BEHAVIOR

Increased competitiveness and aggressive behavior are often associated with hormonal changes occurring around puberty, a biological change that may lower the threshold for several significant sex-related behavior patterns, including intermale and interfemale aggression. While lowering the threshold for general activity, urine marking, and aggressive behavior, the threshold for pain and fear may be elevated under the influence of these various hormones.

Stress Hormones and Aggression

The effects of endogenous hormones on aggressive behavior are evident in wild canids. A lower threshold for aggressive behavior is exhibited by both male and female wolves during the annual mating season, when both sexes show an increased tendency to engage in sex-related aggressive behavior (Derix et al., 1993). This sharp increase in aggressive behavior is probably mediated by a number of interacting hormonal systems. The alpha female can be particularly intolerant and hostile toward her female subordinates. McLeod et al. (1995) have shown that the upsurge of aggressive activity among captive wolves is especially stressful (by cortisol measures) on the lowest-ranking female and the second-ranking male.

Increased corticosteroid levels may play an indirect role in regulating sexual and competitive activity among wolves. Only the dominant female comes into full estrus and whelps young. Estrus in subordinate females is suppressed by some external cause, possibly as the result of the dominant female's continuous harassment and badgering before, during, and after the mating season. Estrus may be blocked by stress-mediated mechanisms involving corticosteroid secretions or related physiological mechanisms, such as stress-mediated suppression of luteinizing hormone (Sapolsky, 1990, 1994). In addition to impeding reproductive activity in subordinate females, stress produced by aggressive interaction between wolves appears to reduce the sex drive of subordinate males, as well. Consequently, the increase of aggressive interaction during the mating season may serve to "disable" rivals sexually and competitively, while helping to achieve an optimal physiological state for reproduction in the dominant or alpha pair.

It is interesting to note in this regard that Sapolsky (1990) found that dominant males among free-ranging olive baboons showed distinct differences in cortisol concentrations, depending on the presence or absence of five personality traits. Dominant baboons were most likely to have optimally low cortisol concentrations, if (1) they were able to differentiate between threats and neutral interaction, (2) they initiated the fight with the threatening rival, (3) they won the fight they initiated, (4) they exhibited differentiated behavior after winning or losing a fight, and (5) they redirected aggression toward another baboon when they lost a fight. Dominant males not exhibiting these traits tended to have cortisol levels similar to those of subordinate males.

Sex Hormones: Estrogen, Testosterone, and Progesterone

Estrogen (estradiol) levels are highest during proestrus, with progesterone levels increasing as the female enters estrus. Progesterone appears to exercise a modulatory effect over estrogen, and only after estrogen levels begin to fall will the female become receptive toward the male. Also, as estrus is approached, circulating testosterone in female dogs reaches plasma levels that are comparable to those in male dogs (Olsen et al., 1984). The various sex hormones are closely related steroidal compounds, with testosterone being easily biosynthesized from progesterone and estradiol synthesized from testosterone (Johnson, 1998).

Estrogen affects dog behavior in many ways: it increases general activity levels, promotes increased urine output and marking, increases vocalization, and stimulates nervous arousal in female dogs (Hart, 1985). All of these changes are the result of estrogen's threshold-lowering effects on the female brain, especially involving target areas mediating the expression of proestrus sexual behavior needed to attract a mate. Progesterone, on the other hand, appears to exercise an opposite effect to that of estrogen by generally elevating behavioral thresholds and asserting a calming effect on dogs and enhancing their receptivity to intimate contact. In high doses, progesterone may even induce general anesthesia. Not all practitioners agree on the anti-aggression effects of progesterone. For example, Overall (1997) directly implicates progesterone as an aggression-facilitating hormone, noting that "high levels of aggression in hamsters are associated with the presence of progesterone" (97). Although progesterone may facilitate certain forms of aggression under the influence of certain hormonal environments in certain species (Archer, 1988), the general contention that progesterone promotes aggressive behavior does not appear to be supported by the weight of experimental evidence (Kislak and Beach, 1955; Fraile et al., 1987) and the clinical impressions of many practitioners who use progesterone to control aggressive behavior in dogs. Several laboratory and clinical reports have noted the threshold-elevating effects of progesterone on aggression in both male (testosterone environment) and female (estrogen environment) animals, including intact dogs (Voith, 1980c; Joby et al., 1984) and other domestic species exhibiting undesirable aggressive behavior (Hart, 1985; Houpt, 1991). As of 1991, Houpt described the progestins as the "most effective pharmacological treatment of aggression now available" (66). Progestins in the form of megestrol acetate (Ovaban) or long-lasting injections of medroxyprogesterone (Depo-Provera) *were* frequently administered to control aggression in dogs. Unfortunately, progestins produce a number of potential side effects, including diabetes mellitus, mammary tumors, sterility in intact males, and excessive weight gain. Coupled with the growing popularity of psychotropics, the use of progestins has become much less common. In combination with appropriate behavior modification, however, progestin therapy remains a viable short-term adjunctive treatment for the control of some forms of intractable intermale aggression and other sexually dimorphic behavior problems (Hart and Eckstein, 1998).

Adult sensitivity to androgens and estrogens may be influenced by perinatal exposure to these sexual hormones. Simon and Whalen (1987) found that female mice treated with testosterone or estrogen on the day of birth exhibited an enhanced responsiveness to the hormone upon reaching adulthood. Testosterone-treated mice showed increased aggressiveness in response to testosterone but not to estrogen, whereas estrogen-treated mice selectively responded to estrogen but not to testosterone.

Male and female sexual hormones play an important regulatory role in the expression of sex-related intraspecific aggression. Whether such hormones play a significant role in the expression of interspecific aggression (e.g., toward people) remains an open question. Although testosterone has been often implicated as a facilitating hormone, its role in the expression of aggressive behavior is anything but clear and straightforward. Both androgens and estrogens appear to facilitate aggression, especially during the mating season. Perhaps the facilitative effects of sex hormones on aggression are mediated indirectly by the activation of sex-related emotions and drives, making aggression most likely to occur in the presence of species-typical triggers shown by conspecifics operating under the influence of similar hormonal changes.

Effects of Castration on Aggressive Behavior

The importance of sexual hormones for the modulation of aggressive behavior has long been recognized. However, the effect of hormones on dog behavior is ambiguous and highly variable. Endogenous sexual hormones appear to play a role in the development of some behavior problems (Borchelt, 1983; Wright and Nesselrote, 1987). The relationship between androgens and unwanted behavior is especially evident in the case of aggression, where male dogs present much more often than females—as much as 90% more often by some estimates (Voith and Borchelt, 1982). In general, males also present more frequently than females with other common behavior problems (Hart and Hart, 1985a), including playfulness, destructiveness, snapping at children, territorial defense, and general activity excesses. According to the Harts' study, females are more trainable, easier to house train, and more affectionate. Areas where no significant differences between the sexes were found include watchdog barking, nuisance barking, and general excitability. Voith and Borchelt (1996) reported similar findings indicating that male dogs present more frequently with behavior problems than females (Figure 6.3).

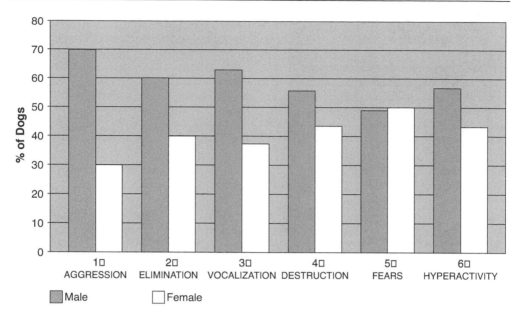

FIG. 6.3. Distribution of behavior problems by sex (N = 1718). Males tend to present more often with various common behavior complaints, which suggests the presence of a hormonal influence underlying the development of some behavior problems. From Voith and Borchelt (1996).

From such data, one might suppose that a more or less direct causal connection exists between the presence of male hormones and increased tendency to behave aggressively. However, such a robust causal relationship between hormones and aggression does not appear to exist. This lack of a definitive cause-effect relationship is evident in the highly variable effect of castration on behavior. Contrary to common belief, castration often fails to affect offensive and defensive aggression significantly; neither does it typically have a significant effect on a dog's general activity level. In general, castration appears to exert its strongest influence over sexually dimorphic behavior patterns, such as intermale aggression, urine marking, mounting, and roaming. Neilson and coworkers (1997) found that such behavior was reduced between 50% and 90% following castration.

Many studies have been performed to evaluate the effects of castration on male behavior. For instance, Beach (1970) carried out a series of experiments investigating the effects of castration on the sexual behavior of dogs.

The dogs included in his study were experienced copulators. If testosterone predominantly controls or mediates the expression of copulatory behavior, then one would expect to observe a sharp decline in sexual activity in castrated dogs. However, Beach found that castration had limited effects, with no apparent effect on sexual response latency or mounting frequency in the dogs he observed over the study period, though he did find a reduced frequency of intromission and more brief durations of coital lock.

These findings are consistent with the effects observed after castration on other sexually dimorphic male behavior patterns like aggression, roaming, urinary scent marking, mounting, and intermale fighting. Although such behavior patterns are not always entirely eliminated by castration, their frequency and magnitude may be reduced—occasionally very significantly so. In the case of agonistic displays, one should expect a slight general modulation in the direction of reduction, especially in terms of the intensity/duration of episodes and the tendency for aggression to escalate. Also, the denouement phase following an episode may be much more steep following castration than before. The effect of castration is one of degree and subtlety—an effect that is often unobserved and unappreciated by the owner.

Some hormonal factor probably exists in the etiology of dominance aggression, since males exhibit the behavior problem more often than females, but the cause and source of this effect may be largely independent of a dog's adult sexual status. The most likely mechanism for the effect of hormones on aggressive behavior is androgen-mediated perinatal differentiation of neural tissue. Early ontogenetic exposure to sex hormones may facilitate the elaboration of sexually dimorphic circuits modulating respective threshold differences between males and females for the display of aggressive behavior as adults.

If testosterone actually plays a significant role in the expression of aggression, one might reasonably expect to see increased signs of it between 6 to 8 months of age, when dogs undergo an endogenous surge of androgen activity (Hart, 1985). Although many dogs do appear to go through an *adolescent adjustment phase* around this period, it is not a statistically significant time frame for the expression of dominance-related aggression, although dogs may become more competitive and difficult and become more aggressive toward other male dogs. Tinbergen (1958/1969) describes some of these apparent and dramatic effects of the adolescent hormonal surge observed among free-ranging huskies in Greenland:

> We followed the behavior of two young males carefully and found, to our surprise, that when they were about eight months old they suddenly began to join their pack in fights with their neighbors. In the very same week their trespassing upon other territories became a thing of the past. And it was probably no coincidence that in that same week both made their first attempts to mate with a female in their own pack. (34)

Castration is often recommended as a means for controlling dominance-related and other forms of aggression (Borchelt and Voith,

1986). The most commonly cited study concerning the therapeutic efficacy of castration on behavior was performed by Hopkins and colleagues (1976) (Figure 6.4). Unfortunately, the study examined a very small sample of dogs (N = 42) and was poorly controlled. The authors noted striking improvement in dogs exhibiting various behavior problems, including roaming (16 dogs, 90% improved), mounting (15 dogs, 67% improved), intermale fighting (8 dogs, 62% improved), and urine scent marking (10 dogs, 50% improved). Both territorial aggression (8 dogs) and fear-related aggression (4 dogs) showed no improvement following castration: "The subjective reports of the present study substantiate the contentions by others that only aggressive behavior toward other males is altered by castration" (1110). One potential source of error in the study was the fact that most of the dogs (37 of 42) involved were castrated to curb an unwanted behavior problem in the first place, perhaps biasing the owners' observations to some extent in the direction of a placebo effect. The owners might have also picked up a few tips on how to control their dog's unwanted behavior, thereby confounding the results. Additional support for the putative benefits of castration on dominance-related aggression have been reported by Neilson and colleagues (1997), who found that 25% of dogs exhibiting aggression toward family members improved between 50% and 90% after castration.

Finally, testosterone appears to be released following competitive victories, whereas a decrease of circulating testosterone follows defeats (Kreutz et al., 1972). The differential increase or decrease of testosterone may affect the relative physical size (anabolic effect) of dominant and subordinate animals, lower aggression thresholds, and increase the magnitude of aggressive behavior. Increased testosterone levels may also provide a source of positive reinforcement for the successful combatant, perhaps promoting feelings of well-being and elation that occur as the result of the victory. Testosterone appears to facilitate aggressive arousal and preparatory reflexes conducive to agonistic success. For example, the direct stare and focused readiness commonly

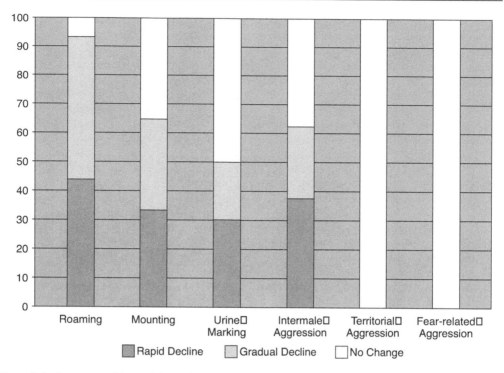

FIG. 6.4. Percentage of dogs exhibiting behavior changes involving various problems following castration. After Hopkins et al. (1976).

preceding dominance contests may be mediated by testosterone. Many studies involving a variety of species have shown that testosterone enhances selective attention in the direction of the target while simultaneously reducing distraction to extraneous stimuli (Archer, 1988). Attention control is a significant factor in the modification of such behavior. Once attention is frozen on the target, it is very difficult to disrupt or divert it, making it of utmost importance to capture the dog's attention during the earliest stages of aggressive arousal. In addition to possibly reducing the reward value of successful aggressive competition, castration may serve to reduce preparatory arousal and decrease the dog's ability to focus its attention fully on the target of attack, thereby making it more easy to divert or disrupt the dog's agonistic intentions and direct the dog into incompatible counterconditioning activities. Consequently, although castration alone may not eliminate aggression, it may make aggression problems more responsive to management and control efforts.

Effects of Prepubertal Castration on Behavior

Some veterinarians and humane groups have promoted early castration as a viable population and behavioral control measure, claiming that prepubertal castration produces superior effects over the current practice of performing castration and spay surgeries at 6 months of age. The evidence supporting this opinion is mixed and controversial. For example, on the pro side of the debate, Lieberman (1987) reports findings based on the results of a questionnaire generated by the Medford, Oregon, SPCA spay and neuter program. The study collected and compared information on about 400 dogs that had been castrated at different ages. The sample was divided into two groups: (1) 200 puppies castrated at 6 to 12 weeks of age, and (2) 200 puppies castrated after 6 months of age. According to Lieberman's survey, the male dog's unwanted sexual and aggressive behaviors were significantly reduced by prepubertal castration when compared to the group of dogs castrated after 6 months of age. If valid, these findings contradict the observation by Hopkins and colleagues (1976) that the "age of the dog does not seem to have a pronounced influence on the effectiveness of the operation" (1110).

On the con side, Lieberman's findings have been challenged by a controlled study carried out by Salmeri and coworkers (1991), who found that puppies castrated at both 7 weeks and 7 months exhibited little positive difference in significant behavioral parameters (for example, barking, playfulness, aggression toward other dogs, affection toward people, and outgoing nature)—*all significant traits were unaffected by castration.* The only behavioral traits influenced by castration were excitability and general activity, but both in a direction opposite to what one might expect; that is, *dogs castrated early in life tended to become more excitable and active than intact controls.* Even in cases involving intermale fighting, few dogs exhibited significant improvement after castration, although the tendency to fight appears to have been modulated to some extent. Perhaps castrates are less attractive as aggressive opponents for intact males. Finally, Jagoe and Serpell (1988) question the effectiveness of prepubertal castration in 6- to 12-week-old puppies, arguing that the surgery may be detrimental to a dog's health, but they present no significant evidence to support their concern and warning. Although the scientific evidence is mixed, the selective use of early castration might be seriously considered in puppies exhibiting signs of excessive aggression at an early age.

Effects of Spaying on Female Aggressive Behavior

Voith and Borchelt (1982) reported observing a tendency of some female dogs to exhibit an increase in dominance-related aggressive behavior after spaying. The authors speculate that female dogs displaying such tendencies may have been exposed to fetal androgenization, resulting in their malelike behavioral characteristics (see *Perinatal Androgenization* in Chapter 7). Spaying may predispose such dogs to express these undesirable androgynous traits. O'Farrell and Peachey (1990) observed a similar effect in a subgroup of spayed female dogs. They compared the behavior of 150 spayed females with a matched (breed and age) control group of 150 nonspayed females. Spayed females showed a significant increase in dominance-related aggression following surgery, especially if they were under 1 year of age and had exhibited aggressive behavior prior to spaying. In addition, Podberscek and Serpell (1996) have reported that females spayed *before* exhibiting aggression were more likely to exhibit aggression toward children.

Progestin as a Testosterone Antagonist

Joby and colleagues (1984) performed a series of studies to investigate the effects of oral progestins on the behavior of intact male dogs. The sample included 163 dogs with a variety of behavior problems, ranging from dominance aggression to destructiveness. The dogs were administered a daily dose of megestrol acetate (1 mg/kg or 4 mg/kg—30 dogs required the higher dose) over the course of 2 or 3 weeks of treatment, depending on the dog's response to treatment. Most of the dogs exhibited more than one unwanted behavior problem. Of the 163 dogs presented for treatment, 123 (75%) showed improvement at the conclusion of a brief exposure to megestrol acetate. An interesting aspect of the study is the broad effect that progestin treatment had on remote behaviors not directly related to a sexual motivation, such as dominance-related aggression (79% improved), fear-related aggression (71%), destructiveness (79%), and excitability (73%). The primary side effects reported (in 36 dogs) by the authors was an increase in appetite and lethargy. After 3 months off medication, many of the dogs continued to exhibit lasting improvement, although some had relapsed somewhat. Recidivism was especially evident in the case of dominance aggression and household urine marking. The broad benefits of progestin are probably due to its general tranquilizing and anesthetic effects (Knol and Egberink-Alink, 1989a,b).

Note: Although the authors reported minimal side effects, the use of progestin therapy is now widely criticized because of the availability of alternative medications and the potential for serious side effects resulting from long-term use of such hormones.

Pseudopregnancy

Pseudopregnancy or *pseudocyesis* is a hormone-mediated condition that may reduce functional thresholds for aggressive behavior. Pseudopregnancy occurs in female dogs, usually 6 to 8 weeks after estrus, but in some cases not presenting for 4 or 5 months after estrus. In addition to mammary enlargement or lactation, various behavioral signs may present with the condition, including toy adopting, nesting behavior, hyperactivity, destructiveness, and aggression. Aggression thresholds may be generally lowered during the period of pseudopregnancy, with aggressive behavior being particularly likely to occur when the dog's nesting area or toy surrogates are approached. Destructiveness involving digging into sofas and carpeting may also occur during pseudopregnancy. Voith (1980b) has speculated that pseudopregnancy may have served an adaptive function for the dog's ancestors. She argues that the physical and behavioral changes associated with pseudopregnancy may be the result of evolutionary pressures favoring the communal care of young by closely related females belonging to the mother's group. Spaying is commonly recommended in the literature to control the problem (Houpt, 1991); however, spaying a dog while she is still exhibiting signs of pseudopregnancy may significantly protract the condition (Voith, 1980b), perhaps causing it to persist for years in some cases (Harvey et al., 1999). Consequently, spaying should be undertaken only after signs of pseudopregnancy have disappeared (approximately 4 to 6 weeks). Further, some females may develop signs of pseudopregnancy only after spaying, perhaps helping to explain some of the increased incidence of aggression in females after the surgery. In this regard, Borchelt (1983) found that spayed females were significantly more likely to engage in possessive aggression than intact counterparts. Further, in the only cases involving dominance aggression in intact females, it was later discovered that the females were under the influence of pseudopregnancy. Symptoms of pseudopregnancy are often controlled with sex hormones [e.g., progestins (Hart and Hart, 1985a)].

NUTRITION AND AGGRESSION

A great deal of speculation exists concerning the effects of nutrition on behavior, but little scientific knowledge is known about these effects. Animal behavior consultants commonly cite this or that nutritional imbalance as being responsible for causing or predisposing dogs to a exhibit a particular behavioral problem. Recommendations ranging from supplemental B complex for aggressive behavior to massive doses of calcium and other minerals for destructiveness have never been demonstrated clinically or in the laboratory. Campbell (1992), for example, claims that a positive correlation exists between relative protein/carbohydrate proportions in a dog's diet and general excitability levels. High protein levels supposedly decrease excitability while at the same time producing various benefits such as increased trainability. In the opposite direction, high carbohydrate levels are believed to increase excitability and promote distractibility. In addition, he recommends supplementing his stress diet with B complex as nutritional "insurance," even though the dog appears healthy without it. Unfortunately, no experimental data are presented to support these various recommendations or the hypotheses on which they are founded.

Over the past several years, a growing concern has been expressed regarding the effects of food coloring and chemical preservatives on the development of hyperactivity and other behavior problems (see *Dietary Factors and Hyperactivity* in Chapter 5). One result of this concern has been the production of a new generation of diets containing fewer additives—a change in dog food manufacturing that can do no harm, but the potential good of such diets is not clearly known or demonstrated. Research on this topic is scanty and, at present, little scientific evidence exists showing a direct causal relationship between food additives and the incidence of behavior problems in dogs.

However, some evidence does suggest that adjusting dietary protein levels may provide a viable means for influencing the behavioral thresholds of some forms of aggressive behavior (see *Diet and Serotonin Activity* in Volume

1, Chapter 3). For example, Mugford (1987) reported observing a significant decrease in aggressive behavior in a group of golden retrievers after they were placed on a low-protein diet. More recently, a multiclinic study that compared the effects of low-protein versus high-protein diets on aggressive behavior in dogs found that reducing dietary protein levels exerted a beneficial influence in dogs exhibiting territory-related aggression with fear (Dodman et al., 1996). The strongest evidence for a linkage between aggression and dietary protein levels has come from basic brain research. Numerous studies have indicated that dietary protein levels significantly affect the amount of tryptophan reaching the brain for the manufacture of serotonin (Spring, 1986; Christensen, 1996). Paradoxically, high levels of circulating protein in the blood may deprive the brain of adequate tryptophan. This effect is due to a transport mechanism responsible for the selective transfer of nutrients from the blood into the brain. When the blood contains high levels of protein, other relatively more abundant circulating amino acids compete with tryptophan for a limited number of transport molecules, thereby causing an impediment of tryptophan transport into the brain. This situation can be nutritionally modified by simultaneously lowering dietary protein levels while increasing the intake of carbohydrates. The ingestion of carbohydrate-laden foods stimulates the secretion of insulin. Insulin biochemically alters competing amino acids, causing them to move into surrounding muscle tissue. The net result is that tryptophan obtains a numerical advantage over other amino acids competing for limited transport channels providing passage through the blood-brain barrier.

Serotonin serves many important functions as a neurotransmitter, especially the management of stress, impulse control, and mood regulation. Decreased serotonin activity is associated with depression and increased irritability. Many antidepressant psychotropics are believed to work by increasing serotonergic activity. When serotonin levels are low, dogs may become more impulsive and irritable and exhibit a lowered threshold for aggressive behavior. Diets adjusted toward decreased protein intake (less than 18%) coupled with increased carbohydrate intake appear to exercise a mild threshold-raising influence, perhaps by enhancing serotonin-mediated impulse control and improving the brain's ability to manage stress. Recently, DeNapoli and colleagues (2000) have reported evidence suggesting that supplementation of the canine diet with tryptophan may exercise a significant modulatory effect over certain forms of aggressive behavior. In the case of dominance aggression, tryptophan supplementation of high-protein diets yielded a significant decrease in aggression scores. In the case of territorial aggression, scores were most strongly reduced in dogs that were fed a low-protein diet supplemented with tryptophan. Although this research is promising, increasing nutritional tryptophan levels may not necessarily result in an appreciable increase of serotonin production. Above a certain point, the rate-limiting factor, tryptophan hydroxylase, is saturated and unable to support further synthesis of 5-hydroxytryptophan (5-HTP)—the immediate precursor of serotonin (5-HT) (Christensen, 1996). Given the aforementioned limitation, supplementing the protocol diet with 5-HTP might have proved significantly more efficacious for enhancing serotonin production. In addition to being more directly and efficiently converted into serotonin than tryptophan, 5-HTP moves more freely through the blood-brain barrier (not needing to compete for transport molecules). Furthermore, unlike tryptophan, which remains banned from over-the-counter sale, 5-HTP is readily available and sold at health food stores (Murray, 1998)—a significant consideration if 5-HTP is ultimately shown to exert a beneficial effect on aggression problems in the dog.

ROLE OF INTEGRATED COMPLIANCE AND OBEDIENCE TRAINING

Most treatment programs for aggression problems incorporate some element of obedience training (Tortora, 1983; Blackshaw, 1991; Clark and Boyer, 1993; Reisner, 1997) or nonconfrontational compliance training (Line and Voith, 1986; Campbell, 1992; Overall, 1997). According to Tortora (1983), the benefits of obedience training depend on treated dogs learning that safety can always be obtained by engaging in cooperative behavior. Similarly, Clark and Boyer (1993) have argued that obedience training promotes a "feeling of security" as the result of establishing clear lines of communication and social boundaries by selectively and consistently applying incentives and appropriate deterrents to guide and shape dog behavior. The efficacy of obedience training as a therapeutic tool has been confirmed by Blackshaw (1991), who reported a high success rate involving dominance and territorial aggression by introducing proper restraint techniques and obedience training as her primary form of behavioral intervention. Even those individuals who appear to discount the preventative value of obedience training as a *placebo,* exerting "neither positive nor negative effects on the incidence of behavior problems" (Cameron, 1997:271), may nonetheless recommend such training because "obedience training provides tools for owners to use in modifying pet behavior" (271). Finally, nonconfrontational compliance training utilizes the most simple obedience exercises (e.g., sit and sit-stay) and positive reinforcement to achieve secondary control over the expression of aggressive behavior (Voith, 1980a; Uchida et al., 1997).

Despite the apparent therapeutic efficacy of obedience and nonconfrontational compliance training, the role of such activities for the prevention of behavior problems remains controversial. Although the literature is conflicted and equivocal on the preventative value of training, many authors, nonetheless, suggest that training does appear to exert a strong preventative influence. For example, Overall (1997), an advocate of preventative compliance training, has claimed that dogs require *rules* and need a rule-based social structure to communicate and cooperate with one another and with humans, claiming that her type of compliance training (a highly intrusive variation on Voith's "nothing in life is free" program) provides a means for "preventing such problems and in treating all forms of behavioral problems" (410).

But the question remains: Does obedience or compliance training serve to prevent problems, especially aggression problems? With respect to obedience training, Voith and colleagues (1992) suggest that it may not perform a preventative function. In a study involving the analysis of 711 questionnaires filled out by dog owners visiting a veterinary hospital clinic, they found that obedience training (as well as spoiling activities and anthropomorphic attitudes) showed no significant correlation with a wide spectrum of behavior problems, including aggression. A subsequent study performed by Podberscek and Serpell (1996) also failed to show a linkage between obedience training and the incidence of aggression problems in English cocker spaniels (N = 596). Finally, in a case-controlled study involving 178 matched pairs of biting and nonbiting dogs, Gershman and colleagues (1994) failed to detect a significant statistical relationship between obedience training and the incidence of aggressive behavior.

More recently, upon analyzing the data extracted from a large sample (N = 2018), Goodloe and Borchelt (1998) reported that a preventative relationship *does* appear to exist between a history of obedience training and the occurrence of a variety behavior problems, including aggression. Obedience training was significantly correlated with a lower incidence of aggression in all categories analyzed, except aggression toward unfamiliar dogs. They also found that obedience training was generally correlated with better-behaved dogs in two complementary directions: a decrease of undesirable behavior and an increase of desirable behavior. These findings suggest that training may help guide and refine a dog's adaptation to domestic life, making it more successful and problem free. In addition to the obvious benefits of establishing limits and control, the authors suggest that the benefits of training may be related to various incidental aspects of interaction that are associated with the training process, including increased time spent with the dog, added exposure and socialization resulting from class attendance, and a better appreciation and understanding of dog behavior. This study appears to contradict the earlier findings of Voith and colleagues (1992), which failed to identify a beneficial relationship between obedience training and the incidence of behavior problems. Goodloe and Borchelt note that the larger sample of respondents used by them may have provided a better statistical pool for detecting the beneficial influences of obedience training. They suggest that the earlier study performed by Voith and colleagues may have been too small to detect these correlations. Finally, Patronek (1996) has reported that dogs that participated in obedience classes were much less likely to be relinquished by their owners to an animal shelter.

Given the evident therapeutic value of obedience and compliance training, it is a bit astonishing that such training would not exert a more consistent and strong preventative influence over the development of aggression problems. This impasse is of considerable significance, since most treatment programs for aggression (especially dominance-related aggression) depend, in part, on some variant of obedience or compliance training. Behaviorally speaking, the treatment applied in advance (preventative training) should exert some mitigating influence over the problem, for the very same reasons that it presumably reverses it. Logically, in fact, one should expect the preventative effect to be far more robust and persuasive than the treatment effect, since the therapeutic influence must exert enough power to reverse already established aggressive behavior and prevent its reoccurrence (behavioral momentum). Further, most treatment programs are founded on the behavior-modifying effects of learning. Learning does not just occur when guided by an expert's recommendations or under the owners conscious efforts, but proceeds continuously insofar as a dog lives and interacts with its environment:

> One cannot choose to either employ or ignore the empirically established rules of learning. Much like the law of gravity, the laws of learning are always in effect. Thus, the question is not whether to use the laws of learning, but rather how to use them effectively. (Spreat and Spreat, 1982:593)

Given the apparently robust effect of behavior therapy, on the one hand, and the continuous influence of learning on the other, it is difficult to imagine how such things as obedience training, spoiling activities, and anthropomorphic attitudes would not have a significant effect on behavioral adaptation and the incidence of behavior problems.

PART 2: CHILDREN, DOGS, AND AGGRESSION

PREVENTING PROBLEMS

Children are often implicated in the development of serious dog behavior problems, especially those involving hyperactivity and aggressiveness. Many consultants recommend that a family not acquire a dog until the children are at least 6 or 7 years of age. This recommendation is based on a widely held assumption that children under this age lack sufficient maturity to treat a dog properly and safely. However, a child's age is not always a reliable marker of maturity. Older children may be more irresponsible and abusive toward a dog than their age would seem to indicate. In addition, younger children can be taught to interact with a canine companion safely and affectionately, often surpassing the ability of insensitive adults! Such matters depend on individual cases and on the parent's willingness to explain and demonstrate acceptable ways of behaving around a dog. In addition, the parent must provide adequate incentives and deterrents to ensure compliance by the child.

Sources of Conflict and Tension Between Children and Dogs

In the case of difficult children of any age, teasing and abusing the family dog is a prescription for disaster. Such behavior is often employed as a manipulative attention-seeking ploy and annoyance for the parent. Some older children see the dog as an easy and ever-available target for the release of pent-up frustration and redirected anger. Not surprisingly, abusive treatment of the dog often occurs after the child has been punished by parents or by a teacher at school. In a rather bizarre and unsettling report exploring the psychosocial benefits of dog companionship for children, Bossard (1944) seriously recommends that dogs be used as ready objects for such hostile "personal needs" involving ego frustration and gratification:

> If things have gone wrong, and you feel like kicking some one, there is Waldo, waiting for you. If you have been ordered about by the boss all day, you can go home and order the dog about. If mother has made you do what you did not want to, you can now work on the dog. Long observation of children's behavior with domestic animals convinces me that this is a very important function. Often the child has been the victim of commands, "directives," shouts, orders, all day long. How soul-satisfying now to take the dog for a walk and order him about! This is a most therapeutic procedure. (411)

Recommendations like those of Bossard neglect to appreciate fully that a dog is a feeling victim, albeit silent and forbearing, until at last it is pushed to the limits of its tolerance and forced to defend itself with the familiar devastation for both the child and the dog.

Bossard also suggests that the family dog be used for sex education, arguing that "the external physical differences of sex can be seen, identified, and discussed, without hesitation or inhibition on the part of either parent or child" (411). Unfortunately, this sort of pedagogy may, in addition, facilitate abusive handling and treatment when a child is left alone to investigate and study the subject on their own. Inquisitive children may secretly offend their canine companions in forbidden ways—extracurricular activity that Bossard might have regarded as a vital and informative outlet for childhood sexual fantasies.

The incidence of such aberrant behavior among preadolescent children and the impact it has on dogs is not known. More information is available concerning the incidence of cynophilia/zoophilia among adolescent children. Kinsey and colleagues (1948, 1953) estimated that approximately 8% of the urban male population had experienced some sexual contact with an animal, whereas a surprising 40% to 50% of adolescent boys living in rural environments reported having sexual contact with domestic animals. Among adolescent urban women, 3.6% reported having sexual contact with animals, mainly (74%) involving dogs. Overall, the researchers conclude that sexual interaction between humans and dogs is relatively rare.

Children exhibiting abusive behavior toward the family dog should be referred to a child psychologist for evaluation (Ascione et al., 2000). Such activity may presage the development of more serious sadistic and violent behavior later in life. Many violent offenders abused animals as children. Also, animal-abusive children may themselves be the victims of similar abuse in the home. There are reports (Ascione et al., 2000) of findings of others indicating that pet abuse and neglect frequently present together. In one study mentioned, children exposed to sexual abuse were significantly more likely to abuse animals (27–35%) than nonabused counterparts (5%). Unfortunately, research is still lacking, but anecdotal reports and psychological case studies point to a significant relationship between child abuse and animal abuse.

Establishing Limits and Boundaries

To prevent problems, children must learn how to respectfully handle and care for their dogs. These efforts should include instruction involving appropriate and inappropriate play. Parents often assume that children instinctively know how to behave properly toward dogs. This wishful viewpoint is not always true, and some dogs are intolerant of play, just as some children are disinterested in the play of dogs. Further, children and dogs play in species-typical ways, containing movement messages that are only partially understood by each other and responded to as intended. Although significant evolutionary continuity informs the play habits of children and dogs, there are important differences in the way each initiates, interprets, and modulates their respective play activities (Rooney et al., 2000).

These fundamental behavioral differences are probably the source of many failures of children and dogs to get along together successfully. Under the guidance of a vigilant parent, both the child and the dog can learn how to play constructively with each other and avoid the risk of their playful efforts escalating into problems. This is not always an easy process, but with perseverance and consistency the child (and the dog) can be taught to respect proper social boundaries and limits. Most importantly, the parent must be careful to set a good example for the child by avoiding inappropriate play and disciplinary efforts.

Another beneficial socializing influence on dogs and children is training. First and foremost, dogs should undergo sufficient training to establish the basic social boundaries: no jump, bite, chase, bolt, or pull. Once these boundaries are set, children can easily interact with their dogs on a friendly level and reinforce cooperative behavior with affection, food, and toys. Children should participate in the training process and practice with their dogs on a daily basis. Rewards of all kinds can be used by children to gain a surprising degree of control over their dogs. The primary benefit of such training is the provision of a foundation for effective interaction between the children and dogs based on enhanced communication, cooperation, compliance, and compromise. In addition, according to Levinson (1980), many subtle psychological benefits may be obtained by allowing children to participate in training activities:

> Part of acquiring autonomy is the taking over of control of one's behavior, the development of self-disciplining and impulse control. The ability to delay gratification, to exercise patience, to carry out responsibilities, to recognize and defer to the needs of others on occasion are all part of being a self directing human being. A child who is responsible for the well-being and training of a pet has to exhibit all these capacities. He is also trying to inculcate some of the abilities in his pet, who must wait to be fed or walked, will not always be played with on demand, must learn not to damage furnishings, etc. Of course, the more self-mastery the child has acquired the better he can train his pet, but the very act of trying to train his pet successfully will reinforce self-control to some extent. . . . Through trial and error in teaching his pet new tricks, the child discovers that he must at times control the frustration he feels when his pet is not learning as quickly as he would like. Through bitter experience he learns that scolding and punishment will only serve to delay or impede the pet's learning. As the child develops more tolerance for his pet's difficulties, he may become more tolerant of his own

inability to master his lessons, less inclined to view himself as "stupid" or "bad." (69)

Even under the most favorable circumstances, children may be tempted to test limits with their canine companions. Such interaction might actually help children to build an empathetic appreciation of how their behavior impacts on others. Optimally, the dog offers itself as a living being with which the child can explore and *test* the effects of affectionate and caring treatment. However, even innocent behaviors like hugging and holding may be interpreted by a dog as threatening gestures, particularly while it is sleeping or eating (Voith, 1981). Teaching children not to disturb dogs engaged in these activities goes some way toward preventing unnecessary dog-bite incidents. Also, whenever possible, conscientious efforts should be made to decrease the amount of screaming and rushing around the dog. In the case of busy households, an open crate can be provided to the dog as a haven of security within the otherwise chaotic maelstrom of household activities.

In addition to training, children should be taught to avoid engaging dogs in improper and provocative play like roughhousing, chase-and-evade jousts, and inappropriate tug-of-war games. Exposing dogs to daily agitational play and excessive teasing may result in the development of adjustment problems, especially competitive excesses and hyperactivity. Children constantly teasing, screaming, and running wildly through the house are bound to unnerve even the most calm and docile dog. Such behavior on the child's part increases the dog's irritability while simultaneously lowering his threshold for aggression. Consulting trainers should draw attention to the dangers of such "play" and candidly suggest to owners ways of teaching their children better ways of behaving around dogs. Ideally, parent-owners should patiently guide children by explaining how such behavior adversely affects dogs. Children should be instructed to leave sleeping and eating dogs alone and not to tease them with toys or disturb them when they possess one. On the positive side, children should be taught alternative games like ball play and hide 'n seek. Finally, children should be explicitly taught how to touch and handle dogs properly in a calming and reassuring manner.

DOG AND BABY

A common reason for dog owners to seek professional advice is to learn how to introduce a baby *safely* into a household with a resident dog. Expectant parents seeking such information are often concerned about how the dog might react to the presence of an infant, but they are often especially apprehensive about the possibility that the dog might actually bite or otherwise injure the child. These fears may be based on unfounded worries or express legitimate concerns about the dog's behavior, based on previous overt displays of aggression toward family members, guests, or other animals. Even in those cases where no evidence of previous aggression exists, the expectant parent may still harbor reasonable fears about their dog's potential behavior toward the baby, based on more subtle behavioral signs and temperament traits.

Of course, the worst secret fear is that the dog might actually attack or kill the infant. Although this is a remote possibility, fatal dog attacks on babies are statistically rare and very unlikely if the owner takes the most basic precautions. Unfortunately, there exists an irrational and widespread exaggeration of the risks involved, making some owners unnecessarily fearful about the possibility of an aggressive incident. This perception may be a by-product of the way in which periodic serious or fatal dog attacks are handled by the news media. The occurrence of such horrifying incidents receive inordinate (and often irresponsible) national and international coverage. Such reports are shocking to the public. The dog is a cultural symbol of devotion, fidelity, and protection and, when a fatal attack occurs, it strikes a deep and discordant chord of curiosity and horror. It is not difficult to understand how such reports stimulate unnecessary foreboding about the family dog's reaction to the arrival of a new baby. Regrettably, the result of such misunderstanding is often the unnecessary relinquishment of a healthy and friendly dog to an animal shelter, thereby exposing it to a potentially tragic and unjustifiable fate.

Recognizing that such apprehensions probably exist (unconsciously or consciously) in the minds of many parents, dog behavior counselors should allay or dispel such fears by explaining that dogs rarely attack or kill babies. Nonetheless, commonsense precautions should be taken to make the transition an easy and uneventful one for both the dog and the infant. Although most dogs represent a minimal risk to infant children and ultimately make suitable companions, some dogs are simply too dangerous to be in close contact with young children and should be placed into a home without children. Many owners express fears that the dog will resent the baby, perhaps *acting out* toward the infant as the result of sibling rivalry or jealousy. These owners need to be reassured that the dog is not likely to behave aggressively toward the infant as the result of jealously, but excessive *rivalry* for the owner's attention may increase the risk of problems arising as the result of competition for the owner's attention and contact. Although the vast majority of dogs are not likely to attack or otherwise hurt a baby, a dog does represent some degree of risk to a helpless infant and, therefore, should be evaluated and receive sufficient training *before* the baby comes into the home, rather than waiting until problems arise. These situations are often very complicated and should receive the utmost care and professional attention.

EVALUATING THE RISK

The average dog owner is often unable to assess objectively their dog's potential threat to the infant. Consequently, an important service rendered by dog behavior consultants is to provide an assessment of the various risks involved and to advise owners on how to minimize them. This can be a very uncomfortable and onerous responsibility, since a number of serious decisions have to be made that may dramatically affect a dog's future, based largely on a consultant's findings and recommendations. Furthermore, although many risk factors have been identified (Voith, 1984; Wright, 1985; Riegger and Guntzelman, 1990; Mathews and Lattal, 1994), no evaluation procedure currently exists that provides a *certain* determination of risk. Ultimately, such assessments rely on available scientific information, a history of aggressive behavior, and, most importantly, *gut* feelings about the dog and the situation.

The telephone interview provides valuable information about the dog and the family situation. An important goal of the initial interview is to develop a preliminary risk assessment of the immediate danger of bringing an infant into the home. The information obtained should include (at least) the following: the dog's sex and status, age, breed or mix, general activity level, training history, past socialization with children, evidence of predatory behavior toward small animals, history (e.g., place, frequency, and persons involved) of aggressive behavior toward people, type of aggression involved (e.g., dominance related, fear related, predatory), and history (e.g., place, frequency, and dogs involved) of aggressive behavior toward other dogs. Initial findings like these provide a risk profile based on salient behavioral, physical, and temperament factors.

The following profiles exemplify the opposing directions of high risk and low risk:

High-risk profile: A 2-year-old male (intact) dog with minimal previous contact with children. When exposed to children, the dog exhibits signs of increased irritability and nervousness. The dog has not received significant training, bolts out of control if given a chance, guards (growls and snaps) over food and toys, threatens guests (must be leashed for their protection), and has a history of chasing and killing small animals.

Low-risk profile: A 1½-year-old female (spayed) with a gentle disposition toward children with whom she has had steady contact. The dog attended puppy classes and has received 10 weeks of obedience training, she is playful and affectionate toward people and other dogs, enjoys ball play and brings the ball back, exhibits an enthusiastic greeting toward everyone (animals and humans alike), and never guards food or toys.

Obviously, most family dogs fall somewhere between these two extreme profiles, with a few exceptional dogs situated above and below them. Although the hypothetical dog profiled in the high-risk category has never actually bitten anyone, he still represents a serious potential threat to a baby. Generally, rather than tolerate the dangers posed by a dog with a high-risk profile, the owner is advised to rehome the dog and to consult further with their veterinarian about other courses of action to consider. Clearly, anticipating such problems and rehoming the high-risk dog into a home without children would be preferable to waiting until a definitive incident occurs, perhaps leaving only one recourse available—euthanasia.

In such cases, astute counselors make it a practice to error on the side of safety and caution, rather than to make a grave mistake that could result in serious injuries and catastrophic consequences for the victim and the trainer alike, potentially including very serious legal and professional repercussions. Unfortunately, the behavioral risk presented by high-risk dogs to children may not be significantly alleviated by the most conscientious and intensive training efforts. Again, rather than waiting until it is too late, it is far better for all involved to rehome high-risk dogs and to discourage their owners from pursuing behavior modification and training. In addition to the risk factors listed in Table 6.3, some dogs may become progressively irritable and intolerant of contact as they grow older, either as the result of physical disease and discomfort or due to geriatric cognitive deficits. Interestingly, female dogs are twice as likely as males to exhibit geriatric or *late onset* aggressiveness (Hart and Hart, 1997). Also, according to this research, male dogs are more likely to become less aggressive as they age than are female counterparts.

In addition to evaluating the dog, it is important to consider the family situation, as well. This is particularly important in *borderline* cases where a successful transition will depend on the family's ability to faithfully carry out the various instructions provided to them. One especially problematic situation involves families that are divided about the dog's continued residency in the home. In such cases, one owner may be very fond of the dog and willing to assume the full responsibility for its training, but the other spouse may be overtly hostile toward the idea or secretly harbor serious misgivings and actually prefer that the dog be rehomed or euthanized. The reluctant partner might even go along with the idea of training the dog, often to

Table 6.3. Significant risk factors for aggression toward children

Lack of significant obedience training, especially in highly active, controlling, or independent dogs that resist efforts to control them.

Little or no significant socialization with children, especially if combined with evidence of fear or past aggression toward children.

Possession-related aggression over food, toys, and places.

Overly sensitive to touch or exhibit obvious signs of fear when approached with outstretched hands.

Fearful and slow to adapt to new situations, especially if the dog becomes avoidant or aggressive toward nonthreatening contact with children.

A history of preying on small animals, especially if it includes killing after the chase.

History of dominance-related aggression, especially in cases where the dog exhibits aggression when awakened from sleep.

Dogs that react to minimal frustration with aggression.

Dogs kept outdoors or chained most of the time.

placate the determined spouse defending the dog. When all is said and done, though, he or she may refuse to recognize the dog's progress, ultimately demanding that the dog leave despite good progress. This is a no-win situation that can be detected and avoided by a skillful counselor during the initial interview with the family.

The natural and easy way that dogs and children appear to get along may produce a perilous misunderstanding and complacency about the risks involved when introducing a newborn infant to the resident dog. As a result of this unwise perception, the infant may be put at great risk by being brought home and presented to the dog without much advance preparation to make the transition more safe and uneventful. On the other extreme, some dog owners are irrationally fearful of what the dog might do to the newborn child, even though it has never exhibited any real evidence of being a significant risk. Instead of working with the dog, they simply remove the "threat" from the home.

Preventing Bites

The child and dog have enjoyed an age-old comradeship. While reading W. Fowler Bucke's (1903) study of children's attitudes toward dogs, one is struck by the perennial and universal way children perceive and appre-

ciate dogs. Unfortunately, children do not always interpret correctly the risks involved. Many situations involving bites are obviously evoked by children by placing dogs under some form of physical or mental duress. One of Bucke's young correspondents wrote,

> During the summer he had sore ears. One day I was playing near the door. Mother had just said, "Be careful, do not pull Bowler's sore ears." I did not heed mother's word, but went on climbing up his back by holding on to his ears. The poor dog endured the pain as long as he could, and suddenly snapped at me, biting my lower lip. When the doctor came I was lying on the sofa near the window. The dog came and looked in the window, and gave a pitiful whine, and for several days went about with his head down, and his tail between his legs. I begged father not to kill him, as he threatened to do. (493)

Many attacks delivered by family dogs upon children are produced by similar causes; that is, the dog bites only under provocative and easily avoidable circumstances. The bites involved are typically well directed and inhibited, occurring once, and have a self-protective character and purpose. Dogs that undergo daily abuse at the hands of their *own* child companions may be incredibly forbearing and may never attempt to bite *them,* but, woe, let another child enter the house unexpectedly or approach the dog in a startling way, and a very serious attack may occur.

How can dog bites be prevented? An adequate answer to this question involves addressing at least three equally important areas:

1. Educate the child about the dangers of mistreatment and teach him or her how to interact appropriately with the family dog and other dogs.
2. Provide the dog with adequate training and socialization around children and strangers.
3. Reward breeding efforts that emphasize temperament and intelligence over good looks.

One of the most frequently cited causes for the apparent increase in aggressive behavior in recent years is the dog world's favorite whipping boy and black sheep—the *puppy mill.* Although a convenient and worthy target of blame for some of the modern dog's plight, the puppy-mill hypothesis can hardly account for all of the dog's problems. Dogs acquired from pet stores represent only a small fraction of the total dog population, with approximately 7% of all dogs registered by the American Kennel Club being obtained through that venue (Shook, 1992).

As destructive as the puppy-mill situation is, it can hardly shoulder all of the blame for the alleged degeneracy afflicting purebred dogs (Lemonick, 1994). Other equally unscrupulous breeding practices for show and profit have also played their part. Although dogs acquired from pet stores often have behavior problems, their contribution to the aggression problem is eclipsed by dogs derived from other sources, including those bought from professional and hobbyist breeders. Reisner and colleagues (1994) at Cornell University, for example, found that dogs purchased from pet stores represent only 9% of the total number of dogs with serious dominance-related aggression problems. On the other hand, dogs bred by breeders constituted 68% (professional, 24%; and hobbyists, 44%) of the 109 cases of dominance aggression presented for treatment.

Aggressive behavior is influenced by an amalgam of acquired and biological factors. Consequently, if the problem of dog aggression is to be addressed, it will take a cooperative effort consisting of responsible breeding, competent training, and education. Responsible breeders can begin by placing an equal or greater emphasis on temperament and function, rather than focusing too much attention on form and good looks. Also, breeding should encourage traits conducive to harmonious family life, rather than perpetuating traditional and obsolete functions that have lost their usefulness. Finally, in addition to sound breeding practices, a dog's innate potential can be fully actualized only by the beneficial influence of early and lifelong training, aimed at perfecting the dog's social and domestic adaptation to modern circumstances and demands.

REFERENCES

Adams GJ and Clark WT (1989). The prevalence of behavioural problems in domestic dogs: A survey of 105 dog owners. *Aust Vet Pract,* 19:135–137.

Allen C and Bekoff M (1996). Intentionality, social play, and definition. In M Bekoff and D Jamieson (Eds), *Readings in Animal Cognition.* Cambridge, MA: MIT Press.

Allman J and Brothers L (1994). Faces, fear, and the amygdala. *Nature,* 372:613–614.

American Veterinary Medical Association (AVMA) (1997). *U.S. Pet Ownership and Demographic Sourcebook.* Schaumberg, IL: AVMA, Center for Information Management.

Archer J (1988). *The Behavioural Biology of Aggression.* New York: Cambridge University Press.

Arnsten AF (1998). The biology of being frazzled. *Science,* 280:1711–1712.

Ascione FR, Kaufman ME, and Brooks SM (2000). Animal abuse and developmental psychopathology: Recent research, programmatic, and theoretical issues and challenges for the future. In AH Fine (Ed), *Handbook on Animal-assisted Therapy: Theoretical Foundations and Guidelines for Practice.* New York: Academic.

Azrin NH, Hutchinson RR, and McLaughlin R (1965). The opportunity for aggression as an operant reinforcer during aversive stimulation. *J Exp Anal Behav,* 8:171–180.

Azrin NH, Hutchinson RR, and Hake DF (1967). Attack, avoidance, and escape reactions to aversive shock. *J Exp Anal Behav,* 10:131–148.

Beach FA (1970). Coital behavior in dogs: VI. Long-term effects of castration upon mating in the male. *J Comp Physiol Psychol (Monogr),* 70:1–32.

Beaver BV (1983). Clinical classification of canine aggression. *Appl Anim Ethol,* 10:35–43.

Beck AL, Loring H, and Lockwood R (1975). The ecology of dog bite injury in St. Louis, Missouri. *Public Health Rep,* 90:262–267.

Blackshaw JK (1991). An overview of types of aggressive behaviour in dogs and methods of treatment. *Appl Anim Behav Sci,* 30:351–361.

Borchelt PL (1983). Aggressive behavior of dogs kept as companion animals: Classification and influence of sex, reproductive status, and breed. *Appl Anim Ethol* 10:45–61.

Borchelt PL and Voith VL (1982). Classification of animal behavior problems. *Vet Clin N Am Symp Anim Behav,* 12:625–635.

Borchelt PL and Voith VL (1986). Dominance aggression in dogs. *Compend Continuing Educ Pract Vet,* 8:36–44.

Borchelt PL, Lockwood R, Beck AM, and Voith VL (1983). Attacks by packs of dogs involving predation on human beings. *Public Health Rep,* 98:57–66.

Bossard JHS (1944). The mental hygiene of owning a dog. *Ment Hyg (Arlington VA),* 28:408–413.

Brogan TV, Bratton SL, Dowd DM, and Hegenbarth MA (1995). Severe dog bites in children. *Pediatrics,* 96:947–950.

Bucke WF (1903). Cyno-psychoses: Children's thoughts, reactions, and feelings toward pet dogs. *J Genet Psychol,* 10:459–513.

Cameron DB (1997). Canine dominance-associated aggression: Concepts, incidence, and treatment in a private practice. *Appl Anim Behav Sci,* 52:265–274.

Campbell WE (1992). *Behavior Problems in Dogs.* Goleta, CA: American Veterinary.

Christensen L (1996). *Diet-Behavior Relationships: Focus on Depression.* Washington, DC: American Psychological Association.

Chun Y-T, Berkelhamer JE, and Herold TE (1982). Dog bites in children less than 4 years old. *Pediatrics,* 69:119–120.

Clark GI and Boyer WN (1993). The effects of dog obedience training and behavioural counselling upon the human-canine relationship. *Appl Anim Behav Sci,* 37:147–159.

DeNapoli JS, Dodman NH, Shuster L, Rand WM, and Gross KL (2000). Effect of dietary protein content and tryptophan supplementation on dominance aggression, territorial aggression, and hyperactivity in dogs. *JAVMA,* 217:504-508.

Derix R, Van Hoof J, De Vries H, and Wensing J (1993). Male and female mating competition in wolves: Female suppression vs male intervention. *Behaviour,* 127:141–171

DiNardo PA, Guzy LT, and Bak RM (1988). Anxiety response patterns and ethological factors in dog-fearful and non-fearful subjects. *Behav Res Ther,* 26:245–251.

Dodd WJ (1992). Thyroid can alter behavior. *Dog World,* Oct:40–42.

Dodman NH and Mertens PA (1995). Animal behavior case of the month. *JAVMA,* 207:1168–1171.

Dodman NH, Reisner I, Shuster L, et al. (1996). Effect of dietary protein content on behavior in dogs. *JAVMA,* 208:376–379.

Doogan S and Thomas GV (1992). Origins of fear of dogs in adults and children: The role of conditioning processes and prior familiarity with dogs. *Behav Res Ther* 30:387–394.

Fonberg E (1988). Dominance and aggression. *Int J Neurosci,* 41:201–213.

Fraile IG, McEwen BS, and Pfaff DW (1987). Progesterone inhibition of aggressive behavior in hamsters. *Physiol Behav,* 39:225–229.

Fuller JL and Clark LD (1966). Genetic and treatment factors modifying the postisolation syndrome in dogs. *J Comp Physiol Psychol,* 61:251–257.

Gershman KA, Sacks JJ, and Wright JC (1994). Which dogs bite? A case-control study of risk factors. *Pediatrics,* 93:913–917.

Ginsburg HJ and Miller SM (1982). Sex differences in children's risk-taking behavior. *Child Dev,* 53:426–428.

Golab GC (1998). New task force addresses canine aggression. *JAVMA,* 213:1097, 1108.

Goodloe LP and Borchelt PL (1998). Companion dog temperament traits. *J Appl Anim Welfare Sci,* 1:303–338.

Harris D, Imperato PJ, and Oken B (1974). Dog bites: An unrecognized epidemic. *Bull NY Acad Med,* 50:981–1000.

Hart BL (1980). *Canine Behavior (A Practitioner Monograph).* Santa Barbara, CA: Veterinary Practice.

Hart BL (1985). *The Behavior of Domestic Animals.* New York: Freeman.

Hart BL and Eckstein RA (1998). Progestins: Indications for male-typical problem behaviors. In N Dodman and L Shuster (Eds), *Psychopharmacology of Animal Behavior Disorders.* Malden, MA: Blackwell Science.

Hart BL and Hart LA (1985a). *Canine and Feline Behavioral Therapy.* Philadelphia: Lea and Febiger.

Hart BL and Hart LA (1985b). Selecting pet dogs on the basis of cluster analysis of breed behavior profiles and gender. *JAVMA,* 186:1181–1185.

Hart BL and Hart LA (1997). Selecting, raising, and caring for dogs to avoid problem aggression. *JAVMA,* 210:1129–1134.

Harvey MJA, Dale S, Lindley S, and Waterson MM (1999). A study of the aetiology of pseudopregnancy in the bitch and the effect of cabergoline therapy. *Vet Rec,* 144:433–436.

Hölderlin F (1966). *Poems and Fragments,* M Hamburger (Trans). Ann Arbor: University of Michigan Press.

Holliday TA, Cunningham JG, and Gutnick MJ (1970). Comparative clinical and electroencephalographic studies of canine epilepsy. *Epilepsia,* 11:281–292.

Hopkins SG, Schubert TA, and Hart BL (1976). Castration of adult male dogs: Effects on roaming, aggression, urine marking, and mounting. *JAVMA,* 168:1108–1110.

Houpt KA (1991). *Domestic Animal Behavior.* Ames: Iowa State University Press.

Hutchinson RR, Renfrew JW, and Young GA (1971). Effects of long-term shock and associated stimuli on aggressive and manual responses. *J Exp Anal Behav,* 15:141-166.

Insurance Information Institute (1999). Dog bite liability. http://www.iii.org/inside.pl5?individuals=other_stuff=/individuals/other_stuff/dog-bite.html.

Jagoe JA and Serpell JA (1988). Optimum time for neutering. *Vet Rec,* 122:447.

Joby R, Jemmett JE, and Miller ASH (1984). The control of undesirable behaviour in male dogs using megestrol acetate. *J Small Anim Pract,* 25:567–572.

Johnson LR (1998). *Essential Medical Physiology,* 2nd Ed. Philadelphia: Lippincott-Raven.

Jones BA and Beck AM (1984). Unreported dog bites and attitudes towards dogs. In Anderson RK, Hart BL and Hart LA (Eds). *The Pet Connection: Its Influence on Our Health and Quality of Life.* Minneapolis: University of Minnesota.

Kinsey AC, Pomeroy WB, and Martin CE (1948). *Sexual Behavior in the Human Male.* Philadelphia: WB Saunders.

Kinsey AC, Pomeroy WB, Martin CE, and Gebhard PH (1953). *Sexual Behavior in the Human Female.* Philadelphia: WB Saunders.

Kislak JW and Beach FA (1955). Inhibition of aggressiveness by ovarian hormones. *Endocrinology,* 56:684–692.

Knol BW and Egberink-Alink ST (1989a). Androgens, progestagens and agonistic behaviour: A review. *Vet Q,* 11:94–101.

Knol BW and Egberink-Alink ST (1989b). Treatment of problem behaviour in dogs and cats by castration and progestagen administration: A review. *Vet Q,* 11:102–107.

Konorski J (1967). *Integrative Activity of the Brain: An Interdisciplinary Approach.* Chicago: University of Chicago Press.

Kreutz LE, Rose RM, and Jennings JR (1972). Suppression of plasma testosterone levels and psychological stress. *Arch Gen Psychiatry,* 26:479–483.

Krushinskii LV (1960). *Animal Behavior: Its Normal and Abnormal Development.* New York: Consultants Bureau.

Lehman HC (1928). Child's attitude toward the dog versus the cat. *J Genet Psychol,* 35:67–72.

Lemonick MD (1994). A terrible beauty: An obsessive focus on show-ring looks is crippling, sometimes fatally, America's purebred dogs. *Time,* Dec 12:65–70.

Levinson BM (1980). The child and his pet: A world of nonverbal communication. In SA Corson, EO Corson, and JA Alexander (Eds), *Ethology and Nonverbal Communication in Mental Health.* New York: Pergamon.

Lieberman LL (1987). A case for neutering pups and kittens at two months of age. *JAVMA,* 191:518–521.

Line S and Voith VL (1986). Dominance aggression of dogs towards people: Behavior profile and response to treatment. *Appl Anim Behav Sci,* 16:77–83.

Lockwood R (1996). The ethology and epidemiology of canine aggression. In J Serpell (Ed), *The Domestic Dog: Its Evolution, Behaviour, and Interaction with People.* New York: Cambridge University Press.

Marx MB, Stallones L, Garrity TF, and Johnson TP (1988). Demographics of pet ownership among U.S. adults 21 to 64 years of age. *Anthrozoös,* 2:33–37.

Mathews JR and Lattal KA (1994). A behavioral analysis of dog bites to children. *Dev Behav Pediatr,* 15:44–52.

McLeod PJ, Moger WH, Ryon J, et al. (1995). The relation between urinary cortisol levels and social behavior in captive timber wolves. *Can J Zool,* 74:209–216.

Mendl M (1999). Performing under pressure: Stress and cognitive function. *Appl Anim Behav Sci,* 65:221–244.

Moyer KE (1968). Kinds of aggression and their physiological basis. *Commun Behav Biol [A],* 2:65–87.

Moyer KE (1971). A preliminary physiological model of aggressive behavior. In BE Eletherian and JP Scott (Eds), *The Physiology of Aggression.* New York, Plenum.

Mugford RA (1984). Aggressive behaviour in the English cocker spaniel. *Vet Annu,* 24:310–314.

Mugford RA (1987). The influence of nutrition on canine behavior. *J Small Anim Pract,* 28:1046–1085.

Murray M (1998). *5-HTP: The Natural Way to Overcome Depression, Obesity, and Insomnia.* New York: Bantam.

Neilson JC, Eckstein RA, and Hart BL (1997). Effects of castration on problem behaviors in male dogs with reference to age and duration of behavior. *JAVMA,* 211:180–182.

O'Farrell V (1986). *Manual of Canine Behavior.* Cheltenham, UK: British Small Animal Veterinary Association.

O'Farrell V and Peachey E (1990). Behavioural effects of ovariohysterectomy on bitches. *J Small Anim Pract,* 31:595–598.

Olsen PN, Husted PW, Allen TA, and Nett TM (1984). Reproductive endocrinology and physiology of the bitch and queen. *Vet Clin North Am Small Anim Pract,* 14:927–946.

Overall K (1997). *Clinical Behavioral Medicine for Small Animals.* St Louis: CV Mosby.

Panksepp J (1998). *Affective Neuroscience: The Foundations of Human and Animal Emotions.* New York: Oxford University Press.

Parrish HM, Clack FB, Brobst D, and Mock JF (1959). Epidemiology of dog bites. *Public Health Rep,* 74:891–903.

Patronek GJ, Glickman LT, Beck AM, et al.(1996). Special report: Risk factors for relinquishment of dogs to an animal shelter. *JAVMA,* 209:572–581.

Pet Food Institute (PFI) (1999). *PFI Fact Sheet.* Washington, DC: PFI.

Pinckney LE and Kennedy LA (1982). Traumatic deaths from dog attacks in the United States. *Pediatrics,* 69:193–196.

Podberscek AL and Serpell JA (1996). The English cocker spaniel: Preliminary findings on aggressive behavior. *Appl Anim Behav Sci,* 47:75–89.

Podberscek AL and Serpell JA (1997). Environmental influences on the expression of aggressive behaviour in English cocker spaniels. *Appl Anim Behav Sci,* 52:215–227.

Podberscek AL, Blackshaw JK, and Nixon JW (1990). The incidence of dog attacks on children treated at a city hospital. *Aust Vet J,* 67:79–80.

Polsky RH (1993). Does thyroid dysfunction cause behavioral problems. *Canine Pract,* 18:6–8.

Price EO (1999). Behavioral development in animals undergoing domestication. *Appl Anim Behav Sci,* 65:245–271.

Quartermain D, Stone EA, and Charbonneau G (1996). Acute stress disrupts risk assessment behavior in mice. *Physiol Behav,* 59:937–940.

Reinhard D (1978). Aggressive behavior associated with hypothyroidism. *Canine Pract,* 5:69–70.

Reisner IR (1997). Assessment, management, and prognosis of canine dominance-related aggression. *Vet Clin North Am Prog Companion Anim Behav,* 27:479–495.

Reisner IR, Erb HN, and Houpt KA (1994). Risk factors for behavior-related euthanasia among dominant-aggressive dogs: 110 cases (1989–1992). *JAVMA,* 205:855–863.

Riegger MH and Guntzelman J (1990). Prevention and amelioration of stress and consequences of interaction between children and dogs. *JAVMA,* 196:1781–1785.

Rooney NJ, Bradshaw JWS, and Robinson IH (2000). A comparison of dog-dog and dog-human play behaviour. *Appl Anim Behav Sci,* 66:235–248.

Sacks JJ, Sattin RW, and Bonzo SE (1989). Dog bite—related fatalities from 1979 through 1988. *JAMA,* 262:1489–1492.

Sacks JJ, Kresnow MJ, and Houston B (1996a). Dog bites: How big a problem. *Injury Prevent,* 2:52–54.

Sacks JJ, Lockwood R, Hornreich J, and Sattin RW (1996b). Fatal dog attacks, 1989–1994. *Pediatrics,* 97:891–895.

Salmeri KR, Bloomber MS, Scruggs SL, and Shille V (1991). Gonadectomy in immature dogs: Effects on skeletal, physical, and behavioral development. *JAVMA,* 198:1193–1203.

Sapolsky RM (1990). Stress in the wild. *Sci Am,* 262:116–123.

Sapolsky RM (1994). *Why Zebras Don't Get Ulcers.* New York: WH Freeman.

Scott JP (1992). Aggression: Functions and control in social systems. *Aggressive Behav,* 18:1–20.

Shook L (1992). *The Puppy Report: How to Select a Healthy, Happy Dog.* New York: Ballantine.

Siegel A and Edinger H (1981). Neural control of aggression and rage behavior. In PJ Morgane and J Panksepp (Eds), *Handbook of the Hypothalamus,* Vol 3, Part B: *Behavioral Studies of the Hypothalamus.* New York: Marcel Dekker.

Simon NG and Whalen RE (1987). Sexual differentiation of androgen-sensitive and estrogen-sensitive regulatory systems for aggressive behavior. *Horm Behav,* 21:493–500.

Spreat S and Spreat SR (1982). Learning principles. *Vet Clin North Am Small Anim Pract,* 12:593–606.

Spring B (1986). Effects of foods and nutrients on the behavior of normal individuals. In RJ Wurtman and JJ Wurtman (Eds), *Nutrition and the Brain,* 7:1–47.

State Farm Insurance (1999). Dog bites fact sheet. http://www.statefarm.com/media/release/bitfac.htm.

Thorne FC (1944). The inheritance of shyness in dogs. *J Genet Psychol,* 65:275–279.

Tinbergen N (1958/1969). *Curious Naturalists.* New York: Natural History Library Anchor Books.

Tortora DF (1983). Safety training: The elimination of avoidance-motivated aggression in dog. *J Exp Psychol [Gen],* 112:176–214.

Tortora DF (1984). Safety training: The elimination avoidance-motivated aggression in dogs. *Aust Vet Pract,* 14:70–74.

Uchida Y, Dodman N, DeNapoli J, and Aronson L (1997). Characterization and treatment of 20 canine dominance aggression cases. *J Vet Med Sci,* 59:397–399.

Ulrich RE and Azrin NH (1962). Reflexive fighting in response to aversive stimulation. *J Exp Anal Behav,* 5:511–520.

US Advisory Board on Child Abuse and Neglect (1995). *A Nation's Shame: Fatal Child Abuse and Neglect in the United States.* Washington, DC: US Department of Health and Human Services.

US Department of Health and Human Services (1999). *Child Maltreatment 1997: Reports from the States to the National Child Abuse and Neglect Data System.* Washington, DC: US Government Printing Office.

Voith VL (1980a). Aggressive behavior and dominance. In BL Hart (Ed), *Canine Behavior.* Culver City, CA: Veterinary Practice.

Voith VL (1980b). Functional significance of pseudocyesis. *Mod Vet Pract,* 61:75–77.

Voith VL (1980c). Intermale aggression in dogs. *Mod Vet Pract,* 61:256–258.

Voith VL (1980c). Aggressive behavior and dominance. In BL Hart (Ed), *Canine Behavior.* Culver City, CA: Veterinary Practice.

Voith VL (1981). An approach to ameliorating aggressive behavior of dogs toward children. *Mod Vet Pract,* 62:67–70.

Voith VL (1984). Procedures for introducing a baby to a dog. *Mod Vet Pract,* 65:539–541.

Voith VL and Borchelt PL (1982). Diagnosis and treatment of dominance aggression in dogs. *Vet Clin North Am Small Anim Pract,* 12:655–663.

Voith VL and Borchelt PL (1985). *Introducing Your Dog to Your New Baby.* Kankakee, IL: Gaines [pamphlet published by the Gaines Dog Food Company for distribution by veterinarians: Gaines, 3 Stuart Drive, PO Box 1007, Kankakee, IL 60902].

Voith VL and Borchelt PL (1996). Elimination behavior and related problems in dogs. In VL Voith and PL Borchelt (Eds), *Readings in Companion Animal Behavior.* Trenton, NJ: Veterinary Learning Systems.

Voith VL, Wright JC, Danneman PJ, et al. (1992). Is there a relationship between canine behavior problems and spoiling activities, anthropomorphism, and obedience training? *Appl Anim Behav Sci,* 34:263–272.

Wells DL and Hepper PG (1997). Pet ownership and adults' view on the use of animals. *Soc Anim,* 5:45–63.

Winkler WG (1977). Human deaths induced by dog bites, United States, 1974–75. *Public Health Rep,* 92:425–429.

Wright JC (1983). The effects of differential rearing on exploratory behavior in puppies. *Appl Anim Ethol,* 10:27–34.

Wright JC (1985). Severe attacks by dogs: Characteristics of the dogs, the victims, and the attack settings. *Public Health Rep,* 100:55–61.

Wright JC (1990). Reported dog bites: Are owned and stray dogs different? *Anthrozoös,* 4:113–119.

Wright JC (1991). Canine aggression toward people: Bite scenarios and prevention. *Vet Clin North Am Adv Companion Anim Behav,* 21:299–314.

Wright JC and Nesselrote MS (1987). Classification of behavior problems in dogs: Distributions of age, breed, sex and reproductive status. *Appl Anim Behav Sci,* 19:169–178.

7

Intraspecific and Territorial Aggression

Lo, when two dogs are fighting in the streets,
With a third dog one of the two dogs meets;
With angry teeth he bites him to the bone,
And this dog smarts for what that dog has done.

HENRY FIELDING, *TOM THUMB THE GREAT* (1918)

PART 1: INTRASPECIFIC AGGRESSION

Competitive interaction between dogs results from a variety of complex social and territorial interests. Many of the same issues affecting aggression toward humans (interspecific) also affect aggression exhibited between dogs (intraspecific). But, unlike interspecific threats and attacks, intraspecific aggression also appears to be motivated to some extent by sexual-reproductive imperatives. Dog fighting

203

occurs under two broad circumstances: (1) between dogs not sharing the same household (nonresident directed) and (2) between dogs sharing the same home (resident directed). Most interdog aggression takes place between dogs of the same sex.

ETIOLOGY AND ASSESSMENT

Fighting is common among dogs and often results in serious and expensive injuries to combatants and to people, who are frequently bitten while attempting to separate gnashing and thrashing antagonists. The behavior is particularly prevalent among male dogs, but female dogs may also become determined fighters, especially females that live together in the same household. Urban dogs appear to be relatively more likely to develop a fighting problem, with most dog fights occurring between dogs walked off-leash in the late afternoon or night (Roll and Unshelm, 1997). The higher incidence of fighting among this particular population of dogs may occur because of the close daily contact they have while being walked on narrow sidewalks or exercised together in city parks. For obvious reasons, the powerful working breeds, especially shepherding dogs, are most commonly involved in fights that result in injuries requiring veterinary attention, but severe fighting is certainly not limited to such breeds. Intraspecific intolerance is recognized as a typical feature of terrier-type breeds (Scott and Fuller, 1965). Sherman and colleagues (1996) found that terriers presented disproportionately with fighting problems but only with respect to nonresident targets. Also, male and female dogs appear to differentiate in terms of the context and targets of intraspecific aggression. The majority of nonresident-directed aggressive episodes involve unfamiliar intact-male dogs obtained from breeders (Roll and Unshelm, 1997), whereas most resident-directed aggression involves spayed-female combatants (Sherman et al., 1996).

Many factors influence the development of intraspecific aggression. Determining the targets and the exact situations where fighting breaks out is useful information. Does a dog exhibit aggression toward all dogs regardless of their sex or status (castrated/spayed)? Does

a dog exclusively fight with members of the same sex? In the case of dogs that live together, does fighting ever occur in the owner's absence? Is fighting more likely to break out in the presence of any particular family member? Answers to questions like these and others are extremely useful for properly evaluating the problem and helping to select the most appropriate course of training and behavior modification. Dogs fight with one another for many different reasons. Although dogs may be biologically inclined to exhibit such behavior, the effects of early socialization, traumatic events involving other dogs, and a dog's history of fighting should be carefully assessed. This is especially significant when evaluating aggression that is highly generalized and targeted against both male and female dogs, regardless of context.

OWNER CHARACTERISTICS OF *AGGRESSORS* AND *VICTIMS*

Roll and Unshelm (1997), who collected and analyzed questionnaire information from dog owners (N = 206) seeking emergency treatment after a dog fight, found clear differences among the owners of aggressors (N = 55) versus the owners of victims (N = 151). Unfortunately, the authors neglected to interpret their findings (see Table 7.1), and it is difficult to see how they might influence the development of interdog aggression. In practice, many owners of aggressors are in active denial with respect to their dog's behavior, often refusing to come to grips with what the dog is doing. They are prone to engage in diverse and capricious interpretations of their dog's aggressiveness in order to avoid the painful recognition that their beloved dog is a public threat and menace. Frequently, their explanations take the form of irrational justifications and rationalizations designed to mitigate the seriousness of the dog's behavior, to make excuses for it, or to lessen the dog's culpability and, perhaps, their own responsibility for it (Sanders, 1999). Other owners may be indifferent or exhibit an unusual degree of tolerance for such behavior. Some may condone the behavior or hesitate to correct it, fearing that such efforts might inadvertently suppress more desirable protective tendencies. These

TABLE 7.1. Owner characteristics of aggressors and victims

Owners of aggressors
  Mostly males who were self-employed or academics aged between 30 and 39 years.
  They tend not to form emotional relationships with their dogs and often report having owned dogs
    for most of their lives.
  They consciously select specific breeds and show interest in protection training (Schutzhund).
  They tend to obtain dogs for security reasons.
  Dogs are often trained through physical force.
  During the fight itself, owners of the aggressor may react impassively and shout at the dog only after the
    fight has come to an end. Many of these owners (40%) show no reaction at all, during or after the fight.

Owners of victims
  Many owners of victims are women who are housewives or pensioners.
  They often keep dogs for the prevention of loneliness and safety.
  They do not tend to select their dogs on the basis of breed considerations.
  Dogs are trained by less forceful means.
  Fewer owners of victims report having owned dogs most of their lives than reported by owners of
    aggressors.
  Owners of victims will often attempt to console their injured dog after a fight.

After Roll and Unshelm (1997).

concerns are not necessarily allayed by explaining that protective aggression and dog fighting are not necessarily linked with each other; in fact, dog-aggressive dogs are usually surprisingly friendly and outgoing toward people. Finally, a special case exists in which the owner secretly takes pride in the dog's dangerous behavior. Such owners appear to project their own aggressive fantasies and insecurities vicariously upon their dog, thereby exploiting and victimizing all involved for the sake of their own perverse and cowardly pleasures.

DOMESTICATION AND DEVELOPMENTAL FACTORS

Phylogenic Influences

The tendency to fight is a phylogenetic or species-typical trait. The tendency predisposes many dogs to engage other dogs of the same sex in agonistic contests, primarily involving ritualized displays and assertions of dominance. In general, however, the trend among the majority of domestic dogs is in the direction of exhibiting maximum tolerance and minimum aggression when interacting with conspecifics. Over many centuries of domestication and selective breeding, the dog's physi-

cal structure, physiology, and behavior have undergone dramatic transformations, resulting in a significant biological divergence from the ancestral prototype on many levels (Frank and Frank, 1982). The dog's appearance and behavior have been strongly influenced by a pervasive process of neoteny, causing it to remain more puppylike as an adult than the wolf. Neoteny has also disrupted the normal developmental expression of various instinctive behavioral and communication systems. Relevant to the present discussion is the finding that these neotenous changes in the dog's appearance may impede its ability to express and receive unambiguous threat and appeasement displays (Goodwin et al., 1997). Besides making dogs appear more puppylike, neotenic changes appear to have elevated fear and aggression thresholds in dogs while simultaneously lowering the threshold for affiliative behavior and play. In most well-socialized dogs, close friendly bonds and playful interaction overshadow and restrain the expression of fear and aggression (Bradshaw and Lea, 1992).

Despite these general trends among the majority of dog breeds, some guard and fighting breeds may have undergone specific genetic changes that cause them to respond abnormally to conspecific agonistic threat and appeasement displays (Lockwood and Rindy,

1987). In such dogs, genetically lowered thresholds for overt damaging attacks appear to take priority over ritualized aggressive contests. Also, guard-type and fighting breeds may have undergone genetic alterations enabling them to tolerate pain at more intense levels of stimulation than the average dog—all factors contributing to their aggressive tenacity and *gameness*. Besides hardness of bite, such breeds often exhibit a notorious unwillingness to let go once the bite is secured, sometimes requiring extreme measures to get them to release their hold (Clifford et al., 1983).

Ontogenic Influences

Playful competition can be observed in young puppies shortly after they enter into the socialization period around week 3 (see *Learning to Relate and Communicate* in Volume 1, Chapter 2). These agonistic activities escalate over the ensuing weeks until much of the interaction between puppies is devoted to aggressive play and sparring. Some litters are more aggressive than others, but all healthy puppies play aggressively with one another. A possible purpose underlying early aggressive contests is the establishment of a hierarchically stratified group, resembling in many important respects an adult pack. While establishing relative dominance among littermates appears to be an important function of aggressive play, it also appears to be done for its own sake, that is, for the sheer physical exertion and pleasure of it. As puppies develop, the intensity of their fighting may escalate and involve more than two playful combatants, with puppies aligning themselves cooperatively in order to outnumber and subdue an opponent. Occasionally, the lowest-ranking puppy is at risk of receiving excessive mobbing by the rest of the group and may need to be removed to avoid injury or emotional trauma (Scott and Fuller, 1965).

HORMONAL INFLUENCES

Hormonal activity appears to influence the expression of intraspecific aggression (see *Hormones and Aggressive Behavior* in Chapter 6). Intact males are the most common aggres-

sors and targets of attack (Roll and Unshelm, 1997). An androgen surge in the male dog during the adolescent period between months 6 and 8 (Hart, 1985) may exert a pronounced influence on behavioral thresholds regulating aggressive behavior between dogs. These hormonal changes are frequently associated with the simultaneous appearance of heightened intermale aggressiveness and urine-marking activities. Adult males appear to be particularly intolerant and hostile toward other intact males coming into puberty. Such aggressive challenges and frisks do not usually escalate to the scale of damaging fights, but this rule is definitely not always the case, since not all adolescents subordinate themselves without offering a contest. This increased aggressive interest and targeting of intact adolescents may be under the influence of olfactory pheromonal cues and the often taunting and *uppity* behavior shown by adolescent dogs. Not only are adolescent intact males more attractive as targets, they themselves are much more provocative than castrated counterparts or females. Castrated dogs, in contrast, belonging to this age group are far less likely to attract the aggressive interests of mature intact dogs. In general, castrated dogs appear to be less aggressive toward other male dogs and more apt to submit, rather than fight back, when challenged. Male dogs rarely direct their aggression toward females, except in cases in which the female attacks first. And, even then, the resulting skirmish is often more a picture of confused self-defense than fierce fighting.

Castration and Dog Fighting

Since there appears to be a clear correlation between the development of intermale aggression and adolescent hormonal activity, a preventative measure that ought to be considered is early castration. Hopkins and colleagues (1976) found that 63% of dogs showing intermale aggression exhibited either a rapid decline (38%) or a gradual decline (25%) of fighting activity after castration. More recently, Neilson and coworkers (1997) reported,

> With regard to aggression toward other canine or human members of the family, approximately 25% of dogs can be expected to have a

50 to 90% level of improvement after castration. A comparable reduction in aggression toward unfamiliar dogs or human territorial intruders can be expected in 10 to 15% of dogs after castration. (182)

For optimal preventative effects, the surgery should be carried out sometime between months 5 and 6, although the benefits of castration on such behavior do not depend on a dog's age at the time castration or the duration of the problem. Some evidence suggests that castration performed between weeks 8 and 12 may produce even more pronounced effects (Lieberman, 1987), but the actual benefits of early castration remain controversial. However, this option may be seriously considered in the case of individuals belonging to breeds prone to dog fighting. It must be emphasized, however, that even early castration will not necessarily prevent the development of dog fighting. Many individuals that have undergone preadolescent castration still exhibit strong intermale aggressive tendencies. This effect may be due to perinatal androgenization occurring just before and after birth.

Urine Marking and Intermale Aggression

Although a causal relation between urine-marking behavior and territorial aggression has not been definitively established in dogs (see below), some authorities strongly believe that such a causal relation probably exists. The assumption that urine marking is a causal precursor of territorial aggression has resulted in treatment programs in which dog owners are instructed to discourage their dogs from urine marking away from the home, especially in cases involving interdog aggression (Campbell, 1974; Juarbe-Diaz, 1997). Apparently, following Campbell's logic (although not citing him as her source of information), Juarbe-Diaz (1997) suggests that a major motivation of nonhousehold intermale aggression is the defense of urine-marked territories. Along with Campbell, she recommends constraining such aggressors from eliminating away from the home *territory,* "because this is believed to extend their territory beyond the boundaries of their owner's property" (504). This treatment program is of questionable value, not only because there is no credible evidence

showing that it actually works, but, more importantly, because such restriction is highly intrusive and very difficult to implement. Further, simply because urine marking and intermale aggression appear to occur together in the same dog is not proof that the one habit is causally related to the other or that restricting the one activity will significantly limit the expression of the other. If such a causal link exists, dogs isolated to yards and rarely walked should be much less aggressive toward conspecifics than dogs walked and allowed to urinate freely; this has not been proven to my knowledge. Lastly, Hopkins and coworkers (1976) found no effect of castration on territorial aggression, even though castration exerted a pronounced effect on marking behavior. Other relevant studies have shown only a very slight benefit from castration on aggression related to territorial defense [see Neilson et al. (1997)]. Although increased urine marking and intermale aggression may share a common source of causality at some level of functional organization [see *Arginine-Vasopressin (AVP) and Aggression* in Volume 1, Chapter 3], the frustrative inhibition of one habit will not likely help to suppress the other; on the contrary, such efforts might actually potentiate it, thereby making matters worse. A major source of concern with the recommendation is that the abrupt restriction of urine-marking activity may instigate iatrogenic elimination problems, such as marking inside the house. Finally, urine marking is a normal canine activity that appears to represent a significant source of pleasure and excitement for dogs and, unless significant evidence is made available to support the notion that its restriction can significantly aid in the control of interdog aggression, it would seem advisable to let dogs urinate where they sniff fit to do so—as long as it is done outside of the house.

SOCIALIZATION AND AGGRESSION

An important factor in the development of intraspecific aggression is the quality and quantity of early socialization. Puppies taken too early from the litter (before week 6) may become socially intolerant toward other dogs as adults. Even in cases in which puppies are removed from the litter at an optimal time for secondary socialization with people (e.g., around week 7 or 8), the social learning needed to interact confidently with other dogs is not complete. Subsequent to adoption, the average puppy is only infrequently exposed to other dogs, perhaps further compromising the social skills needed for peaceful interaction. Roll and Unshelm (1997) report that nearly half of the aggressors and victims in their study were described as having few interactions with conspecifics between the ages of 5 weeks to 5 months. Such socialization deficits can be ameliorated by exposing a young puppy to other dogs of its age group through various activities like puppy kindergarten or play groups.

Even when a puppy remains with the litter throughout the socialization period, the experience itself may predispose it in various ways to react aggressively toward other dogs as an adult, especially unfamiliar dogs perceived as not belonging to its social group. This is particularly true in the case of puppies situated on either extreme of the dominance hierarchy. An *omega* subordinate, having undergone excessive or traumatic badgering by higher-ranking littermates, may consequently become progressively agitated and defensive toward other dogs. Such puppies can be surprisingly difficult to handle and train because of their sharpened reactivity to close social contact. As a result of their early experiences, they may become conditioned to react defensively when approached or touched. On the other hand, an *alpha* puppy may be influenced adversely by an opposite set of early social experiences, especially the successes it experienced while threatening and subordinating littermates. As an adult, the *alpha* puppy may be more prone to exhibit intolerance toward male conspecifics and actions perceived as *status* threats. Socially controlling or *dominant* puppies have been socialized to be aggressive and unyielding—early learning that often must be countered with remedial training. The most socially adaptable puppies are those that fall somewhere in the middle of the dominance hierarchy. Such puppies know how to assert themselves effectively and to occupy dominant roles or, conversely, they can submit and play subordinate roles when it is in their best interest to do so.

Early Trauma and Fighting

Many fighting problems stem from unpredicted attacks perpetrated by strange dogs. Although most adult dogs are gentle toward young puppies, some are not so inclined and may trounce defenseless youngsters, sometimes causing a lasting fearful psychological impression, making the victims wary of such contacts in the future. Such experiences appear to underlie the later development of some forms of intraspecific aggression. Puppies exposed to such attacks are susceptible to develop a prejudice against other dogs belonging to the aggressor's breed type or generalize more broadly in terms of the aggressor's size and color or simply learn to react defensively to all unfamiliar dogs. Many owners report a single surprise attack as the sole precipitating cause of their dog's fighting problem. Affected dogs appear to strike preemptively in an effort to assume the defensive advantage of a forceful offense. Such dogs, affected by the belief that they cannot predict when an attack might occur, may become increasingly vigilant and treat every encounter as though it represented a serious threat.

Territorial Agitation

Some dogs have developed intense aggressive attitudes toward other dogs as the result of territorial intrusion or violation. This is especially the case in dogs restrained on a chain and stake or kept behind fencing exposed to passing dogs. Dog fighting along fence lines is a common problem. Both males and females engage in this behavior, but it is a particular favorite of intact males, especially when the target is another male dog. The fence line is very problematic when it is shared with a neighboring dog, since it simultaneously demarcates the *intruder's* territorial boundary as well as the defender's. In nature, such situations rarely, if ever, develop. Territory is safely ensconced deep within a home range that is regularly inspected for intrusion. Under natural conditions, distant scent marking and various remote activities such as vocalizations and obvious evidence of pack residency like past kills and fecal deposits serve to ward off all but the most persistent intruders. Such territorial devices serve to prevent inadvertent territorial overlapping between neighboring animals and, thereby, prevent unnecessary intergroup agitation, competition, and the potential for dangerous fighting.

Under domestic conditions, these territorial mechanisms are frequently ignored or violated, leading to heightened reactivity and the constant threat of serious attacks. In the case of fence fighting, intense aggression is frequently seen because both dogs claim the same boundary as their own. Since nothing is ever resolved one way or the other and both remain protected from each other, fighting escalates and becomes ritualized, frustrative, and very persistent. Many fence fighters develop various compulsive weaving, whirling, and fence-running habits. Although dogs have broken teeth on chain-link fencing and experienced other superficial injuries as the result of such fighting, the real problem involves kindling effects and the fostering of more general aggressive reactivity and aggressive biasing toward other dogs.

The agitation of daily fence fighting and the heightened aggressive arousal associated with it stress dogs, as well as facilitate the development of various undesirable behaviors: hypervigilance, hyperactivity, frustrative oral and somatic activities (chewing and digging at fence lines), and excessive barking. In addition, such unrestrained behavior is at risk of being redirected toward nearby people or dogs. When more than one dog is defending a fence line against intrusion, the situation can easily escalate into an outbreak of fighting between erstwhile defenders. Furthermore, unchecked aggressiveness near fence lines may inadvertently encourage dogs to become aggressive toward children and others walking nearby. The influence of fence fighting on territorial defense is discussed in greater detail in Part 2 of this chapter (see *Sources of Territorial Agitation: Fences and Chains*).

VIRAGO SYNDROME

While fighting behavior problems are most typically associated with male dogs, female dogs may also engage other dogs (male and female) in aggressive contests. This is especially the case with females living together in the same home. Females tend to establish a separate dominance hierarchy from that of males. Interfemale aggression is often intense and frequently involves injury. Causal factors appear to involve reproductive rights and privileges of dominance. Among wolves, only the alpha female is permitted to procreate. The alpha female appears to protect this privilege by hounding and harassing other mature females. This bickering and agitation appears to psychologically stress potential rivals, thus preventing them from entering a receptive and fertile estrus (see *Stress Hormones and Aggression* in Chapter 6). At such times as these, intense conflicts may flare up and grow into overt and damaging dominance fights. This pattern of birth control does not always work, however. In those cases where a subordinate interloper mates successfully, the punishment may be severe—her death. Wolves rarely fight to the death, but this is one situation where such fighting has been observed at least among captive wolves (e.g., Wolf Park, Battle Ground, Indiana). Breeders should be careful when breeding a subordinate female that lives in a situation with a more dominant female.

Aggression Between Opposite Sexes

Although resident-directed aggression between opposite-sex combatants is less common, when it does occur females are twice as likely to initiate attacks against male dogs than male dogs are to initiate attacks against females (Sherman et al., 1996). The mildest form of such fighting occurs when an unreceptive female rebuffs the advances of an unwanted suitor. The male usually accepts the rejection without retaliation, although he may persist in his seductive adventures until more fully convinced of her sincerity. Occasionally, however, a male may answer in kind, sparking a more serious battle of wills that may escalate into serious fighting. Another source of intersexual agonistic behavior can be observed when two puppies of the opposite sex are raised together. Although larger and, perhaps, more aggressive in general terms, the male is often pitifully subordinated by the relentless harrying of the more dominant female. The inclination for females to attack or excessively dominate conspecific males is here referred to as the *virago syndrome*. As an adult, a viraginous female may engage the opposite sex in earnest fighting but not to the exclusion of members of her own sex, which she will also readily fight. This is a somewhat disconcerting situation for a male that does not recognize the female as a target for aggression and may be nonplused by her intentions. As a result, many males halfheartedly defend themselves, give ground, fumble over themselves, and simply retreat if they can. Such safe and successful consequences may be very reinforcing for a victorious female, encouraging her to instigate other aggressive challenges when encountering male dogs. Although many males do give ground, even very dominant males that would readily fight if it were another male making such trouble, she will eventually encounter a male that will not back down, with great potential for a serious and damaging fight.

Few unlimited generalities can be made about virago females other than their tendency to fight male dogs. Many are somewhat larger than others of their breed, and they often have a masculine appearance, exhibit some malelike behavior patterns, and are frequently aggressive in other ways besides dog fighting, including aggressive behavior exhibited toward people. Virago females urinate more frequently than is usually the female's custom, sometimes raising their leg in an effort to squirt onto vertical surfaces.

Perinatal Androgenization

One potential etiological basis for the development of the virago syndrome and other forms of heightened intraspecific aggression in females may stem from prenatal influences brought about by vagrant testosterone in amniotic fluids. Strong experimental evidence suggests that female embryos situated between males in the uterus are more likely to develop malelike aggressive tendencies and scent-marking patterns than are counterparts otherwise situated. Although this effect has not been directly demonstrated in dogs, it has been observed experimentally in mice and guinea pigs (Knol and Egberink-Alink, 1989). Some suggestive evidence regarding the effects

of perinatal androgenization of female dogs has been reported by Coppola [1986—see Borchelt and Voith (1996)]. Among 14 female dogs presenting with dominance aggression and an increase of malelike behavior after spaying, he found that female aggressors were more likely to have been from litters predominantly composed of male puppies. Supportive evidence for this hypothesis has been reported by Beach and colleagues (1982), who exposed female dogs to testosterone prenatally and postnatally in an effort to determine the long-term effects of early androgenization on adult agonistic behavior. The researchers subsequently tested the androgenized or *pseudohermaphroditic* females for relative dominance ranking in dyadic pairings with adult intact males and spayed females. The paired dogs competed against one another for access and control of a bone. When male dogs were paired with spayed females, the former controlled the bone in 78 of 100 encounters. The androgenized females were similarly effective against spayed females, controlling the bone in 70 of 100 encounters but were only 39% of the time successful against intact males. When the androgenized females were already in possession of the bone and then challenged, they did not fare much better than spayed females against the males' effort to expropriate the prize. One significant difference did emerge, however: the androgenized females were much more aggressive, threatening males in 78% of the encounters compared to 20% of the time by spayed females:

> Males were threatened by P [pseudohermaphroditic] possessors in 78% of the tests compared with 20% for the F [spayed females] possessors. In 12 of 61 tests, a P possessor and a M challenger fought vigorously, but in all instances the M emerged as victor. . .. The aggressive behavior of P possessors was maladaptive in that it did not constitute successful defense. Although they always lost the bone, several Ps engaged in fights repeatedly. This was the outcome of strong reluctance to yield possession and a heightened tendency toward contentious behavior. (873)

Clearly, perinatal exposure to testosterone enhanced the pseudohermaphroditic females' dominance ranking over spayed females but not toward intact males. The observation by

Beach and colleagues that androgenized females are more aggressive and ready to fight maladaptively is of some significance to the role of testosterone in the expression of competitive aggression. Incidentally, androgenized females eliminate in the familiar raised-leg fashion of male dogs.

AGGRESSION BETWEEN DOGS SHARING THE SAME HOUSEHOLD

The majority of aggressive episodes involving dogs sharing the same residence are initiated by the youngest and most recently obtained member of the group. Statistically, as already mentioned, females are more likely than males to fight with one another when living in the same household. Also, aggression between resident dogs frequently results in more serious injuries to the combatants than observed in the case of nonresident fighting (Sherman et al., 1996).

In domestic situations involving two or more dogs, ritualized fighting is a common occurrence. This is especially the case where the dogs are of the same sex. Three basic forms of aggressive interaction can be observed among dogs sharing the same residence: (1) aggressive play that involves many of the behavioral components involved in actual fighting but without the intention to subdue or injure the opponent; (2) actual dominance fighting clearly designed to subordinate the opponent but without injuring it; and, lastly, (3) overt and damaging fighting intended to both subdue and injure the opponent. All three forms of fighting are involved in the establishment and maintenance of relative social dominance between individuals sharing the same home territory.

Most dogs sharing the same household establish remarkably stable dominance relations, needing only infrequent dominance threats and ritualized quarrels to maintain the status quo. Even so, fighting between resident dogs is a common complaint. The causes for such fighting are complicated and varied. Some authorities have speculated that the primary cause of instability is owner interference (Hart and Hart, 1985). In such cases, owners may feel sorry for the subordinate "under-dog," which they may feel obligated to protect from the "bullying" dominant dog. This protective role may include punishing the more dominant dog while pouring affectionate consolation and comfort onto the subordinate. From the perspective of the combatants, it appears as though the meddling owner is taking sides, perhaps conspiring with the subordinate to overturn the dominant dog's position. The effect of such extraneous interference not only narrows the relative social status existing between the dogs, it may destabilize the situation and set off serious dominance contests whenever the owner is present (Hart, 1977). The owner's alignment with the subordinate antagonist may gradually forge an unwitting social alliance under which the subordinate is inadvertently encouraged and obliged to challenge the dominant dog's authority, at least whenever the owner is present. On the other hand, the dominant dog may progressively *feel* uncertain about the turn of events and shore up its compromised position by resorting to more frequent and damaging attacks, potentially resulting in serious injury to both the misled upstart and the interfering owner. Under such destabilized conditions, what began as a rare ritualized contest over dominance may develop into a serious pattern of escalating aggression between the dogs. Since such contests are never allowed to run a natural course, hostilities are kept at a high pitch of readiness, with the potential for an outbreak of fighting whenever the combatants meet in the presence of the owner. Because overt aggression invariably causes both combatants discomfort, they may, over the course of several fights, begin to view each other as conditioned aversive stimuli. Aversion, the close cousin of fear, causes the combatants to lose aggression-inhibiting affection for one another, further disinhibiting aggressive hostilities and setting the stage for injurious and potentially deadly fights. It is interesting to note that such dogs rarely fight when left alone, but this cannot be relied on in every case, especially where a high degree of interactive tension is present and where a history of serious fighting already exists. As part of their treatment program, some authorities have recommended leaving resident aggressors together when the owner is absent (McKeown and Luescher, 1988), based on a questionable assumption that such dogs will not fight in the owner's absence. Besides the significant risk involved when the owner returns to potentially aggressive dogs vying for attention, resident combatants do occasionally fight when the owner is absent. Sherman and colleagues (1996), for example, found that 12 pairs of dogs (N = 73 cases) involved in household fighting fought at least one time during the owner's absence. Leaving resident aggressors alone together may result in very serious injury, so the practice should be avoided.

PREVENTION

Many breeds appear to be naturally preadapted to live in peaceful coexistence with other dogs and require little socialization to prevent problems. As previously noted, however, some dogs (especially the traditional fighting breeds) appear to be preadapted to *show* aggression toward other dogs as they mature and may require intensive socialization and training to gain control over their aggressive propensities. For these dogs, the appearance of another male dog represents a powerful releasing signal, triggering a very intense aggressive response. Further, although such behavior can be controlled through training, such dogs may never be completely trustworthy around other dogs.

The most important function of socialization for puppies is to encourage the development of repertoire of playful competitive behaviors. Aggressive play is composed of noninjurious agonistic sequences and species-typical cutoff, threat, and appeasement displays, with which dogs learn how to compromise, control, or defer to an opponent without aggression. Through such interaction, puppies learn that competition does not necessarily result in aggressive conflict. In addition to contact with other puppies, thoughtful efforts should also be made to expose puppies safely to other dogs of various ages. Exposure, however, is not enough to ensure a beneficial result. Socialization is a two-edged learning process and, depending on the sort of interaction involved, can result in either a positive or a negative outcome. Obviously, the benefit or damage produced by socialization depends on the sort of things that happen to puppies while they are exposed to other dogs. Socialization efforts can either lead to greater trust and security or result in increased mistrust and aggressiveness. A puppy should be exposed to other dogs under various environmental conditions and at various locations, but these encounters should always be carefully controlled and supervised. Unfortunately, in uncontrolled situations (e.g., the dog park), the threat of an all-out attack by a poorly socialized and aggressive dog is always possible. Some adult dogs are grossly disorganized in the way they play, whereas others are simply intolerant of puppies; in either case, such exposure may exert a lasting adverse impression on a puppy's attitude toward other dogs.

PART 2: TERRITORIAL DEFENSE

The concepts of territory and territorial defense are commonly appealed to in order to help explain certain forms of canine aggression. Defining precisely what territory is and in what sense a dog defends it is highly problematic, however. Some authors have entirely rejected the construct of territoriality. Moyer (1976), for example, writes,

> The definitions of territorial aggression frequently infer unobservable, anthropomorphic motivational states. These motivational states are projected to the animal and treated as though they were established observations. Territoriality has come to refer to a complex of diverse behavior patterns that vary widely across animal species and within species depending on the animal's sex, the characteristics of the intruder, the season of the year, the developmental stages of the animal, as well as a variety of environmental variables. (226)

The expression of territorial defense varies considerably among animal species, and there is little consensus about what *territory* actually means. The most generally accepted construct of territory is *a defended area*. A difficulty with this definition involves how one can reasonably differentiate territorial defense from protective aggression (Askew, 1996). Borchelt (1983) suggests that the term *protective* is more descriptive and useful than the notion of territorial defense. He argues that dogs aggressively protect household members (humans and other dogs)—not a territory. Although the concept of protectiveness may solve some problems, Borchelt does not explain how one can be sure that the dog is specifically motivated to protect *others,* rather than simply responding to species-typical threat triggers, such as unfamiliarity or unwelcome approach-proximity (a territorial dimension). One way to test the hypothesis is to challenge the dog in the presence of a stranger or when alone. If the dog responds aggressively, it diminishes the likelihood that it is doing so to protect others belonging to the household. In any case, all protective aggression occurs within some *territorial* frame of reference—a given that is consistent with the *defended area* construct of territory. One way of analyzing how territorial defense and protectiveness may be related to each other is by appealing to distal and proximal causes. Intrusion upon territory may elicit preparatory aggressive arousal (distal influence), whereas close approach-proximity (proximal influence) may evoke a consummatory aggressive response. According to this analysis, intrusion upon territory represents an establishing operation making aggression more likely to occur and, should it occur, result in reinforcement if the intruder is expelled as the result of the aggressive action.

Self-defense and group-defense seem to be inextricably bound up with the defense of territory, that is, the space occupied by the group. After all, without the existence of a territory there is no place for the group to exist and, vice versa, without a group there is no territory to defend. Even the individual animal needs to *claim* a personal space and defend it against intrusion in order to maintain its safety and security. On a most basic level, territory and group defense cannot be adequately understood without reference to the other—the group and the territory within which it exists are mutually dependent constructs, just as the description of a circle depends on reference to both its perimeter and area. In some sense, the decision to emphasize territorial versus social variables depends on the focus of one's analysis. However, what is needed is an integrated analysis—a kind of behavioral geometry that simultaneously addresses both

social and territorial variables. Social competition and territorial defense may operate within a single matrix of control-seeking vectors extending over both social (vertical) and territorial (horizontal) space. Among wolves, for instance, this territorial responsibility falls on the alpha and his deputies. When a breech in the territorial integrity of the pack occurs, it is the alpha that leads the defense and engages the intruding interloper; although lower-ranking members may participate in the rout, it is the alpha that is clearly in charge and leading the way.

CONTROL-VECTOR ANALYSIS OF TERRITORY

Need Tensions and Control-vector Analysis

On a very fundamental level, all behavior exhibits the character of spatiotemporal directionality; that is, behavior possesses both temporal sequentiality (e.g., attention-intention-action) and orderly spatial points of reference (e.g., sees bird flying by, physically orients toward it, and finally jumps at the bird). Within this context, motivational interests may be conceptualized as need tensions, having particular goals or target objectives located within the animal's local space. To obtain goal satisfaction through the acquisition of these target objectives, an animal must change or control the environment in some way. Need tensions, in combination with their specific target objectives, form control-seeking vectors of variable magnitude that behaviorally converge upon relevant resources, places, and activities located in the environment [see Lewin (1936)]. The sum area containing these various resources, places, and activities represents an animal's social and territorial space. One way of understanding aggression is to analyze it in terms of competing control vectors belonging to *outsider* and *insider* conspecifics conflicting or colliding with each other over the same target resource. The group's living space is defended by deflecting, displacing, or destroying outsider control-seeking vectors that threaten its social and territorial space. Such defense not only protects the integrity of the group's space, it also preserves and reinforces the more or less stable control-vector relations or *politics* operating within the group itself.

Control vectors are not only characterized by having directionality associated with need tensions, they also possess physiobehavioral properties such as inertia, momentum, velocity, and force. The probable outcome of conflict between two competing control vectors depends on the combined power of these properties exhibited by competitors. In other words, a more forceful control vector, exhibiting a high degree of momentum and velocity, will certainly deflect or displace a control vector possessing less-powerful vector properties. Control vectors possessing the same power vying over the same location or resource will result in momentary unstable equilibrium.

Under the influence of growing levels of destabilizing anxiety and frustration, however, unstable equilibrium between competitors may result in one of four possible outcomes: (1) attack-fight (competitor displaced with potential for injury), (2) attack-retreat (competitor displaced with no injury), (3) cutoff or *lateral escape* (simultaneous deflection of both control vectors), or (4) threat-appeasement (competitor deflected from location or resource) (Figure 7.1). Under the influence of increased anxiety (reduced appetitive need tension) unstable equilibrium is most likely to result in lateral escape or appeasement, whereas under the increasing influence of frustration (enhanced appetitive need tension) overt combat is more likely to occur.

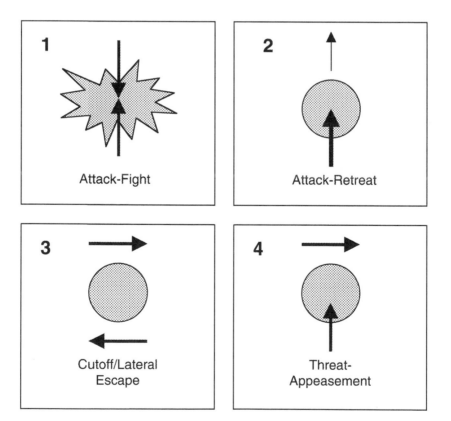

FIG. 7.1. Various control-vector conflict outcomes. (1) Equal control-vector magnitudes and need tensions under the influence of frustration over the same resource, with the result of attack and fight. (2) Control vectors of unequal magnitude but with equal need tensions converging on the same resource, resulting in attack and retreat. (3 and 4) Outcomes of unstable equilibrium (control vectors exhibiting equal magnitude and need tensions) under the influence of mutual anxiety (3) and increasing anxiety (4, *top arrow*) and increasing frustration (4, *bottom arrow*).

Horizontal and Vertical Organization of Social Space

Potentially disruptive interaction between group members exhibiting competitive control-seeking vectors is allayed by the exchange of ritualized threat-appeasement displays—displays designed to maintain adequate distance between *insiders* on both vertical (dominance hierarchy) and horizontal (personal living space) axes of social space (Figure 7.2). The center of territory for a domestic dog is within the home, presumably located precisely where the dog habitually rests or sleeps. At this central zone, the vertical social distancing effects of relative social status are most evident and potentially troublesome. As the result of organizing both horizontal and vertical aspects of group space, serious competition between insiders and their various control-seeking vectors is mitigated. According to this analysis, deference occurs when one individual's control-seeking vectors yield to the control-

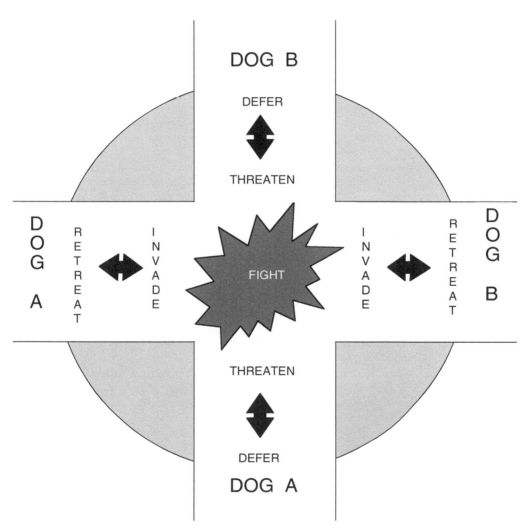

FIG. 7.2. The social space and interaction of a dyad over some common resource. The *vertical axis* of the cross represents the dominance hierarchy, and the *horizontal axis* represents territorial and personal space imperatives. Note that aggression is most likely to occur when both dog A and dog B are simultaneously threatening each other over the same resource or location.

seeking vectors of another by virtue of cooperation (alliance), deflection (ritual threat), or displacement (attack). The *dominant* leader, or alpha, can assert control-seeking vectors in any direction along both vertical and horizontal axes of the group's social space, while yielding to none.

Calhoun's Rat Universe

Of interest with respect to the foregoing vector analysis of territory and social organization are the experimental population ecology studies of Calhoun (1962) [see also Papero (1990)]. In one study, Calhoun captured wild rats and housed them in large enclosures or *universes* with access to unlimited food and protection against predation. Under protected conditions in which unlimited food was provided and predation prevented, he hypothesized that growth rates would be significantly inhibited as the result of social interaction developing under such conditions of abundance and safety. Calhoun made several important discoveries with respect to the development of territory and anomalous social behavior emerging under the influence of adverse environmental conditions. As the population of rats grew, more dominant individuals (corresponding to insiders) took up residency in one quadrant of the habitat, where they eventually established highly stable territories among themselves. As the population of this quadrant increased, weaker individuals (outsiders) were driven out and forced to migrate into other areas of the habitat. These migrant rats were typically low-ranking males. Over time, large numbers of these migrant males formed a colony quadrant of their own. Although more than enough food was provided to feed all the rats, the more dominant rats seized and protected the food, forcing the lower-ranking migrant males to *steal* opportunities to eat while the dominant males were either absent or sleeping.

In contrast to the more orderly quadrant belonging to high-ranking insider rats, the quadrant occupied by low-ranking outsiders was highly chaotic, with no individual rats being able to establish a viable territory of their own. As a result, the few females living in this quadrant were unable to breed and

reproduce successfully. When in estrus, females were hounded by packs of male rats, all of whom made efforts to mount and copulate. Calhoun estimated that a female in estrus might be mounted as many as 1000 times in a single night. As a result, such females appeared highly stressed and were much less able to conceive and raise healthy rat pups. This picture was in sharp contrast to the high-ranking females living within the more orderly quadrant controlled by insider males. Under the protection of dominant insider males, insider females were better able to reproduce successfully and raise their young within the security of well-defended territories. Even though the enclosure was large enough to support as many as 5000 rats, Calhoun found at the conclusion of the study that only 150 rats had survived.

Detailing all of the ways in which control-vector analysis might be used to explain Calhoun's findings is not within the immediate scope of the present discussion, but a few points of convergence and interest should be emphasized. Theoretically, when control-vector conflicts reach a density that the group space can no longer support them, the group may experience general unrest and break up into *insider* and *outsider* subgroups, with each exhibiting their own internal and external control-seeking vectors. In the case of Calhoun's rat colony, only the insider rats developed a territory that was defended against the intrusion of outsiders. Even though there was more than enough food available for both insiders and outsiders, the stronger control-vector magnitudes of dominant insiders deflected or displaced outsiders from the common feeding area. Also, it is interesting that the outsiders were unable to form stable control-vector relations among themselves (dominance relations). This failure may have been due to their inability to control access to food and, most importantly, establish and defend nesting areas. The nesting area is presumably the center of territory and the point where vertical social space is first organized as the result of littermate interactions among themselves and the mother. Without a stable horizontal living space and central nesting area, the organization of vertical social space into stable dominant-subordinate status relations is not possible. Further, without the organization of stable status relations between dominant individuals and subordinates, there is little chance of forming territories within which productive nesting sites might be possible.

HOW TERRITORY IS ESTABLISHED AND DEFENDED

Despite Moyer's misgivings, the concepts of territory and territorial defense remain useful empirical and heuristic constructs for understanding certain aspects of dog behavior. Besides overt territorial-group defense, dogs exhibit other habits that seem intended to communicate both social and territorial messages (e.g., urine marking and alarm or threat barking), perhaps advertising the group's presence or denoting some territorial implication, such as a warning to intruders that the area is occupied. Further, although group protection is undoubtedly a significant variable motivating territorial defense, many dogs exhibit intense aggressive arousal at doors, property boundaries, when chained, or when otherwise exposed to trigger situations presumably related to territory, whether the group is present or not. These observations suggest that the violation of territory in some way triggers or potentiates aggressive behavior independently of the presence or absence of a group to protect. Perhaps the violation of territorial boundaries functions as an establishing operation, preparing a dog to act effectively in defense of itself or its social group.

The propensity to defend personal space and surrounding territory against intrusion by outside conspecifics is a very common feature shared by a great many animal species. This so-called *territorial imperative* is grounded on several ecological and survival needs: resource conservation, population control and dispersion, reproductive needs, group protection, and social unity. The maintenance of territory involves several sensory modalities and methods of communication. Perhaps the most familiar forms of territorial advertisement among dogs are scratching earth, urine marking, and barking. Although territory is an area that is aggressively defended against intrusion, the ultimate

function of territory may be to reduce aggression between competing conspecific groups. The establishment and defense of territory appear to parallel the aggression-reducing effects of status established among individuals sharing the same territory. Among most territorial species, the usual targets of territorial defense are conspecifics of the same sex, but other species may also be the object of attack. Even though the same sexes may share a territory by belonging to the same group, they do so by the establishment of vertical space, that is, the formation of a dominance hierarchy. In conjunction, territorial advertisements and dominance displays serve to reduce actual fighting between conspecific outsiders and conspecific insiders, respectively. The evolutionary success of territorial behavior is evidenced by its wide phylogenetic distribution and the tremendous variability that it presents from species to species (Klopfer, 1969).

Urine-marking Behavior

The habit of urine marking appears to be intensely engrossing, especially for socially dominant or aggressive dogs. Many dogs spend their entire walk outdoors doing little more than performing this intriguing ritual. Although primarily a male prerogative, females may also urine mark in a malelike fashion but rarely do so upon vertical surfaces, as is the common habit of male dogs. Mature dogs, like wolves, urine mark conspicuous objects by lifting and crooking their rear leg before squirting a small amount of urine onto a suitable object. Although this method of depositing urine is the most common, other variations are also used (see Figure 9.1), including a modified squatting form where dogs crouch slightly downward with one leg turned outward or slightly elevated (Anisko, 1976).

Urine-marking behavior is usually preceded by olfactory investigation of previously marked areas. At least one apparent motivation for this behavior is to identify and over-mark areas scented by intruders. Many dogs lick the area being investigated, perhaps, to "freshen" it for closer scrutiny or to introduce a sample of it into the vomeronasal organ for pheromonal analysis [see *Vomeronasal Organ (VNO)* in Volume 1, Chapter 4]. Occasionally, when a site proves particularly interesting, a dog may exhibit a flehmenlike behavior known as *tonguing* in which the tongue is rapidly and repeatedly pushed up against the roof of the mouth. Tonguing is sometimes associated with chattering teeth and profuse foaming of the mouth. After marking, many dogs make conspicuous scratching movements with their front and rear feet. These movements not only scar the ground but also cast dirt and debris several feet behind the marker, perhaps imbuing the material with identifying odors from scent glands located in the feet. It has been speculated that such scratching is done to spread the odor of urine, but this is not convincing, since the urine mark is rarely disturbed by the action. A more plausible explanation for the behavior is that it may serve to augment and amplify the scent mark visually, thereby providing additional clues and information about the marker's size, weight, state of health, general vigor, and other such details not readily exacted from the scent mark alone. Fox (1971) notes that such scratching is particularly likely when the dog is aggressively aroused by the presence of a strange dog.

Urine Marking and Territory

One theory of urine-marking behavior is that it helps to space aggressive individuals, thereby reducing competition over limited resources or mates. According to this general notion, chemosensory cues are integrated with other socially significant signals serving various roles in the regulation (e.g., increase, decrease, or maintain) of social distance between individuals and between conspecific groups. Dogs, in general, do not avoid areas marked by other dogs, although it would not be surprising in the case of particularly aggressive dogs to find some avoidance exhibited by dogs that had been previously attacked or worried by the urine marker. The urine-marking behavior of dogs often involves marking over previously established scent marks—a habit that appears to be highly provocative in its own right.

According to Anisko (1976), odors associated with urine marking may play a significant role in "the establishment and maintenance of dominance hierarchies and pair bonds, thereby stabilizing social organization" (291–292). Marking by urinating near or over areas previously visited by other dogs may function to secure or dominate the olfactory environment. An active social interchange results from the activity—a kind of urinary challenge and personal advertisement of the marker's presence. According to Bekoff (1979), the most likely time for a male dog to mark is after observing another dog marking. Socially dominant dogs appear to mark much more frequently than subordinate ones. Dunbar and Carmichael (1981) also found that male dogs are especially attracted to the urine deposits of other male dogs (especially strangers), tending to urinate more frequently on areas marked by dogs unfamiliar to them.

Although a great deal of speculation attributes a territorial function to urinary-scent marking by dogs, the empirical evidence is scant and conflicting. Many authorities have disputed the value of urine-marking behavior for establishing territory by dogs (Scott, 1967; Bekoff, 1979). Voith and Borchelt (1985) succinctly state the case against attributing a territorial function to urine-marking behavior:

> The term *marking behavior* is often used with the implication that it is territorial. This presumption elicits several problems. In the animal behavior literature, territorial behavior denotes defense of a well demarcated area. The relationship between territoriality and marking in dogs as well as many other animals is unclear. Many animals, particularly dogs, do not limit their marking behavior to their territorial boundaries. They mark multiple locations within the territory as well as areas other than the territory. Additionally, scent marking does not keep other animals out of territories. Dogs typically enter other dogs' territories to urine mark. (540)

Evidence for a Territorial Function of Urine-marking Behavior

Actually, some field evidence does support the notion that urinary-scent marking may play a functional role in the establishment of territorial boundaries consistent with the aforementioned rather stringent criteria, at least in some populations of dogs. For example, Tinbergen (1951/1969, 1958/1969) made ethological observations of huskies in Greenland that support the notion that dogs do establish and defend stable territories. Huskies belonging to small pack groups consisting of 5 to 10 members communally defend and drive off intruders. They are also purported to have an "exact and detailed knowledge" of the extent of their neighbors' home territories and avoid areas where attacks are likely occur:

> The most interesting aspect of their behaviour was the fact that these packs defended group territories. All members of a pack joined in fighting other dogs off, the males being more aggressive than the females. This tendency to join forces when attacking strange dogs was the more striking since within each pack relations were far from friendly. . .. The clashes between neighboring packs were extremely interesting to watch. If they met at the boundary between their two territories, where the issues were even, neither group attacked. The males, and more particularly the leaders, growled at each other, and every now and then they lifted a leg and urinated—"planting a scent flag" as it can be called, for this is a means of staking out a territory and advertising it by smell. The state of tension in these strongly aroused, yet inhibited, champions also showed itself in acts which, in their similarity to human behaviour, were a source of endless amusement to us: they took it out on their own pack and the unfortunate dog of low rank who happened to come too near was growled at, or even severely mauled. (1958/1969:30–31)

In addition, Tinbergen found that young huskies did not participate in territorial disputes. Prepubertal dogs appear to lack a concept of territoriality, frequently violating neighboring areas defended by other huskies in spite of their harsh reprisals. Further, the dogs appear unable to learn where they can safely go and cannot go. Tinbergen (1951/1969) comments that "their stupidity in this respect is amazing" (150). As they reach sexual maturity at approximately 8 months of age, they appear to immediately understand, recognizing the topography of surrounding territories, and thereby learn to

avoid attacks. He observed in the case of two dogs that several significant developmental changes took place within the course of 1 week, including the first copulation, first active defense of territory, and first avoidance of strange territory. These cumulative field observations seem to give credible support to the notion that dogs—given sufficient opportunity—establish and defend territorial boundaries.

Studies of stray and feral dog populations also suggest that dogs do establish stable groups and defend territory against intruders. For example, Font (1987), who studied a group of stray dogs in Valencia, Spain, found that stray dogs form stable social affiliations, involving the establishment of a dominance hierarchy and the group-coordinated defense of a communal territory. These observations appear to conflict with earlier findings by Beck (1973), which suggested that urban stray dogs form only loosely defined and temporary group affiliations. More recently, Boitani and colleagues (1996) reported that even more active and wolflike patterns of territorial defense and wariness are exhibited by feral dogs. They describe an incident that strongly suggests that dogs do appreciate the territorial implication of scent marking, at least with respect to the significance of lupine scent marking:

> The presence of wolves may, therefore, be an important factor shaping the dogs' home range and determining its location. . . No dispersal movements were observed, and only few brief excursions outside the usual home range were recorded. We have the impression that the dogs moved as if suddenly attracted by a scent: they went to check out the origin and possibly the nature and consistency of the signal. This impression was reinforced when the dogs went into the northern wolf pack territory at a time wolves are usually in oestrus. The dogs ran into and out of the area without stopping or slowing down, as if aware of the risks of being caught intruding in a wolf area. (238)

Although the role of urine-marking behavior for the establishment of territorial boundaries remains undecided, urine-marking behavior by domestic dogs may have been adapted to serve a more subtle "psychological" function than the explicit demarcation of territorial boundaries. In particular, urine marking may provide dogs with an enhanced sense of confidence while ranging about the neighborhood, making it more familiar and secure. This notion is supported by the observation that puppies eliminate in familiar areas and, later on, at locations previously marked by their parents (Fox, 1971).

Urinary-scent Marking by Wolves

Although the role of urinary-scent marking by dogs for establishing territory is unclear, the activity does appear to serve a territorial function among free-ranging wolves. Peters and Mech (1975), who studied the scent-marking habits of wolves, concluded that scent marking *probably* does help to define territorial boundaries between neighboring packs. One observation they describe is strikingly similar to the incident reported by Boitani and associates. They saw a group of wolves chasing a deer that the pack had just severely wounded. The deer evaded capture by running into the territory of a neighboring pack. The trailing wolves gave up their chase as the deer moved into the adjacent territory. According to the authors, this behavior was out of keeping with the wolf's normal persistence in the pursuit of wounded prey, thereby suggesting that some territorial mechanism may have been at work. Unfortunately, they do not show how scent-mark identification might have played a vital role in the foregoing case. Other bits of circumstantial and anecdotal evidence (subject to much interpretation) are presented in support of the hypothesis. Surprisingly, even among wolves, the case has not been proven beyond doubt that urinary-scent marking is performed to delineate territorial boundaries. Nonetheless, it does seem reasonable to attribute a significant territorial function to scent marking by wolves.

Other studies investigating scent-marking behavior by wolves have shown that it is strongly influenced by both hormonal and social factors, especially relative social status (Asa et al., 1985). Among captive wolves, only dominant males and dominant females urine mark (with an exception of subordinates that

are competing for higher status). Urine-marking postures reflect an individual's relative dominance. Additionally, marking behavior increases seasonally corresponding to periods of increased sexual activity and raised testosterone levels. However, seasonal variations of testosterone levels have little effect on the urine-marking activity of subordinate males, suggesting that social status modulates hormonal influences responsible for mediating the expression of such behavior (Asa et al., 1990).

Barking and Territory

In addition to urine marking, territory may be defended through vocal alarms and threats (acoustic marking). Dogs exhibit various forms of both alarm and threat vocalization as a means to draw attention to, or to ward off, intruders. Not only do auditory signals provide information about the approximate distance and direction of the vocalizer, they also provide biologically significant information about the identity of the sender (Heffner, 1976). A recent study of canine growling suggests that *formants* or frequency patterns contained in a growl may give receivers vital information about the sender as a potential opponent, with smaller and larger dogs producing distinctive auditory formants (Riede and Fitch, 1999). In addition to the size of the opponent, growling variations appear to express important information about the sender's readiness to attack, degree of confidence, or willingness to submit. Whereas low-frequency, broad-band growling is associated with threats, high-frequency whining is most often associated with submission. Social and territorial threat displays incorporate a variety of sensory modalities to help amplify and disambiguate the sender's intention and meaning.

Alarm barking is highly valued by most dog owners but may represent a nuisance to neighbors (Senn and Lewin, 1975). Such barking behavior warns the group of a pending threat, as well as countering the intruder's advances further into the home territory; that is, barking appears to serve a dual territorial and group-defense function. Alarm barking is usually sustained as long as an intruder remains present. It is rhythmically organized with brief pauses of silence of various lengths apparently used to follow the intruder's movements. A less loud and sustained alarm-barking sequence takes place when a dog is surprised by an outside stimulus that it cannot immediately identify as an intruder. Surprise or startle barking involves low-volume "woof, woof" sounds followed by a brief period of silence and more energetic alarm barking, if warranted. Threat barking frequently develops out of alarm barking, especially in situations in which an intruder continues to advance upon the territory. As barking escalates and becomes more threatening, it takes on a more aggressive and threatening character. Threat barking may be interspersed with bouts of growling, snarling, lunging, or snapping at the intruder. If the intruder continues to advance, the dog may either launch an attack or flee from the situation, perhaps continuing its threat barking from the advantage of a more secure position.

FREE-FLOATING TERRITORY

The operative definition of territory is *a defended area.* This definition is neither limited in terms of the size of the area nor is it qualified by the amount of time that the area has been occupied. Accordingly, territory can be either small or large or defended over short or long periods (Immelmann, 1980). Some highly dominant dogs appear to take possession of any area in which they happen to be and will defend it against the intrusion of other dogs or people. When such dogs are first introduced to a new area, they often immediately set out to urine mark the entire perimeter of the area systematically before taking interest in other activities. The mere fact of *being* somewhere is sufficient for such dogs to prompt energetic efforts to establish a territorial presence over the area and to defend it against the intrusion of other male dogs and people. A territorial imperative appears to follow or *float* with such dogs, moving fluidly from one place to the next with great ease. Each new area is secured and defended with an equal aggressive tenacity.

Some of the peculiar territorial adaptations (e.g., free-floating territorial defense) and associated hypertrophied behavior patterns (e.g., barking and urine marking) may be the result of artificial pressures placed on dogs during domestication. Under the influence of domestication, natural pressures conducive to the organization of species-typical territorial defensive behavior are absent. Domestic dogs are neither required to hunt for their own food, locate mates, nor rear their young under adverse natural conditions. In fact, not only are dogs unique in that they do not hunt for a living or form lasting pair bonds with their mate, male dogs are the only canids that do not contribute to the care of their progeny. The absence of such pressures as these may help to explain some of the unusual aspects and variations of canine territoriality:

> The term "territorial" aggression is applicable to species in which the actual securing and holding of territory has adaptive advantage. In the domestic dog, the function of this behavior has apparently generalized or been selected to include protection of significant persons in the dog's social unit as well as places in the environment. (Borchelt, 1983:58)

An important effect of domestication is the alteration of behavioral thresholds controlling freeze, flight, and fight responses. Selective breeding has exercised a pronounced influence on the development of breed-specific variations in territorial defense by artificially enhancing or diminishing relevant traits and behavioral thresholds (Price, 1998).

TERRITORIAL AGGRESSION VERSUS GROUP PROTECTION

In practice, it is often difficult to differentiate defensive aggression from territorial aggression (Askew, 1996). One useful way to differentiate defensive aggression from territorial aggression is to determine whether fear is present as a significant motivational variable, and whether behaviors indicative of territorial motivation (e.g., barking and marking) are present or absent. Dogs exhibiting strong territorial aggressive tendencies are typically more assertive and confident. Also, the contexts of aggression are often highly specified, involving other male dogs and unfamiliar human targets intruding on significant territorial boundaries or areas. Territorial aggression involving a high degree of assertiveness can also be differentiated from defensive aggression by the latter's response to behavioral intervention. Defensive behavior is often highly responsive to behavior modification, whereas assertive territorial aggression may strongly resist training efforts. Territorial aggression and group protection cannot be entirely differentiated, because they are mutually dependent constructs. Group protection is the prerogative of a highly dominant dog that appears to respond to territorial intrusion as an establishing operation for the expression of assertive and threatening behavior toward the intruder. Aggression with respect to the protection of others (e.g., children) may be a generalized form of maternal-paternal aggression.

VARIABLES INFLUENCING TERRITORIAL AGGRESSION

Canine territorial aggression is inextricably entwined with the development and protection of the group's integrity as a social and cooperative unit. Protective behavior both establishes territorial boundaries and sets limits between the group and other conspecifics or people not belonging to it. A number of social and environmental factors facilitate social distancing and influence the character of territorial aggression in dogs. Among the most important of these are frustrative restraint, frequency of territorial violation, social facilitation, crowding, and ambience.

Frustration and Restraint

Confinement in the house, behind a fence, or tied to a chain tends to invigorate territorial behavior. Unlike wolves and feral dogs, a domestic dog's freedom of movement is artificially constrained and limited by both physical and social barriers. Such constraints not only define the boundary of a dog's home territory, they also prevent escape to safety in case of danger. These artificial boundaries are often vigorously defended against intrusion. Under conditions of confinement in which a dog's freedom of movement is constrained, it may feel trapped, vulnerable, frustrated, agitated, and thereby become progressively more and more vigilant and aggressive toward the potential threat of intruding strangers and vagrant dogs. In general, the effect of frustrative restraint is to invigorate or distort the species-typical defensive tendencies present in dogs.

Fences, doors, and windows are particularly problematic, since these barriers simultaneously define a dog's territorial boundary, with the potential intruder located just on the other side, leaving little room for other options to present themselves or develop. Defending what little space is left before the territory is breached becomes critically important for a confined dog, especially if escape is not a viable option. There is no buffer zone or room to negotiate other courses of action under such circumstances of territorial intrusion. This state of affairs is especially problematic for dogs exhibiting relatively low fear thresholds and defensive aggression. The resulting defensive behavior of such dogs is often frenetic, compulsive, and extreme. Under situations in which escape is not possible, fearful dogs possessing a strong tendency to engage in defensive aggression are often highly vigilant and prepared to threaten or attack strangers intruding upon their domain. Aggressive tensions and wariness around disputed boundaries (e.g., doorways and fences) can reach compulsive levels.

Finally, some evidence suggests that frustration over food may increase territorial aggression. Jagoe and Serpell (1996) found that dogs fed after their owners showed significantly more territorial aggression than dogs fed before their owners. Speculating, they attributed this tendency to feeding schedule-induced differences of general arousal. They also noted that making a dog wait may alter its perception of the value of food, perhaps making it more defensive over food when confronted with intruding strangers. These explanations are a bit of a stretch given the limited data presented, but it may be important from a husbandry and preventative perspective to feed dogs *before* rather than after the family eats—in opposition to the advice of some trainers and behavioral counselors regarding the benefits of feeding the dog in a reverse order (Rogerson, 1988; Seksel, 1997). Further, contrary to the opinion of Rogerson about order of feeding, Jagoe and Serpell found no evidence indicating that feeding the dog before the owners ate increased the risk of the dog developing dominance-related aggression.

Effect of Frequent Territorial Intrusion

Dog bites are a common cause of injury to mail carriers, with 2851 of them having been bitten in 1995 (U.S. Postal Service statistic). The daily intrusion of mail *violating* the territorial integrity of the door is often the object of fierce aggression, with the dog attacking and tearing up the mail as it is pushed through the letter slot. The mail carrier's daily "intrusion" upon the dog's home territory may gradually heighten its aggressive efforts into a frenzy. Serious problems have developed out of this perceived intrusion and violation of territory. During such encounters, dogs have crashed through glass windows for the opportunity to attack a mail carrier, even ignoring the chemical-spray deterrents used for defense against such occurrences. Since mail carriers are common targets for territorial aggression (Beck et al., 1975), special precautions should be taken to prevent such aggression from developing. A couple of simple measures often help to prevent or reduce such tensions: (1) let the dog regularly meet and accept treats from the mail carrier, (2) when a mail slot is used have the mail carrier insert a biscuit with the mail for the dog's pleasure, and (3) consistently discourage aggressive displays. In extreme cases, the mail should delivered to a mailbox located some distance away from the front door.

Sources of Territorial Agitation: Fences and Chains

Territorial defensive excesses are often expressed in a compulsive form along fences toward other dogs and passersby. Konrad Lorenz reports a comic incident involving territorial aggression between two dogs *defending the same fence line* (Lorenz, 1954). He describes how these two enthusiastic fence

fighters were surprised to discover one day that a portion of their shared fence had been removed for repairs. The two dogs, accustomed to run along the fence carrying on a spirited exchange of threat and counterthreat, found themselves face to face without an intervening barrier between them. After a brief stay of hostilities, the erstwhile combatants broke the lull of bewilderment by retreating back to the part of the fence still standing to continue their battle safely. Unfortunately, this amusing anecdote defines the extreme exception rather than the rule. Most fence fighters would readily welcome the opportunity to engage in actual fighting, often jumping over or digging under fences to do so. In addition, serious attacks have been delivered on innocent children and adults reaching through fences or car windows to pet a dog— attacks that sometimes occur without much warning or indication of the dog's aggressive intentions. Children playing near a fence or in view of a chained dog are common sources of agitation, and measures should be taken to prevent such contact and stimulation. This situation is compounded when children actually tease and taunt a dog. Many cases involving the chasing of bicycles and cars appear to involve similar territorial issues.

The invigoration of aggression by restraint can be seen in an exaggerated form in situations where a dog is habitually restrained on a chain and stake. Some of the most severe and *deadly* canine attacks toward humans have been launched by chained dogs or dogs that have broken free of their chain. Sacks and colleagues (1989) reported that among pet-related mortalities that 28% resulted when a child approached too close to a chained dog. In 36% of these cases, the children were killed after gaining unauthorized access to a fenced area containing the dog. Among stray dogs, 35.7% of the fatal attacks were delivered by a dog that had escaped a fence, pen, or other form of restraint. The following is a typical report:

HAMILTON, Ohio, Nov. 18 (UPI)—Butler County Animal Shelter officials will determine Monday whether a Siberian husky and a chow will be destroyed for attacking and killing 7-year-old Ethan Fricke.

The 3-year-old husky and 18-month-old chow killed Fricke at the child's uncle's home in Ross while his parents, and other relatives were attending a Saturday baby shower.

The uncle, Nick Toon, said he warned the boy not to play with the dogs unless an adult was present.

"I tried to explain to him that even though they are friendly, they could hurt him because they are bigger and stronger than he is," Toon told the *Cincinnati Enquirer.*

Sheriff Don Gabbard said the boy was playing alone and went into a fenced area of Toon's backyard where the dogs were chained.

Gabbard said one, or both dogs, bit the child, severing an artery in his neck.

Sheriff's deputies say Fricke died less than one-hour after being attacked.

"If the decision is to destroy them, I will agree with that," Toon said, "But I would like to say to others who own chow dogs that they shouldn't run out and destroy them because of this. A lot of people will say they are vicious, but they are not. This was just an accident."

A service for Fricke was scheduled Wednesday at the Fairfield West Baptist Church.

Moral: A chained, intact, male dog is a statistical menace to public safety.

Social Facilitation and Crowding

Dogs living in communal situations are subject to additional pressures that may intensify territorial defensiveness. A well-know factor augmenting territorial aggression is social facilitation. The mere presence of another dog alters the strength of shared or allelomimetic behavior, including group-coordinated territorial defense. Most dogs are much more aggressive when in companionship with other dogs acting out aggressively. This fact is commonly employed by police and military-dog trainers who frequently agitate dogs in group (line agitation) to build confidence and aggressiveness. Under the influence of social facilitation, dogs tend to intensify their behavioral efforts beyond the magnitudes that they would exhibit if alone. When social facilitation is combined with crowded circumstances, especially involving untrained or poorly socialized dogs, the situation is ripe for the outbreak of frequent and potentially serious displays of territorial aggression. Dogs, unlike other species, appear to accommodate crowded conditions without exhibiting a significant increase in agonistic behavior, especially in circumstances where a stable dominance hierarchy has been established among group members before they are exposed to crowded conditions (Pettijohn et al., 1980).

Ambience

Pettijohn (1978) reported interesting findings concerning the relative effects of various environmental influences on the expression of agonistic behavior among male Telomian dogs. Although not specifically concerned with territorial aggression, the study nonetheless provides obvious environmental management strategies that may have practical implications for manipulating aggressive thresholds. He observed changes in agonistic interaction under the influence of various environmental conditions, including a control room (same as home pen—3.0 × 3.5 meters kept at 21°C), cold room (10°C), bright light (floodlights placed in the corners of the room), dim light (lights turned off and windows covered), and small space (room reduced to 3.0 × 1.8 meters). The dogs were all 7 months of age. He found that the total number of attacks, vocalizations, and retreats were most significantly influenced by the amount of light present in the test situation. Dim light increased agonistic interaction by 32%, whereas bright light decreased it by 28% relative to agonistic behavior occurring under normal lighting conditions. These results are striking and pronounced, but it is unclear how relative light intensity might affect the expression of aggressive behavior.

Stressful exposure to loud and sustained noises may also lower thresholds for the exhibition of offensive aggression, perhaps as the result of increasing irritability. Some dogs appear to have a greater tendency to exhibit aggressive behavior during or immediately after noisy household repairs. Two dogs come to mind where sound stress appears to have played a significant role. In one case, involving an adult male Labrador retriever, workmen used a jackhammer to remove an asphalt driveway. During the 2 days while the work was being done, the dog observed the various activities from the vantage of the front porch and did not show any signs of agitation or aggression. At the end of the second day, however, when a workman approached the front door, the dog darted at to him and bit him on the leg. In another case, an adult male Labrador mix was left outside in a garden while workmen were occupied grinding down several tree stumps. After several hours, the dog approached and threatened one of the workmen, backing him across the yard with threatening barks and lunges. Neither dog exhibited threatening behavior before or after the aforementioned incidents. As a general rule, when work is being done that produces loud noises, dogs should be kept indoors and insulated from such stimulation.

PART 3: FEAR-RELATED AGGRESSION

FEAR AND AGGRESSION

Fear is a major motivational factor in the expression and inhibition of aggression. The role of fear is a bit complicated and equivocal, since fear usually inhibits aggression under most circumstances involving moderate levels of fearful arousal. For example, trainers of circus animals, especially those working with large cats, put their lives at risk on the assumption that fear can inhibit aggression. Such training with cracker-whips, blank guns, and various threatening props deliberately serves to evoke and carefully balance the opposing tendencies of flight or fight in such animals. Essentially, such training proceeds to establish control by alternately evoking fear and aggression. Whether flight or attack occurs during such challenges depends on past training and relative thresholds for running away (*flight distance*) or holding ground (*critical distance*). Under conditions of abrupt and intense aversive arousal, both fear and anger may be simultaneously evoked—a potentially lethal circumstance for large-cat trainers. Under such conditions, efforts to suppress aggressive behavior by punishment may not reduce aggression but instead precipitate a spiraling escalation of fear and anger. Such efforts are especially problematic in cases in which dogs lack a safe alternative with which to control the evocative situation.

Fear and Avoidance-motivated Aggression

Fearful territorial defense occurs in situations involving intense threatening arousal that cannot be otherwise escaped, that is, when flight is blocked. When threatened, dogs in such situations attack only as a last resort and then only if their freedom of movement is blocked. Fearful aggression is not employed to defend a territorial boundary but to establish a route of escape from an otherwise inescapable and threatening situation. As a result of successful escape, however, dogs may learn to attack more easily (threshold lowered) in the future under the influence of similar circumstance and territorial triggers. Avoidance-motivated aggression (AMA) develops in situations where a dog has learned that aggression will likely work to control some threatening situation. Although defensive aggression theoretically stands opposite to offensive aggression on the agonistic continuum, AMA is often difficult to distinguish from offensive aggression, especially as the dog becomes progressively confident in its ability to control the threatening situation through aggression. In an important sense, aggression, whether it occurs to secure escape or to defend some resource or area, is motivationally unified under the construct of control. Control-related aggression includes aggression occurring under the influence of escalating adversity that thwarts a dog's ability to control an attractive situation or impedes its ability to escape or avoid an aversive one. In other words, a frustrated or anxious dog may assert itself aggressively to secure or alter a motivationally aversive situation. Interestingly in this regard, defensive and offensive aggression may be alternately present in the same dog. Functionally speaking, most forms of dominance- and fear-related aggression are motivated to establish control over a frustrating or threatening social situation.

Fear and Territorial Aggression

Fear-related aggression is highly directional, situationally specific, often precipitated by a territorial intrusion, and highly predictable. Fear-related aggression often occurs under an inhibitory influence, with the target receiving ample preliminary signs and threats before an inhibited attack is launched. This feature is frequently lacking in *dominance aggressors,* who may attack without noticeable warning and deliver a hard, *angry* bite. A fearful dog usually attacks in an inhibited and nervous manner, biting only hard enough and long enough to escape the feared situation. The target may be children, adults, or other dogs (frequently without respect to sex), and such attacks occur under a variety of provocative circumstances. Obviously, reducing fear is central to effective behavioral control and modification of fear-related territorial aggression. However, in addition to fear-reduction efforts, fearful aggressors need to learn more constructive ways to control evocative social transactions and territorial transitions without responding aggressively.

A strong association exists between territorial aggression and fear. In fact, fear-related aggression is commonly misinterpreted as territorial aggression. Interestingly, both fear-related and territorial aggression are unaffected by castration (Hopkins et al., 1976), perhaps reflecting a similar motivational substrate shared by the two forms of aggression. Fearful dogs are frequently nervous and reactive during territorial transitions (e.g., meeting guests at the door) or under circumstances in which their personal space is limited or their movements are constrained. Such dogs may engage in sustained, frenetic barking efforts, perhaps while simultaneously backing away from the unwanted advance of guests. A fearful dog's reactions are particularly intense in situations involving close confinement. For example, extreme reactions (e.g., sustained barking, lunging, growling, and air snapping) are commonly observed among such dogs when they are approached while restrained or confined (e.g., in a crate or automobile, or on leash). These dogs are probably more worried about defending themselves than defending their territory, but arbitrarily separating these defensive constructs is not useful. Although a dog may react aggressively to defend itself, the trigger is often related to a threat of territorial intrusion. Identifying these territorial triggers, altering them, or changing the dog's expectations with respect to them are important aspects of the behavioral management of such problems.

REFERENCES

Anisko JJ (1976). Communication by chemical signals in Canidae. In RL Doty (Ed), *Mammalian Olfaction, Reproductive Processes, and Behavior.* New York: Academic.

Asa C, Mech LD, and Seal US (1985). The use of urine, faeces, and anal-gland secretions in scent-marking by a captive wolf (*Canis lupus*) pack. *Anim Behav,* 33:1034–1036.

Asa CS, Mech LD, Seal US, and Plotka ED (1990): The influence of social and endocrine factors on urine-marking by captive wolves (*Canis lupus*). *Horm Behav,* 24:497–509.

Askew HR (1996). *Treatment of Behavior Problems in Dogs and Cats: A Guide for the Small Animal Veterinarian.* Cambridge, MA: Blackwell Science.

Beach FA, Buehler MG, and Dunbar IF (1982). Competitive behavior in male, female, and pseudohermaphroditic female dogs. *J Comp Physiol Psychol,* 96:855–874.

Beck AM (1973). *The Ecology of Stray Dogs: A Study of Free-ranging Urban Animals.* Baltimore: York.

Beck AL, Loring H, and Lockwood R (1975). The ecology of dog bite injury in St. Louis, Missouri. *Public Health Rep,* 90:262–267.

Bekoff M (1979). Scent-marking by free-ranging domestic dogs: Olfactory and visual components. *Biol Behav,* 4:123–139.

Boitani L, Francisci F, and Ciucci P (1996). Population biology and ecology of feral dogs in central Italy. In J Serpell (Ed), *The Domestic Dog: Its Evolution, Behaviour, and Interaction with People.* New York: Cambridge University Press.

Borchelt PL (1983). Aggressive behavior of dogs kept as companion animals: Classification and influence of sex, reproductive status, and breed. *Appl Anim Ethol* 10:45–61.

Borchelt PL and Voith VL (1996). Dominance aggression in dogs (Update). In VL Voith and PL Borchelt (Eds), *Readings in Companion Animal Behavior.* Trenton, NJ: Veterinary Learning Systems.

Bradshaw JWS and Lea AM (1992). Dyadic interactions between domestic dogs. *Anthrozoös,* 5:245–253.

Calhoun JB (1962). Population density and social pathology. *Sci Am,* 206:139–148.

Campbell WE (1974). Dog-fighting dogs. *Mod Vet Pract,* Oct:813–816.

Clifford DH, Boatfield MP, and Rubright J (1983). Observations on the fighting dogs. *JAVMA,* 183:654–657.

Coppolla MC (1986). Dominance aggression in dogs [Master's thesis]. Department of Psychology, Hunter College, New York, NY.

Dunbar I and Carmichael M (1981). The response of male dogs to urine from other males. *Behav Neural Biol*, 31:465–470.

Fielding, Henry (1918). *The Tragedy of Tragedies or The Life and Death of Tom Thumb the Great* (H. Scriblerus Secundus). New Haven, CT: Yale University Press.

Font E (1987). Spacing and social organization: Urban stray dogs revisited. *Appl Anim Behav Sci*, 17:319–328.

Fox MW (1971). *Behaviour of Wolves, Dogs and Related Canids*. New York: Harper and Row.

Frank H and Frank MG (1982). On the effects of domestication on canine social development and behavior. *Appl Anim Ethol*, 8:507–525.

Goodwin D, Bradshaw JWS, and Wickens SM (1997). Paedomorphosis affects agonistic visual signals of domestic dogs. *Anim Behav*, 53:297–304.

Hart BL (1977). Fighting between dogs in the owner's presence. *Canine Pract*, 4:19–21.

Hart BL (1985). *The Behavior of Domestic Animals*. New York: WH Freeman.

Hart BL and Hart LA (1985). *Canine and Feline Behavioral Therapy*. Philadelphia: Lea and Febiger.

Heffner HE (1975). Perception of biologically meaningful sounds by dogs. *J Acoust Soc Am*, 58:S124.

Hopkins SG, Schubert TA, and Hart BL (1976). Castration of adult male dogs: Effects on roaming, aggression, urine marking, and mounting. *JAVMA*, 168:1108–1110.

Immelmann K (1980). *Introduction to Ethology*. New York: Plenum.

Jagoe JA and Serpell JA (1996). Owner characteristics and interactions and the prevalence of canine behaviour problems. *Appl Anim Behav Sci*, 47:31–42.

Juarbe-Diaz S (1997). Social dynamics and behavior problems in multiple-dog households. *Vet Clin North Am Prog Companion Anim Behav*, 27:497–514.

Klopfer PH (1969). *Habitats and Territories: A Study of the Use of Space by Animals*. New York: Basic.

Knol BW and Egberink-Alink ST (1989). Androgens, progestagens and agonistic behaviour: A review. *Vet Q*, 11:94–101.

Lewin K (1936). *Principles of Topological Psychology*. New York: McGraw-Hill.

Lieberman LL (1987). A case for neutering pups and kittens at two months of age. *JAVMA*, 191:518–521.

Lockwood R and Rindy K (1987). Are "pit bulls" different? An analysis of the pit bull terrier controversy. *Anthrozoös*, 1:2–8.

Lorenz K (1954). *Man Meets Dog*. Boston: Houghton Mifflin.

McKeown D and Luescher A (1988). Canine competitive aggression: A clinical case of "sibling rivalry." *Can Vet J*, 29:395–396.

Moyer KE (1976). *The Psychobiology of Aggression*. New York: Harper and Row.

Neilson JC, Eckstein RA, and Hart BL (1997). Effects of castration on problem behaviors in male dogs with reference to age and duration of behavior. *JAVMA*, 211:180–182.

Papero DV (1990). *Bowen Family System Theory*. Boston: Allyn and Bacon.

Pettijohn TF (1978). Environment and agonistic behavior in male Telomian dogs. *Psychol Rep*, 42:1146.

Pettijohn TF, Davis KL, and Scott JP (1980). Influence of living area space on agonistic interaction in Telomian dogs. *Behav Neural Biol*, 28:343–349.

Peters RP and Mech DL (1975). Scent-marking in wolves. *Am Sci*, 63:628–637.

Price EO (1998). Behavioral genetics and the process of animal domestication. In T Grandin (Ed), *Genetics and the Behavior of Domestic Animals*. New York: Academic.

Riede T and Fitch T (1999). Vocal tract length and acoustics of vocalization in the domestic dog (*Canis familiaris*). *J Exp Biol*, 202:2859–2867.

Roll A and Unshelm J (1997). Aggressive conflicts amongst dogs and factors affecting them. *Appl Anim Behav Sci*, 52:229–242.

Rogerson J (1988). *Your Dog: Its Development, Behaviour, and Training*. London: Popular.

Sacks JJ, Sattin RW, and Bonzo SE (1989). Dog bite-related fatalities from 1979 through 1988. *JAMA*, 262:1489–1492.

Sanders CR (1999). *Understanding Dogs: Living and Working with Canine Companions*. Philadelphia: Temple University Press.

Scott JP (1967). The evolution of social behavior in dogs and wolves. *Am Zool*, 7:373–381.

Scott JP and Fuller JL (1965). *Genetics and the Social Behavior of the Dog*. Chicago: University of Chicago Press.

Senn CL and Lewin JD (1975). Barking dogs as an environmental problem. *JAVMA*, 166:1065–1068.

Seksel K (1997). Puppy socialization classes. *Vet Clin North Am Prog Companion Anim Behav,* 27:465–477.

Sherman CK, Reisner IR, Taliaferro LA, and Houpt KA (1996). Characteristics, treatment, and outcome of 99 cases of aggression between dogs. *Appl Anim Behav Sci,* 47:91–108.

Tinbergen N (1951/1969). *The Study of Instinct.* Oxford: Oxford University Press (reprint).

Tinbergen N (1958/1969). *Curious Naturalists.* New York: Natural History Library Anchor Books (reprint).

US Postal Service (1996). Postal news (Press Release 51). http://www.usps.gov/news/press/96/96051new.htm.

Voith VL and Borchelt PL (1985). Elimination behavior and related problems in dogs. In VL Voith and PL Bercholt (Eds), *Readings in Companion Animal Behavior.* Trenton, NJ: Veterinary Learning Systems.

8

Social Competition and Aggression

Animals can be both sociable and aggressive. At first sight the two seem impossible to
reconcile, for if a fellow species member can arouse both friendly impulses of
attraction and those of repulsion one might expect the result to be insoluble conflict.
And it is true that all animals living in closed groups have had to resolve this problem.
In order to do so a number of inventions have proved necessary. Among other things,
rites that appease and establish bonds had to be evolved. Aggressive animals that live
in groups are always busy keeping the peace.

IRENÄUS EIBL-EIBESFELDT, *Love and Hate: The Natural History of Behavior Patterns* (1971)

ASSESSMENT AND IDENTIFICATION

Dominance aggression is often described as the
most common behavior problem presented for
treatment to behavior specialists and counselors (Landsberg, 1991) (Figure 8.1). Most
dogs fitting this category either have threatened or have actually bitten a family member.
Dominance-related aggression is generally
identified by two criteria present at the time of
attack: (1) a perceived threat (e.g., gesture, posture, or contact) and (2) intrusion upon a situation occupied by the dog (e.g., possessions,
places, and persons). For example, aggressive
attacks may occur when an owner attempts to
restrain or punish (vocally or physically) the
dog or exhibits challenging postures, domi-
nant-appearing gestures (direct eye contact), or
even very subtle or benign actions such as

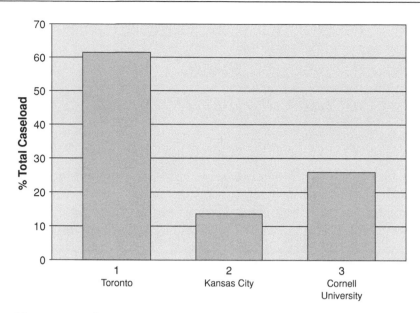

FIG. 8.1. The percentage of cases involving dominance-related aggression for three animal behavior clinics. From Landsberg (1991).

unwelcome petting (contact aversion). Dominance threats or attacks occur under a variety of situations, such as when an owner reaches for toys, food, or other prized possessions located near the dog; when disturbing or attempting to remove the dog from resting areas, especially beds and sofas; when disturbing the dog while in the company of a particular family member (especially when the dog is on the person's lap); and when the dog is put in its crate or the owner attempts to leave the house (Table 8.1).

A distinguishing characteristic of dominance aggression is that it is often situational or object specific and socially selective. For example, it is not uncommon for a dog to be dominant over another dog or family member in one situation but submissive toward them in another. In addition, dogs may exhibit highly selective dominance tendencies, being aggressive, for example, only when in possession of a particular item, while eating, or while in close association with a particular location or person. Aggressive efforts to control a situation appear to be related to motivational factors (biological needs and appetites). Dogs with strong appetitive interests may assert themselves exclusively over food or

chew objects, whereas other dogs with strong attachments toward a particular individual may become aroused only when the object of their affection is approached. Still other dogs may become reactive only when their freedom of movement is momentarily constrained, when various parts of their body are physically manipulated, or when intruded upon while resting or sleeping. The selective nature of these arousal situations suggests an underlying differentiation of motivation with respect to those resources and activities. Consequently, treatment programs should address these functional motivational considerations as well as manage coactive emotional influences that may exert pronounced effects on aggression thresholds. These coactive influences and effects on aggression include

1. Frustrative invigoration of appetitive motivation resulting in lowered thresholds for offensive aggression
2. Increased anxious vigilance and lowered thresholds for defensive aggression
3. Increased contact aversion and lowered thresholds for the elicitation of reflexive aggression in response to discomfort or irritability

TABLE 8.1. Control-related dominance aggression: sources of conflict

Situations	Actions
Locations	
Bed	Aggression may occur if the dog is disturbed while
Furniture	resting or sleeping. Commonly occurs if the dog is
Sleeping area	forcefully removed from furniture or a bed.
Doorways	The dog is prompted to move away from the doorway, touched, or stepped over.
Crate	The dog attacks when forcefully placed into a crate or approached while confined.
Rooms	The dog becomes aggressive as the owner enters or leaves the room or house.
Objects	The dog may become aggressive if approached while
Food	eating, chewing, in possession of some prized
Prized objects	object, or while in close contact with a family
Attachment figure	member. Attacks may occur after the dog has been chased into hiding under furniture or when an item is forcefully removed from the dog's mouth.
Tactile stimulation	In some cases, minimal contact stimulation may
Petting	evoke a strong aggressive response (low-threshold
Hugging	aggression). Aggressive dogs may not show an affectionate response to petting. They are often aloof and emotionally reserved.
Grooming (e.g., touching ears, feet, nails)	Many of these actions may be perceived as a threat by the dog. It is often difficult to differentiate dominance-related, irritable, fear-related, and
Restraint (e.g., lifting, rolling on side, grabbing scruff, clamping muzzle, attempting to put on halter-type collar, forcefully pushing or pulling dog)	avoidance-motivated aggression. All of these forms of aggression fall under the heading of control related and may occur in a variety of situations.
Punishment	
Auditory stimulation	
Reprimanding	The dog may become aggressive (snarling or snapping)
Threatening yelling	when yelled at or reprimanded.
Visual stimulation	The dog may become aggressive when stared at—
Staring	diagnostic for dominance-related aggression. Its
Close eye contact	pupils may exhibit a reddish glow just before an attack.

After Voith and Borchelt (1982).

Although dogs exhibiting dominance aggression may often defend possessions, not all possessive aggression is motivated by social dominance (Borchelt, 1983; Reisner, 1997). Wright (1980) observed among German shepherd puppies that relative social dominance and competitive (possessive) aggression occurs with some apparent degree of independence, depending on the relative familiarity or unfamiliarity of the situation in which the interaction takes place [see *Social versus Competitive (Possessive) Aggression*]. Among wolves, an otherwise submissive individual may actively defend the possession of food against higher-ranking pack members (Mech, 1970). Mech suggests that possession within an *ownership zone* of approximately 1 foot from the wolf's nose gives the possessor rights to defend and control the object against intrusion. In an experiment in which an otherwise submissive wolf was given possession of large piece of meat, the subordinate was able to defend its rights of possession aggressively against higher-ranking pack members that had been starved for 72 hours. Interestingly, after eating half of the meat, the subordinate left the prize and, apparently feeling an obligation to appease the alpha pair, alternately approached both of them with abject submissive postures and gestures seeking reconciliation. From the alpha male, he received very severe growling, snapping, and biting, causing the subordinate to fall and roll into a passive-submission posture. From the alpha female, the active-submission behavior produced regurgitation. These events clearly show that possessive aggression may operate under the influence of motivations other than the assertion of social dominance or rank. Consequently, when occurring independently of other forms of dominance aggression, possessive aggression may be more properly understood in terms of defensive motivations rather than offensive ones.

The dominance aggressor commonly exhibits other forms of aggressive behavior, as well, including territorial defense, intermale fighting, and xenopic (toward strangers) aggression. Many dominance aggressors, however, are quite specialized, threatening and attacking only family members. Other dogs exhibiting dominance aggression may threaten or attack guests after an exciting and disarming show of affection and attention-seeking behavior (Reisner, 1997). Some particularly sensitive and reactive dogs possess an extremely low threshold for the exhibition of disproportionate and damaging aggressive attacks. A low-threshold dominance aggressor may attack during benign dominance challenges involving various movements, postures, or intentions perceived by it as dominance or *control* threats. These perceived challenges include bending over the dog, talking to the dog, putting on or taking off the dog's collar, innocuous eye contact with the dog, or simply petting the dog's head or back. Some interesting experimental evidence suggests that a reflexive defensive reaction may be neu-

rologically hardwired and elicited in response to tactile stimulation (Konorski, 1967). Dogs stimulated by an air puff directed into the ear usually exhibited a strong aggressive response toward the apparatus and would attempt to bite the experimenter's hand if it was nearby. Konorski also reported that decorticated dogs exhibited a stereotypic aggressive response whenever they were touched on the back. These findings suggest the existence of a reflexive mechanism mediating aggressive behavior. Perhaps, in normal subjects, such defensive mechanisms are modulated and controlled (inhibited) by higher cortical centers. In the case of some aggressive dogs, these inhibitory mechanisms may be rendered dysfunctional by physical disease or neurotogenesis. This possibility is especially pertinent in those cases involving a sudden increase in irritability and unpredictable attack occurring while the dog is being petted on the head or back, when being talked to at close quarters, or when the victim playfully blows air into its face.

The evaluation of dominant-aggressive dogs, especially those cases involving episodes of sudden onset or unusual signs, ought to include a thorough veterinary examination. This exam commonly includes various blood panels, urinalysis, and fecal evaluation. In areas endemic with Lyme disease, a Lyme test should also be performed. In addition, thyroid function (Michigan State Test) is assessed in some cases involving atypical presenting signs or other indicators suggesting thyroid involvement [e.g., lethargy, obesity, poor coat quality and alopecia, cold intolerance, and avoidance of exercise (tires quickly)]. Thyroid dysfunction has been considered a relatively rare (Reinhard, 1978) or insignificant (Polsky, 1993) factor in the expression of aggression. However, recently it has been suggested that thyroid insufficiency may play a much more important role than had been previously suspected. Aronson (1998) remarks that one reason for the apparent lack of a positive correlation between aggressive behavior and hypothyroidism might be due to the lack of appropriate testing to detect its presence. Not only has she found a clear link between thyroid insufficiency and aggression, she has also implicated a thyroid factor in the expression of a variety of behavior problems, including generalized fear, separation anxiety, compulsive disorders, hyperactivity, and seizure activity. Although thyroid supplementation may not represent a cure for such problems in hypothyroid patients, it appears to exercise an ameliorative effect:

> While correcting the thyroid imbalance may not provide a complete resolution of the behavior problems, it is an extremely rare animal that shows no improvement, and certainly none shows a deterioration in behavior following treatment. In the future, it is possible that if we test for other endocrine and metabolic parameters, we will discover additional links between systemic conditions and behavior problems. (97)

Some forms of explosive and unpredictable aggressive behavior may be caused by a variety of neuopathologies, including seizure activity (Dodman, 1992). Affected dogs may appear disoriented and exhibit a glazed or deep reddening of the pupils, just before launching into an uninhibited attack. Owners often report that their dogs appear momentarily "possessed" by a paroxysm of aggressive behavior occurring rather independently of identifiable provocation present at the time of attack. Following attacks, dogs may appear dissociated from the event, often acting as though contrite for their behavior. Episodic rage syndrome (sometimes referred to as idiopathic or episodic dyscontrol syndrome) is relatively rare and believed by some authorities to be the result of epileptic seizure activity or damage in limbic areas responsible for the regulaton of aggressive behavior (Voith, 1989). The attacks may occur episodically on a monthly or more frequent basis (Hart and Hart, 1985). Certain breeds appear to exhibit a predisposition for the disorder; English springer spaniels (springer rage syndrome), Bernise mountain dogs, cocker spaniels, St. Bernards, Lhaso apsos, and many other breeds have been reported to exhibit the disorder. Voith (1989) emphasizes the close relationship between unpredictable aggressive attacks and dominance aggression. She notes that such attacks are typically directed toward family members and are provoked under the influence of low levels of stimulation (e.g., petting or ordering the dog to do something). Borchelt and Voith (1985) reported that differential diagnosis can be facilitated by alternately administisitering epileptogenic and antiepileptic

drugs and observing the dog's behavior for aggressive kindling effects or suppression (see *Epilepsy* in Volume 1, Chapter 3). In cases where pathophysiological causes are not identified, episodic attacks would probably be better described and understood in functional terms of *low-threshold dominance aggression* rather than episodic rage syndrome.

The obvious need for accurate diagnostic testing and differential diagnosis of possible underlying disease conditions emphasizes the importance of an active partnership between veterinarians and dog behavior consultants in the resolution of behavior problems. Further, since pharmacological intervention is often employed (especially in severe cases), a consulting veterinarian can prescribe and monitor necessary medications. Ideally, the treatment of dominance aggression should proceed as a team effort, consisting of the client's veterinarian, a consulting veterinary behaviorist, and a professional trainer/behaviorist.

Many authors have emphasized the role of status infringement as a putative cause of dominance aggression, but as will be shown throughout this chapter, what exactly is meant by such notions as social dominance and dominance aggression is far from clear and unambiguous. This is a highly problematic state of affairs, because many of the treatment protocols used to modify this relatively common and dangerous problem are based on assumptions derived from these various theories, especially the belief that treatment efforts should focus on altering a dog's relative status. Unfortunately, however, there is "no convincing evidence" that the usual behavioral treatment programs aimed at reversing the dominance hierarchy actually achieve such changes (Reisner, 1997). Not only are such dogs potentially dangerous, they are also at considerable risk of euthanasia, unless effective behavior modification and training are brought to bear on the problem (Reisner et al., 1994). However, even in cases where appropriate behavior modification is applied, dominance aggression problems are rarely cured. Line and Voith (1986), for example, found that treatment produced some benefit in most dogs (N = 24), but when asked several months later only 1 of 19 dog owners indicated that the aggression problem had been completely suppressed.

CONCEPT OF SOCIAL DOMINANCE

Long ago, Konrad Most (1910/1955) articulated the following influential social-dominance theory of dog aggression:

> In a pack of young dogs fierce fights take place to decide how they are to rank within the pack. And in a pack composed of men and dogs, canine competition for importance in the eyes of the trainer is keen. If this state of affairs is not countered by methods which the canine mind can comprehend, it frequently ends in such animals attacking and seriously injuring not only their trainers, but also other people. As in a pack of dogs, the order of hierarchy in a man and dog combination can only be established by physical force—that is, by an actual struggle in which the man is instantaneously victorious. Such a result can only be brought about by convincing the dog of the absolute physical superiority of the man. (25)

This general theory is familiar to anyone with the most casual exposure to the dog-training literature. Besides the injection of misleading adversarial motivations into the dog's social behavior toward humans, such general explanatory constructions may conceal more by their sweeping generality than they reveal. Such interpretations may also serve to justify inappropriate and abusive training practices. Despite theoretical and empirical problems, Most's dominance theory of aggression is very popular, widely accepted, and sanctified by many respected authorities. In addition, although critical of Most's confrontational philosophy, many contemporary dog behavior consultants embrace the general theory that dogs *normally* form dominance hierarchies among themselves and parallel relations with humans—a system of social organization that determines "which animal has first access to food, resting places, and mates" (Uchida et al., 1997:397). The operative assumption is that dogs view the family as a pack and that they selectively exhibit aggression toward family members, depending on their perceived status. Accordingly, those individuals who are clearly dominant or submissive relative to the dog are believed to be at a significantly reduced risk of suffering an aggressive attack. Only those persons perceived as subordinates

and who happen to challenge or confront the dog are at risk of evoking dominance-motivated attacks.

Although the term *dominance* is used with great alacrity and confidence as an explanatory construct, at a most fundamental level there is considerable confusion about what is meant by the idea. How does social dominance or rank order develop? What is the exact relationship between social dominance and aggressive behavior? Are dominance relations between humans and dogs of the same order as dominance relations between dogs? Is attack and threat antecedent necessities for establishing or maintaining social rank? These general questions and others need careful attention and delineation before an adequate understanding of the relationship between dominance and aggression is possible.

DEFINING DOMINANCE

Social dominance is often treated in the literature as a sort of intervening variable or organismic factor, mediating the expression of aggression under the influence of pertinent stimuli and contexts. In the case of dominance aggression, the attack is the dependent variable, and the various stimuli and contextual conditions under which it occurs represent independent variables. The putative intervening variable is *status* infringement. Other authors have variously described dominance in functional terms, as an emergent attribute or merely as a *post hoc* descriptor. Drews (1993) devised the following operational definition of dominance in order to avoid some of the common pitfalls:

> Dominance is an attribute of the pattern of repeated, agonistic interactions between two individuals, characterized by a consistent outcome in favour of the same dyad member and a default yielding response of its opponent rather than escalation. The status of the consistent winner is dominant and that of the loser subordinate. (308)

There is an important distinction being drawn by this definition: dominance is an attribute of a relationship, not an attribute of an individual animal. Indeed, it is hard to speak of a dog as being dominant, except in relation to some other individual who is subordinate. In other words, dominance is not a personal or biological trait per se but a predictive inference based on a pattern of win-lose contests between two or more animals. The term *dominant* denotes a predictive assumption regarding the most likely outcome of any future competitive event occurring between two contestants. In terms of extremes, the dominance relationship can be termed *rigid* (implying a high probability to any prediction) or *fluid* (implying a low probability to any prediction). Most complex social organizations are structured around a *loose* dominance hierarchy, suggesting that the outcomes of most agonistic encounters are predictable but are not certain. Since dominance is not a trait belonging to an individual, but an *emergent* social attribute arising out of competitive interaction, it is not reasonable to speak of dominance as an inherited trait (Barrette, 1993). Although dominance per se may not be inherited, some characteristics (e.g., size and behavioral thresholds) conducive to competitive success may be heritable.

Many social animals appear to form dominance relations among themselves around situations tending to evoke competition, such as access to food, resting areas, and sexual privileges. For example, if two hungry puppies are presented with a food bowl big enough for only one of them to eat at a time, one of the pair will likely attempt to displace the other by threats or attack (if necessary) to secure exclusive control over the bowl (see *Learning to Compete and Cope* in Volume 1, Chapter 2). During similar future competitive encounters between the two puppies, the loser (now submissive) will tend to yield to the more aggressive winner (now dominant). Among puppies, dominance rank is established through active threats or attack but is subsequently maintained by the mutual exhibition and recognition of species-typical threat and appeasement displays. Social rank order is established to minimize social contests and prevent the outbreak of overt and potentially damaging fighting between competitors, thereby laying a foundation for social order and harmoniously organized group activity (Eibl-Eibesfeldt, 1979).

STRUCTURE OF DOMINANCE RELATIONS

Schjelderup-Ebbe (1935) performed the first systematic studies of social dominance by observing the social exchanges between domestic chickens [see Wilson (1975) for an historical overview]. Chickens form *despotic* or linear *pecking* orders in which the most dominant chicken or *alpha* can peck at all other chickens without fear of reprisal. Ranked just below the top-ranking chicken in the pecking order is the *beta* chicken, who can peck at any other chicken in the group except the alpha, toward which the beta is subordinate. A similar relationship of dominant-subordinate relations is formed among the remaining individuals until a peck status or rank is assigned to all the chickens involved, with the least-dominant or omega chicken receiving pecks from all other chickens belonging to the group, while being unable to peck at any other chicken within the pecking order. In addition to pecking rights, dominant chickens enjoy various privileges associated with status, such as priority access to food and resting places. Also, dominant cocks exercise a sexual advantage over more subordinate competitors for mating privileges. An interesting finding noted by Schjelderup-Ebbe (1935) was that dominant chickens located further down the pecking order were more aggressive toward subordinates than was the alpha *despot* reigning at the top of the hierarchy. The trend toward reduced hostility in dominant chickens was found to occur when their status was improved after placing them into another flock:

> Often when a bird which ranks low in the pecking order in a flock comes to a higher position in another flock, the bird soon becomes strikingly milder in its conduct. If removed to the flock where it again stands low its harsh treatment of its subordinates once more appears. (963)

The linear pecking order is the simplest way in which a dominance hierarchy is organized within a group, but it is not the only

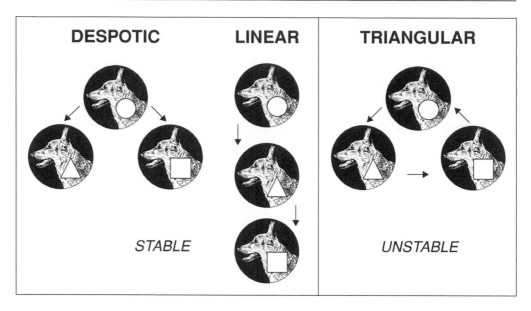

FIG. 8.2. Putative social relations from which dominance hierarchies are organized. Most dominance hierarchies are much more complicated, involving various alliances and contextual influences. After Wilson (1975).

way. In addition to despotic linear structures, triangular and other more complex nonlinear dominance hierarchies exist (Figure 8.2). Among wolves, social ranking is mostly non-linear in structure (Rabb, 1967; Fox, 1973; Lockwood, 1979) (see *Social Dominance and Aggression*). Instead of a neatly defined hierarchy of status relations based on individual competitive success, wolf-pack social organization is affected by other less obvious *political* factors, such as kinship relations (dependent ranking) and various coalitions exerting pressures on the dominance structure.

In the human family situation, in addition to highly unstable triangular relations, parents may form a cooperative coalition under which influence a dog is subordinate, at least while both are present or when the most dominant of the two is present. However, if the less dominant of the two is left alone with the dog, the dog may assume a more dominant (that is, controlling) role. Frequently, a dog is submissive toward both adults but dominant toward children in the family. Ideally, a family coalition should be formed between the parents and children to secure *rank* over the subordinate dog (Netto et al., 1992). Dogs established midway in the dominance hierarchy

(i.e., between adults and children) may behave in a way that parallels Schjelderup-Ebbe's intermediate-ranking chickens, becoming more vigilant and influenced by an enhanced aggressive readiness in relation to *subordinate* family members.

SOCIAL DOMINANCE AND AGGRESSION

To appreciate the role of social dominance as a factor in aggression problems, it is useful to examine some of the ethological findings derived primarily from the study of wolf behavior.

Threat and Appeasement Displays

Both dogs and wolves maintain peaceful social relations by exchanging various species-typical threat (dominant) and appeasement (submissive) displays. Schenkel (1967) has divided submissive displays into two general categories: active and passive. *Active submission* is characterized by increased activity levels and postural diminution, with the tail being carried in a variable carriage and ears held back or twisted in various expressive ways.

Such displays often include active fawning, nuzzling, and licking—*attention-seeking* behavior. Some dogs *grin* or clack their teeth, some may exhibit various pawing motions or crouch down in a play-soliciting bow, and others may crouch with a twist to one side or other, while scooting forward. The tail is often wildly expressive, waving in wide sweeping or whirling motions with the hindquarters moving from side to side. Active-submission displays are observed during greeting between the owner and dog, the dog often jumping up, attempting to push against or lick the returning owner upon his or her mouth—the apparent goal of such behavior (Trumler, 1973). Most so-called attention-seeking behavior by dogs is motivated by active submission. Passive submission is most frequently observed when threats are directed toward the subordinate by the dominant individual. Passive submission involves dramatic reduction of activity (a dog often freezes), averting eye contact, lowering of the head and body onto the ground, and sometimes concluding with a lateral recumbency and exposure of the ventral areas of the chest and the inguinal areas of the abdomen. The ears are pressed back with the tail tucked between the legs. Sometimes, passive submission is associated with submissive urination—an appeasement expression deriving from early reflexive elimination elicited by the mother's lingual stimulation of the anogenital areas (Fox, 1971).

In addition to visual and auditory information, olfactory signals may also play a significant role in communicating social status. Although not yet identified in dogs, releaser pheromones and other sources of olfactory information regulate the expression of aggression and submission in other mammalian species (Sommerville and Broom, 1999). Under intense aversive stimulation, a release of anal sac contents or defecation may occur. Anal secretions may contain chemical or pheromonal alarm signals capable of inhibiting aggression or, perhaps, serving as a chemical-repellent defense aimed at distracting or turning the aggressor away from the attack. Analysis of the pheromonal contents of anal gland secretions [see Preti et al. (1976)] and their various potential effects on canine behavior may be of significant value,

especially with respect to potential antiaggression properties. If found to exert such effects, synthetic-scent homologues could be produced that might offer therapeutic as well as practical benefit as humane inhibitors/repellents for the control of aggressive behavior.

Dominance displays involve various threatening gestures and postures. Low-level threats include a dog standing over or assuming an agonistic T orientation toward its owner or another dog. The dog may rest its head over the opponent's shoulders and proceed to ride up on its back before launching into an attack. Some dogs may grab the skin of the neck (scruff) or attempt to control the opponent's muzzle, especially in the case of adult dogs disciplining puppies. Other dominant displays include body bumping and hip slamming, sometimes forceful enough to knock the opponent off its feet. During displays of increasing threat, a dog's center of gravity appears to shift forward with a stiffening of the body and front legs. Characteristically, a dominant dog sets up squarely facing its opponent and maintains direct eye contact or agonistic stare while poised in a state of increasing readiness: ears are up and turned forward, and its body appears swollen as the result of muscular stiffening and piloerection extending from the neck down to the rump. An aggressively aroused dog may appear to walk on its toes, with the tail carried high and its tip rising above the horizontal line of the back. As the threat escalates, the tail may be held stiffly erect or wagged in short rapid arcs. Just before launching into an attack, the dog may exhibit a threatening growl, snarl, widely bare its teeth by retracting the upper lip up and back (defensive display) or by showing an *agonistic pucker* formed by drawing the commissure of the upper and lower lips forward, thereby wrinkling the muzzle and exposing the teeth (offensive display).

Finally, some dogs may exhibit various equivocal or ambiguous signs, such as pawing the owner, leaning on the owner, placing a paw on the owner's foot, mouthing the owner, jumping up in persistent efforts to get up onto the owner's lap, and obnoxious licking efforts in spite of consistent discouragement. These various behaviors are most often associated with active submission or appeasement but may be used manipulatively to control the owner—efforts referred to as *obnoxious submissiveness*. Various forms of passive resistance may also be used by dogs in an effort to control the owner's actions. These sorts of behaviors can be problematic to correct with punishment, since by doing so they may become worse. Often a combination of instrumental counterconditioning, extinction, and time-out works well to control such behavioral excesses.

Peace-making Theory of Social Dominance

An important goal of dominance relations and the acceptance of dominant and subordinate roles by group members is the maintenance of group harmony and peace. When Lockwood (1979) performed a factor analysis of behavioral and physical traits correlating with dominance status among wolves, he found that the number of threat displays exhibited by pack members showed a low correlation with respect to relative dominance or rank. In other words, dominant wolves are not distinguished by the overall number of threats they exhibit toward other pack members. Of course, dominant individuals are quite capable of asserting and defending their status but do not lightly flaunt their power or engage in superfluous challenges or troublemaking within the pack. Although the initiation of dominance threats was not a significant measure of social status, several other characteristics and traits were found to be correlated with social rank: a high degree of success at controlling food access, heavy body weight, reception of a large percentage of submissive behavior displayed by conspecifics, and a high frequency of scent-marking activity.

Van Hooff and Wensing (1987) have confirmed many of Lockwood's general findings, observing that the most reliable measure of relative status is postural indicators exhibited by interacting wolves. Dominant wolves present themselves in taller postures relative to subordinates, whereas subordinates present themselves to dominant counterparts in postures that accentuate their smallness. Consistent with Lockwood's observations, Van Hooff and Wensing found that threatening or

assaultive behavior was only moderately correlated with dominance, concluding that such behavior may actually belong to a separate behavioral category.

Dominance versus Deference Hierarchy

Although the term *dominance* typically denotes a social relationship based on a regular exchange of species-typical threat and appeasement signals between at least two individuals, the evidence provided by Lockwood and by Van Hooff and Wensing suggests that social rank is not solely or even primarily maintained by threat initiatives exhibited by dominant individuals. For the most part, the dominant animal, or *alpha,* refrains from asserting gratuitous displays of rank, so long as its social priority is recognized and respected by subordinates. Instead of depending on the initiation of threats by the alpha toward subordinates to maintain the group's social hierarchy, such relations appear to be primarily maintained by the deferential active and passive-submission behaviors exhibited by subordinates toward the group leader. Viewed from this perspective, the structure may be more appropriately described as a *deference* hierarchy rather than a dominance hierarchy (Rowell, 1974). According to this notion, the alpha is likely to exhibit dominance threats, only under circumstances in which its status or privileges are disputed, rather than going about unnecessarily challenging and testing subordinate group members. The alpha presumes their subordination, unless they exhibit behavior indicating otherwise. As a general rule, the pack is a peaceful organization, with the highest-ranking individuals being only infrequently involved in serious competitive strafes.

DOMINANCE AND SOCIAL HARMONY

Dog social behavior has often been interpreted and misinterpreted in terms of wolf behavior. Although an alpha wolf is not above an occasional arbitrary assertion of power, a wise lupine leader avoids unnecessary dominance contests and assertions of authority. The establishment of dominance status does not necessarily depend on aggressive competition. Fonberg (1988), for example, found that dominance is often established without any overt exchange of aggression or obvious physical indications of physical superiority. She notes that dominance established without resorting to aggression appears to be more stable than dominance maintained by constant vigilance and display of strength. Instead of relying on force and threat to maintain control, an alpha's authority depends on other group members actively recognizing and deferring to its status and role as their leader. There appears to be a genuine wisdom in this arrangement, since a more intrusive style of control would run the risk of producing unnecessary and disruptive *dominance tensions* within a group. Also, it is not by accident that so many active and passive-submission behaviors in wolves and dogs are also used to express affection. In fact, submissive displays appear to be a composite of fearful and affectionate elements—belying the affiliative origins of such behavior. Affectionate submission reinforces an alpha's status, makes it feel secure in its position of control, facilitates group cohesion and cooperation, and promotes social contentment and well-being.

An alpha's ritualized expressions of dominance, social distancing, and aloofness all encourage a flow of social affection in its direction, thereby consolidating its leadership by popular opinion. The pack follows its leader, not so much out of fear or compulsion, as from a natural attraction and desire to stay in close proximity with an object of affection. Besides facilitating leadership, affection in wolves and dogs is a natural inhibitor of aggressive behavior. The more affection exhibited by subordinates toward their leader, the more secure, peaceful, and lasting its reign of control is likely to be. Although repeated assertions of dominance may reinforce passive submission, such efforts also close social distance and evoke competitive tensions and fear in subordinates. In situations of high levels of such aggressive interaction, one would expect to observe increased agitation, protest, and a greater likelihood of actual fighting.

As long as dominant-subordinate relations are clear-cut, affectionate harmony will properly characterize the interaction of pack members. Disruptive dominance tensions develop

as the result of poor leadership (incompetence) and increased competition between the leader and subordinates. Such competitive interaction has a pronounced influence on the social stability and contentment of the group. Since *only near equals compete,* when excessive competition occurs it signals a narrowing of relative dominance between the leader and subordinates. The direct outcome of competitive interaction is a reduction in affectionate inhibitions and the expression of defiance and aggressive threat by challenging subordinates. During such competitive challenges, the alpha is forced to assert its privilege of rank by escalating aggressive threats toward the disaffected subordinate, which may in turn either submit or counter the alpha's threat with an aggressive counterthreat of its own. At such times, an overt and damaging fight might break out, unless the subordinate submits.

The maintenance of social distance and aloofness plays an important role in the prevention of such tensions. By staying apart and establishing clear symbolic boundaries and limits, an alpha effectively prevents such disruptive agonistic tensions from occurring. When such social boundaries are absent or undefended, the likelihood of competitive tensions and aggression is correspondingly increased. A leader wolf protects its rights and privileges but does not casually intrude on the rights and privileges of subordinates. Even the lowest-ranking subordinate will defend a bone or a piece of food that it has managed to secure for itself. Only a rather incompetent leader would go about challenging and agitating deferential subordinates. In short, the process of maintaining dominance is about regulating social limits and boundaries while making oneself an object of social attention and affection—a leader.

A completely stable group without aggression may not be possible, however. Reportedly, under stable social conditions where agonistic behavior is rarely expressed, aggressive energy may actually *build up* over time, causing the alpha wolf finally, and without much warning or provocation, to attack the omega (lowest) member of the group spontaneously. This sort of aggressive expression has been termed *energy displacement* activity and may represent an adaptive release mechanism controlling the buildup of aggressive energy, perhaps preventing a more disruptive and damaging outburst (Mech, 1970). This general theory, especially in the form of Lorenz's (1966) *psychohydraulic model* of aggression, has been widely criticized. Lorenz argued that aggression reflected the operation of an underlying instinct or appetite for fighting. According to his theory, aggression is motivated by a drive similar in nature to hunger and thirst. He believed that *aggressive energy* accumulates over time, eventually compelling the animal to seek a suitable object upon which to *vent* its aggressive energy. If a species-typical object is not available, the animal may express the aggressive energy in the form of vacuum behavior, perhaps attacking under inappropriate situations or displacing it upon inappropriate objects. Lorenz believed that aggressive energy builds up according to the biological needs of the species, causing some animals to show a greater aggressive drive than others. Others have theorized that social aggression is primarily the result of the inevitable frustration that accumulates as the result of interacting with others competing for the same resources or interfering with one's goal-seeking activities. For example, Dollard and colleagues (1939) argued that "aggression is always a consequence of frustration" (1). Frustration is defined by them as any interference in the performance of goal-seeking activity. Calhoun [see Papero (1990)] describes a similar tendency toward an acquired propensity for aggression as the result of social interaction, but interprets it in terms of a need for the attainment of psychobiological balance between frustration and gratification. According to this theory, under social conditions in which an individual receives too many *gratifying* experiences, it will deliberately seek to trigger agonistic episodes to achieve a more satisfying balance between frustration and gratification. Social contentment is achieved by balancing gratifying and frustrating experiences.

Dominance or Pseudodominance

Many authorities have commented on the degenerative effects of domestication on the social behavior of dogs. In comparison to the robust social dominance and submission rituals exhibited by wolves, the corresponding agonistic behavior patterns in dogs have "disintegrated into an assortment of independent behavioral fragments" (Frank and Frank, 1982:519). Although a dog's social reality is strongly influenced by its wolf-genetic heritage, it is hard to describe faithfully the human-dog relationship in terms of the wolf model of social rank. For one thing, the human-dog relationship is often much more equivocal and complex than captured by the concept of social rank. It is also filled with considerable confusion with respect to the meaning of specific social exchanges between people and dogs and how they should be interpreted.

Most social transactions between people and dogs appear to be organized around playful attention-seeking (active submission) exchanges and following patterns, rather than true dominant-subordinate relations based on the purposeful exchange of threat and appeasement (passive submission) displays. Among highly sociable dogs with elevated fear and aggression thresholds, the impulse to challenge their owners for dominance with a sincere threat or contest probably never passes through their minds. Although not feeling very dominant toward their owners, such dogs probably do not feel very submissive or subordinate either. In such cases, the appearance of competitive tension may simply be the net result of frustrating playful exchanges having little ulterior motivation, being nothing more than play for the sake of play and the immediate pleasures produced by the activity. Fun-loving dogs might get themselves into constant trouble as the result of their playful antics and teasing games, become attention-seeking pests, or possibly form an excessively strong attachment with an overly indulgent owner, but such dogs are unlikely to launch a serious dominance challenge against the owner, except in the most playful and obnoxious sense of the word. In such cases, the appearance of social competition is better described as sham or pseudodominance.

Dominance: Status or Control

Aggression directed toward the owner often occurs as the result of competitive or threatening interaction with the dog. Dogs resort to aggression as a means to establish control over motivationally adverse circumstances generated by the owner. Depending on a dog's success or failure, it may adopt a dominant or subordinate role in relation to its owner and consequently be more likely to threaten or defer to the owner under the influence of similar circumstances in the future. The original causes of aggression are competition or threat, occurring under the influence of loss, discomfort, disturbance, or interference. Under such circumstances, a dog is variably aroused with frustration, anger, or irritability—*establishing operations* that render aggression more likely and provide the motivational bases for its subsequent reinforcement or punishment. If the behavior succeeds, the victim's various gestures, postures, and contact activities present at the time of the attack may be learned as discriminative stimuli controlling future aggressive efforts, especially when the dog is exposed to similar competitive or threatening circumstances. Also, the owner's actions present at the time of attack (approaching, reaching for, or leaning over) may function as conditioned establishing operations (triggers), setting the motivational occasion for the dog to respond aggressively with some expectation of success.

With repeated exposure to such situations, the behavioral thresholds controlling aggression may be lowered, while thresholds regulating the expression of fear may be gradually elevated. These combined motivational influences may cause a dog to become more confident and assertive. As a result, the likelihood of aggression may increase, with its magnitude progressively becoming more vigorous and damaging—all changes occurring as the result of social learning and the alteration of conditioned triggers regulating fear and aggression. If punishment is attempted at such times, the dog's aggressive control efforts may escalate—now intensely invigorated by frustration and rage. If a dog's control efforts are successful, its agonistic behavior may fall under the motivational influence of an additional species-typical incentive: the securement of rank and status. Consequently, the dog may expect its owner to recognize its dominant status and play a submissive role by showing appropriate appeasement and defer-

ence behavior in response to its threats. Further, the dog may become progressively intolerant of intrusion (e.g., while sleeping or eating), resent routine control efforts (e.g., grabbing the dog's collar), and react aggressively toward disciplinary actions carried out by its owner.

Dominance aggression often involves very severe attacks that occur under minimal or no apparent provocation at all—characteristics that nicely fit the control-learning hypothesis and analysis of dominance aggression. The notion of *status* is inextricably bound up with learning and conditioning. Although the recognition and display of status appear to play a significant functional role in the organization of dog social behavior and the maintenance of dominant-subordinate relations, most dominance aggression appears to be the result of social confusion, frustration, irritability, contact aversion, and learning. Rather than being socially dominant, many dominance aggressors simply appear to be socially *incompetent* and unable adaptively to navigate the social and interactive demands placed upon them without biting. In the vast majority of cases involving aggression (Borchelt and Voith, 1986, 1996), the behavior appears to be mostly related to control interests, operating under adverse motivational circumstances involving heightened anger, frustration, or irritability. Although there are many situations in which social status may become a significant factor, aggression is primarily grounded upon control-related efforts. Status and status-related aggression come about as the result of a history of success in threatening or attacking the owner. Essentially, status-related aggression is the conditioned outcome of a history of successful aggressive control efforts.

Locus of Control and Social Attention

The nature of social dominance has been analyzed in a variety of ways. A general characteristic of dominance is locus of control, that is, the initiation of significant social activities. Among wolves the leader is usually responsible for initiating and guiding vital group activities, such as hunting sorties, territorial and group protection, and reproduction. A related notion is focus of attention. Dominant animals appear to attract and control the most attention from group members (Chance, 1967). During greeting displays, for example, the alpha male and female wolf are the object of intense interest and activity. A dog's ability to initiate and control activities and to hold its owner's attention offers interesting possibilities for understanding the notion of pseudodominance. Many pseudodominant dogs express an almost compulsive drive for attention and social recognition. The attention-controlling behaviors involved are frequently of a highly competitive nature (although playful and nonescalating) and are often conflated with hyperactivity. Many of the *games* involved are competitive, involving various taunts and challenges aimed at provoking a response in the owner (Voith, 1980a,b). In many ways, pseudodominant dogs are simply obnoxious subordinates who have not been properly trained to respect appropriate social boundaries.

Schenkel (1967) offers a pithy observation in this regard among wolves: "If the superior is tolerant but fails to display his superiority, the inferior may behave obtrusively" (325). A favorite, rather dominant, attention-controlling game is the familiar "steal a forbidden item and run like hell" routine, thereby evoking an episode of "catch me if you can, stupid" throughout the house. In general, the behaviors involved are designed to maximize the amount and direction of attention toward the dog in a manipulative and controlling mode of interaction. Many other nuisance behaviors fall under this general category, including playful biting at hands and feet, excessive barking, jumping on furniture and guests, pestering antics of various kinds, and other expressions of opportunistic mischief.

Pseudodominant dogs enjoy making a focus of themselves during social encounters and are not adverse to putting on a show for any audience willing to play the role of subordinate *victim*. Dogs that persist in such obtrusive and unwanted behavior, including provocative chase episodes, the initiation of aggressive tug of war games, and rough, uncontrollable play, are expressing a high degree of social competitiveness—a pattern of interaction that may introduce the seed for more serious problems (Netto et al., 1992).

INTERSPECIES SOCIAL DOMINANCE

Harmonious social interaction between people and dogs appears to depend on the establishment of a leader-follower bond. This need is well recognized by most dog behavior authorities and dog owners. A dog's readiness to meet the demands of domestic life is only half provided by its biological predisposition; the other half is provided by the actualizing effects of socialization and training. Without the guidance of a competent leader, a dog's social adjustment may suffer irreparable damage. Although we may sometimes imagine that dogs understand and appreciate our foibles and values, they do not; nor do they appreciate the full consequences of their behavior from our all-too-human perspective. William James (1896/1956) eloquently describes the situation:

> Our dogs, for example, are in our human life but not of it. They witness hourly the outward body of events whose inner meaning cannot, by any possible operation, be revealed to their intelligence,—events in which they themselves often play the cardinal part. My terrier bites a teasing boy, for example, and the father demands damages. The dog may be present at every step of the negotiation, and see the money paid, without an inkling of what it all means, without a suspicion that it has anything to do with him; and he never can know in his natural dog's life. . . In the dog's life we see the world invisible to him because we live in both worlds. In human life, although we only see our world, and his within it yet encompassing both these worlds a still wider world may be there, as unseen by us as our world is by him; and to believe in that world may be the most essential function that our lives in this world have to perform. (57–58)

Konrad Most (1910/1955) echoes these same sentiments:

> We credit him with capacity for thought and with an understanding of human behavior and morality. By introducing the dog into a world which is, in reality, forever closed to him, we prevent ourselves from recognizing the unbridgeable mental gap that exists between man and dog. (3)

As a result of these inherent limitations, a dog's adaptation to domestic life must be con-

stantly guided and shaped by human intervention and training. Suppose for a moment
that the relationship was in reverse, and we as
infants were cast into the midst of a kindly
pack of wolves and somehow managed to survive the ordeal. Consider how confused we
would be by their customs and manner of
doing things. We would never really have a
clue but would nonetheless gradually adjust
to the natural contingencies of reward and
punishment provided by the situation (or per-
ish). A major difference between a dog's fate
and this hypothetical one is that we can serve
a dog's interests and assist in its adaptation by
becoming a rational proxy for it in this
strange world, guiding the dog's choices until
it is adequately socialized and trained to make
the correct choices on its own. To accept our
leadership, a dog must adopt a submissive and
cooperative attitude at a very early stage in its
development and remain that way for the rest
of its life. The majority of dogs appear to
defer to human leadership instinctively; all
that is needed for success is an owner who
embraces his or her responsibility and takes
control. A puppy's affectionate and dependent
attachment is an expression of its natural
inclination to submit to our guidance. A dog's
sense of security and well-being depends on
its owner recognizing these needs and satisfying them with adequate socialization and
training.

Avoiding a persistent "ritualization of confusion" arising from mixed messages and misunderstanding between the owner and dog
begins with the establishment of clear and
definitive social boundaries. Defining oneself
as a leader is accomplished by defending
social limits (e.g., not permitting the dog to
jump up, to bite on hands or clothing, or to
pull on the leash), maintaining appropriate
social distance, and developing a cooperative
relationship based on gentle compliance training and directive measures, when necessary.
As a result of such efforts, the dog will naturally become increasingly affectionate and
cooperative. Leaders avoid engaging dogs in
unnecessary contests of will, but when their
authority is challenged, they provide immediate and definitive actions that leave no room
for doubt about where they stand on the matter. On the other hand, leaders recognize and

reciprocate cooperation with affection and
other attractive consequences. Directive
actions are mostly used as a means to defend
an infringed social boundary, rather than as a
routine means for compelling obedience.
Once these necessary preliminaries are settled,
instructing a dog becomes an easy and enjoyable task because it is oriented toward the
trainer as an affectionate and subordinate follower. Once basic social boundaries are established, other behavioral objectives are rapidly
achieved by differentially presenting or omit-
ting rewards, such as affection, food, play, and
other activities and resources that the dog
may desire to obtain.

Aside from a failure of owners to establish
themselves as leaders, dominance-control tensions often evolve as the result of ineffectual
disciplinary interaction or interference. As
evident by their desire for human contact,
most dogs are innately submissive to their
owners; even in cases where the owners may
fail to play a satisfactory and consistent leadership role, their dogs remain affectionately
submissive. But sometimes such neglected
dogs may become progressively intolerant and
aggressive toward the owner's efforts to control them. Many dominance-related problems
appear to stem from dominance tensions produced by the owner's habitual and ineffectual
efforts to control the dog's behavior. From an
early age onward, dogs are exposed to
repeated and ineffectual efforts to control or
punish them. The problem is compounded
when, failing to secure a dog's compliance,
the owner simply gives up or clumsily
enforces his or her demands. As a result, the
dog may become progressively competitive,
resistant, difficult, and intolerant of control.
Several other negative side effects may ensue
from this pattern of interaction:

1. The owner and dog become locked in a
   pattern of unresolved competition.
2. The stabilizing social distance between the
   owner and dog becomes progressively
   narrowed or obliterated.
3. Unresolved dominance conflicts and
   tensions increase the dog's frustration and
   irritability while simultaneously rendering
   it less submissively affectionate and
   tolerant toward the owner.

Dominance-control tensions and frustration may accumulate as the result of such interaction, until at last a point is reached where a dog becomes intolerant of its owner's irritating or frustrating interference and infringements on its *space*. As the dog becomes more confident and overtly aggressive, its affection and tolerance for contact with the owner may suffer diminishment, as well. It should be noted, however, that many dominance aggressors are highly affectionate toward their owners and may only become intolerant of contact under the influence of specific situations. Upon reaching social maturity, the dog may become progressively aloof, distant, irritable, and resistant to control. If these attitudinal and behavioral changes are not checked, the dog may come to view its owner's efforts to control it as provocative threats. The dog may resort to aggression in an effort to counter the owner's control efforts and to set social boundaries between itself and its ineffectual owner. If the dog does bite, the aggressive actions are likely to go unpunished. Most owners at this point simply back off in shock, only to return later to *reach* the offending dog with placative bribes of affection and food, thereby making matters worse by playing the affiliative role of the subordinate.

Even more potentially damaging, some owners may attempt to punish the behavior, causing the dog to redouble its aggressive efforts, under the escalating influence of pain, fear, and anger. If the dog succeeds in defending itself or perceives that it has controlled the situation by resorting to aggression, it will tend to resort to such behavior under similar circumstances in the future. To defend itself most effectively, the dog may adopt a highly vigilant attitude and learn to react preemptively to previously neutral stimuli associated with such punitive situations—avoidance-motivated aggression. In addition, internal stimuli associated with such provocative situations may trigger establishing operations that prepare the dog to behave in a threatening manner and raise the likelihood that such behavior will undergo significant reinforcement if it succeeds.

According to the foregoing analysis, the dog exhibits aggression because such behavior succeeds in controlling the owner-target. The intrusive actions of the owner function as conditioned establishing operations, triggering motivational changes conducive to the emission of aggressive behavior and setting the stage to reinforce the aggressive behavior strongly, if it succeeds. Reinforcement occurs when the owner is displaced by threat or attack, simultaneously reducing aversive aggressive arousal and replacing it with emotional relief and elative feelings of enhanced well-being and control.

SOCIAL DISTANCE AND POLARITY

Many dominant-aggressive dogs tend to be rather reserved with their affections, often being affection receivers rather than affection givers. Although affection can be a strong inhibitor of aggression (see below), its inhibitory effect depends on the direction of affection, that is, its *polarity*. The subordinate affection giver is much more inhibited about behaving aggressively toward the dominant object of affection than the dominant affection receiver is toward the giver of affection. Fear toward the object of affection is often irrationally suppressed in the affection giver, as is evident, for instance, in the case of an abusive human relationship involving physical battery. This effect is also present in the persistent affection and lack of appropriate fear exhibited by some owners of dominant-aggressive dogs.

A subordinate is urged on by social attraction to stay in relatively close proximity with the leader, an attraction that may paradoxically increase with repeated exposure to the alpha's threats and subsequent reconciliation. The growing leader-follower bond serves both to reduce the future likelihood that the subordinate will challenge the leader and may simultaneously increase the leader's tolerance for contact with the deferential and affectionate subordinate. In both cases, the risk of aggression is decreased by affection; that is, affection reduces the likelihood that the subordinate will act aggressively toward the leader, while the reception of affection renders the leader more tolerant of contact with the subordinate. This ideal arrangement of reciprocal inhibition is not always evident, however. Many dominant dogs appear to be intolerant of contact, even affectionate contact. In such cases, increased affectionate interaction does nothing to encourage tolerance but may, on the contrary, increase intolerance. The effect is analogous to unrequited love between humans, where the lovesick suitor persistently seeks the attentions of a lover, even though the efforts are repeatedly scorned and punished. Although affection is normally highly desirable and conducive to tolerance and reciprocation, under such circumstances the persistent efforts of the suitor (affection giver) may become highly aversive to the object of affection.

The direction of social polarity and attention reflects the cumulative outcomes of agonistic and affiliative exchanges, with affection and attention-seeking behavior (active submission) moving primarily from the subordinate toward the alpha. Social polarity, based on affectionate submission, provides the foundation for orderly group cooperation and organized activity. Early social dependency involving the reception of nurturance and protection gives way to more mature social relationships based on emergent social status and the formation of a leader-follower bond. In essence, social polarity provides a motivational substrate for mediating social stratification and organizing leader-follower roles.

Reversing the direction of social polarity through integrated compliance training, whereby the reception of affection and other rewards is made contingent on subordinate behavior, offers a useful management technique in the treatment of dominance aggression. As a preliminary to such training, dominance aggressors are often ignored for several days until they seek out the owner's contact and actively solicit affection—affection that they must now learn to earn (Campbell, 1992). This may be a very hard recommendation to implement by owners who are profoundly attached to their dogs and unwilling to exchange the immediate pleasures of doting affection for the delayed therapeutic benefits of social distance and integrated compliance

training, that is, owners who are unable to make themselves leaders worthy of canine affection and respect. The power of the *cold shoulder* for managing dog behavior was first reported by George Romanes (1888). The anecdote describes a Skye terrier that had decided with strong aggressive protests not to accept its bath anymore. The owner of the dog happened upon the strategy of withdrawing affection. The effort took several days, but the dog finally relented and accepted her control:

"In process of time this aversion increased so much that all the servants I had refused to perform the ablutions, being in terror of doing so from the ferocity the animal evinced on such occasions. I myself did not choose to undertake the office for though the animal was passionately attached to me, such was his horror of the operation, that even I was not safe. Threats, beating, and starving were all of no avail; he still persisted in his obstinacy. At length I hit upon a new device. Leaving him perfectly free, and not curtailing his liberty in any way, I let him know, by taking no notice of him, that he had offended me. He was usually the companion of my walks, but now I refused to let him accompany me. When I returned home I took no notice of his demonstrative welcome, and when he came looking up at me for caresses when I was engaged either in reading or needlework, I deliberately turned my head aside. This state of things continued for about a week or ten days, and the poor animal looked wretched and forlorn. There was evidently a conflict going on within him, which told visibly on his outward appearance. At length one morning he quietly crept up to me and gave me a look which said plainly as any spoken words could have done, I can stand it no longer; I submit. And submit he did quite quietly and patiently to one of the roughest ablutions it had ever been his lot to experience; for by this time he sorely needed it. After it was over he bounded to me with a joyous bark and wag of his tail, saying unmistakably, 'I know all is right now.' He took his place by my side as his right when I went for my walk, and retained from that time his usually glad and joyous expression of countenance. When the period for the next ablution came round the old spirit of obstinacy resumed its sway for a while, but a single look at my averted countenance was sufficient for him, and he again submitted without a murmur. Must there not have been something akin to the reasoning faculty in the breast of an animal who could thus for ten days carry on such a struggle?"

This strong effect of silent coldness shows that the loss of affectionate regard caused the terrier more suffering than beating, starving, or even the hated bath; and as many analogous cases might be quoted, I have no hesitation in adducing this one as typical of the craving for affectionate regard which is manifested by sensitive dogs [Romanes's comment]. (440–441)

This nice anecdote underscores the efficacy of affection-attention withdrawal for reversing social polarity and enhancing relative dominance.

Despite the ethological appeal of the social polarity hypothesis, it needs to be stressed that the presence of active affection and solicitation of attention is not necessarily a sure indicator of a dog's intention and the risk of aggression. Some dominance aggressors appear to be highly affectionate and excited about contact, only to bite when the owner handles them in the wrong way. Some may enthusiastically greet visitors with intense displays of apparent affection and attention giving, only to bite them as they become more familiar and they attempt to pet or hug them. Others may make themselves the center of affectionate attention and remain nonaggressive, at least until the visitor (or family member) gets up to leave the house. The role of affection and attachment in dominance aggression is complex, and the foregoing is offered as a tentative hypothesis. Perhaps, dogs that show what appears to be authentic affection and attention giving but, nonetheless, bite under the influence of minimal provocation (e.g., upon being petted) are truly of a sociopathic order. In such a case, attention and affectionate displays may be offered in the absence of sincere submissive intentions and other social implications that one might be given to expect. Like the human sociopathic aggressor, the canine sociopathic aggressor may lack true empathy and feeling and more or less *feign* affection and submissive sociability, thereby concealing an aggressive potential. Interestingly, such dogs are often distinguished by an intolerance for frustration and an inability to engage in fluid *give and take* competitive play.

AFFILIATION AND SOCIAL DOMINANCE

An important aspect of group organization is the exchange of affection and the development of affiliative behavior. In addition to offsetting and balancing tensions generated by competitive interaction, social exchanges involving affectionate behavior encourage group cohesion and identity. The importance and function of affiliative bonding between aggressive group members have been emphasized by Lorenz (1964):

Indubitably, ritualized aggressive behaviour is at least one root of bond behaviour. . . . There may be other independent ways in which bond behavior has evolved, but wherever it did, it seems to have done so as a means of controlling aggression, that is to say on the basis of aggressive behaviour preexisting. In the Canidae for instance, in the dog-like carnivore, all gestures and ceremonies of greeting, love and friendship are obviously derived from the expression movements denoting infantile submission. . . . The strongest reason, however, which makes me believe that all bond behaviour has evolved, by way of ritualization, on the basis of intraspecific aggression, lies in an unsuspected correlation between both. We do not know, as yet, of a single organism showing bond behaviour while being devoid of aggression; in a way, this is surprising, as, at a superficial appraisal, one would expect bond behaviour to evolve rather in those highly gregarious creatures which, like many fish and birds, live peacefully in large schools or flocks, but this obviously never happens. . . . Also, there seems to be a strong positive correlation between the strength of intraspecific aggression and that of bond behaviour. . . . No more faithful friendship is known in this class than that which S. Wahburn and I. De Voore have shown to exist among wild baboons, while the symbol of all aggression, the wolf, whom Dante calls the "bestia senza pace" has become "man's best friend," and that not on the grounds of properties developed in the course of domestication. (47–48)

Without a strong social bonding tendency and sense of affiliation, reinforced through species-typical socialization patterns and affectionate exchange, the disruptive effects of agonistic interaction would gradually disperse pack members and destroy the family/pack group. In other words, hierarchically organized animals appear to *love* one another in spite of their ritualized and sometimes fierce competition. Without affection, the social order would rapidly disintegrate into a chaos of disorganized self-interest and individualism. According to Schenkel (1967), among wolves feelings of belonging such as love and intimacy are acquired in the context of forming dominant-subordinate relations:

> There is no doubt that submission is an appeal or effort to friendly social integration, to which the response by the superior is not stereotyped or automatic. Only if the superior, too, is motivated to enter into friendly contact with the inferior, will harmonic social integration really take place. If he responds with non-tolerance, the inferior will not persist in submission. Both components of submission, namely inferiority and "love," can only exist if they meet "generosity," i.e., superiority combined with tolerance or tolerant "love." Both the superiority-inferiority relation and the atmosphere of "love" and intimacy do not rely on automatic responses but are shaped in the social contact as components of "personal" interrelationship. (326)

A representative expression of such group affection is observed in the canid greeting ceremony—an active-submission pattern exhibited by both wolves and dogs. Among dogs, the licking toward the face, presumably done by puppies to elicit regurgitation, is progressively transformed through developmental stages into an appeasement gesture and, ultimately, into a profound expression of canine affection and intimacy.

Affection and Competition

The social behavior of dogs is driven by two antagonistic motivational incentives: affiliation and competition. These complementary interests serve to establish a highly bonded and well-organized family/pack unit. Under normal conditions, these two social motivational systems mutually regulate each other to maintain group order and cohesiveness. In situations where either affiliation or competition oversteps appropriate bounds, one would expect to find corresponding disturbances in the group. For example, without the countervailing effects of affection and affiliative bonding, agonistic behavior would tend to disrupt the normal functioning of the group. Further, in the absence of affection, growing agonistic tensions would gradually disperse group members and destroy the group. Conversely, an excess of affiliative bonding and affectionate restraint would limit beneficial competition, thus preventing the formation of a dominance hierarchy. A group without internal competition and a viable dominance hierarchy would lack effective order, structure, and direction—potentially becoming an amorphous and ineffectual agglomerate of aimless individuals.

An important function of affection and affiliation is to facilitate interactive harmony and tolerance among group members. A few general predictions can be formulated concerning the relative effects of affection and aggression on the organization of canine social behavior. In cases where affectionate bonding is lacking, agonistic behavior should increase along several dimensions. Conversely, as affectionate bonding is rendered more secure and reliable, the incidence of aggressive behavior should correspondingly decrease in frequency and magnitude. Under conditions in which affectionate leader-follower bonding is prominent, one should expect to find increased attention turned toward the owner and a greater willingness for the dog to engage in cooperative behavior. However, in cases where affiliation and affection are conflicted motivationally with excessive frustration and irritability, perhaps as the result of dysfunctional interaction or an absence of leadership, the likelihood of social tension and aggression is increased.

Contact Aversion and Aggression

If affection and affiliative bonding modulate agonistic behavior, how does one explain the appearance of dominance aggression in situations where affectionate interaction between the owner and dog is not lacking? To begin with, although affection giving may foster a strong attachment between the giver-and-receiver dyad, it need not necessarily facilitate affiliative bonding between them (Scott, 1991). Bonding is distinguished from attachment by the presence a shared exchange based on affection, cooperation, and trust. One can form an object attachment to a place, a thing, or an animal without necessarily forming an affiliative bond with it. A bond implies a two-way exchange, whereas an attachment may form and operate in one direction only. Many dog owners form object attachments with their "pet" dogs but fail to form an adequate bond with them. Gratuitous affection may be highly gratifying for the owner to give but be resented by the receiving dog. In some cases, affectionate overtures by the owner may be received by the dog as tactile agitation and interference, resulting in increased irritability and frustration. In other cases, affectionate interaction may be perceived as a threat or source of discomfort. For example, picking up, hugging, and patting a dog may not be perceived by it as a particularly pleasurable or welcome activity. Further, not all dogs enjoy being petted, especially when the petting is delivered by insensitive and clumsy hands. Although a dog may passively accept unsolicited affection, it may gradually become emotionally distressed and resentful of such contact. Thus, what an owner intends as affection may not be received by the dog as affection at all, but rather experienced as an annoyance—an irritating and frustrating annoyance. As the result of unwelcome affection, such dogs may become progressively intolerant of petting or handling and finally act out aggressively to establish social distance.

In summary, some dogs may resent affectionate contact and only tolerate such interaction under clinched teeth. Unwelcome affection may be a significant source of irritability and frustration for such dogs. According to Panksepp (1998), frustration and anger are closely associated in the psychobiology of animals:

> Is the feeling of frustration really substantially different than that of anger? Psychobiological evidence certainly allows us to conclude that they are intimately linked, since manipulations that reduce the effects of frustration, such as antianxiety agents and temporal lobe damage or more restricted amygdaloid lesions, also tend to reduce emotional aggression. Thus, the emotional feeling of frustration may largely reflect the mild arousal of RAGE circuitry, in the same way that anxiety may reflect weak arousal of FEAR circuitry. (192)

If frustration is experienced by a dog as low-grade rage, over time and repeated exposure, the accumulated frustration and irritability arising from unwelcome social contact may gradually lower relevant rage-response thresholds controlling the expression of overt aggression. A contact-aversion interpretation fits a number of the facts associated with dominance aggression:

1. Aggression is often selectively directed.
2. Aggression often takes place in areas associated with affectionate activity (e.g., on sofas and beds).
3. Aggression often occurs under the influence of minimum stimulation, such as when the dog is being reached for in a nonprovocation way.
4. Aggression is often explosive and inappropriate, suggesting an accumulated tension building up over time.
5. Dominance aggressors may become progressively resentful of affectionate contact and resist efforts to elicit play.

This general situation cannot be resolved by simply providing aggressive dogs with more affection. As already noted, giving such dogs affection may not promote affiliation but may instead generate an opposite effect: increased frustration and irritability. The critical factor is to reverse the social polarity between the owner and dog, so that the dog learns to give attention and affection to the owner, rather then receiving it exclusively from the owner. In an important sense, submissive behavior *is* affectionate behavior. Affectionate physical gestures placate the leader, rendering it more benevolent and forbearing with respect to the subordinate's intrusions. Although directing affection and attention toward a dominant individual may have an aggression-reducing or pacifying effect, directing such affection and attention toward a disaffected subordinate may exert an exactly opposite influence, perhaps, in some cases, disabling *status*-related inhibitors that restrain the subordinate from behaving aggressively toward the dominant figure. In other words, making the subordinate the *object* of affection and attention (engaging in submission behavior toward it) may inherently promote annoyance, resentment, and aggressive arousal in the subordinate—an unexpected effect that may actually promote social disruption and disorganization. For example, under natural conditions, an attention- and affection-giving alpha would eventually disinhibit otherwise submissive subordinates to challenge it for social dominance. An interesting possibility is that affection giving by an alpha may be mildly aversive for it, just as receiving affection from a dominant individual may be annoying for a subordinate. Perhaps love is only possible between social equals—the alpha pair.

Reversing Social Polarity and Establishing Leadership

The etiology of dominance aggression is a complicated cluster of inherited traits (especially behavioral thresholds controlling the expression of fear and aggression) and various actualizing experiential influences, including emergent dominance relations. The usual focus on status and the importance of dominance rank and contests between an aggressor and victim-owner overshadows the vital role of social polarity (direction of affiliative interaction) in its management. As previously described, affiliative interaction between a dog and its owner is commonly conflicted in various ways. Where affiliative bonding is secure and affection mutually shared, the probability of overt aggression is much reduced. However, in situations where the dog's affection toward the owner or vice versa is compromised or conflicted by distrust or resentment (contact aversion), the likelihood of agonistic behavior is much increased. Under the influence of distrust or contact aversion, affectionate interaction between the owner and dog may become the source of considerable tension, perhaps causing the dog to become progressively annoyed, intolerant, and aggressive.

This situation can be beneficially influenced in several ways. First and foremost, in the case of a disaffected subordinate, the direction of social polarity must be reversed, so that affection and attention is directed from the dog toward the owner. As Romanes's anecdote suggests, the withdrawal of attention and affection often exercises a pronounced

effect on a dog and its willingness to submit. Requiring a dog to turn its attention actively toward its owner, by withdrawing gratuitous contact and "playing hard to get," offers a viable means for initiating an about-turn in the direction of social polarity. Seeking affection is a step in the right direction toward learning to give it. The owner invites enhanced attention, affection, and other active and passive-submission behaviors by rewarding such activity with highly desirable outcomes. These changes are facilitated by initiating reward-based training activities that possess a high degree of structure, safety (predictability and controllability), and play. Such efforts are designed to promote maximum interactive success while minimizing frustration. As a result of such training activities, the dog learns *how to operate the owner* to satisfy its needs, thereby simultaneously enhancing cooperation, dependency, and submissive tendencies. Furthermore, the dog's success at controlling desirable outcomes by deferring to the owner's contingencies of reinforcement serves to inculcate the notion that cooperation pays off. Interactive success is highly rewarding for both the owner and dog, making the owner a more attractive and effective leader and the dog a more obedient and affectionate follower. Leadership is essential if the owner is to attract the dog's attention, affection, and submission.

An important goal of integrated compliance training is to secure a dog's attention and submission to owner-directed control. As this goal is gradually achieved, the dog learns to defer without resistance or resentment. However, just learning that it can control attractive events is not enough; the dog must also learn that it can control mildly aversive and intrusive ones as well. Physical control and restraint are gradually introduced under highly controlled situations of counterconditioning, response prevention, posture-facilitated subordination, and relaxing massage. Under the structure and control of such training, aggressive impulses may periodically occur, but they are usually inhibited and subside before reaching the critical threshold for attack. Graduated exposure to physical control and restraint helps to improve a dog's ability to control aggressive impulses, while learning to rely on more constructive and cooperative means to control irritating, frustrating, or threatening situations. As a result, in addition to affectionate affiliation, a growing sense of respect and trust may develop toward the owner, in direct proportion to the owner's success in becoming an effective leader through training.

As a buffer of enhanced affection and impulse control is established, the next step in the process involves developing a playful response. As discussed previously, play provides a powerful means for mediating affiliative connectedness with dogs. Unfortunately, dominant-aggressive dogs are not always very interested in play and may resist efforts to elicit such interaction. Dogs unwilling to play may be encouraged by doing things with them that they enjoy and that may gradually be turned toward more playful interaction. Activities that simply require a dog to follow its owner's lead (e.g., a nature walk) or, perhaps, making a game of fetching or finding a hidden treat can provide a foundation for more spontaneous play as the dog learns to relax. An intensive daily exercise program can also produce striking benefits in some dominance aggressors, especially in cases in which comorbid depression is present—depression may make a dog emotionally vulnerable to increased irritability and aggression.

PLAY AND AGGRESSION

Play offers a powerful nonintrusive means to control the direction of social polarity and attention, to balance affection and leadership, and to increase feelings of affiliation and cooperation between people and dogs. Play is relatively incompatible with aggression and fear, although, under the influence of escalating frustration or threat, play may slip over into overt aggression.

What Is Play?

Among potentially aggressive social animals that establish close affiliative relations with one another, play appears to mediate and consolidate *friendships*. Playful interaction among conspecifics appears to take two general forms: some forms of play promote social affiliation and are done apparently for the joy of playing, whereas other forms of play may be used to probe the strength and character of the playful competitor. In terms of behavior, the general qualities associated with play are behavioral openness, curiosity, and flexibility. Playful activity is characterized by an ostensible purposeless purpose in which action is governed by factors independent of serious intent (Immelmann, 1980). Intraspecific play involves the exchange or expression of various species-typical behavior sequences that are emitted out of normal order and in the absence of natural triggers. Playful behavior is often exaggerated and solicitous, random and incomplete, and, in the case of aggressive components, occurs within a safe range of intensity (escalating and abating) over the course of the play episode. In addition, play often involves explicit and inappropriate sexual behavior (e.g., male dogs mounting other males). A large percentage of a dog's play behavior involves competitive components incorporating low-intensity threats and aggressive displays kept within noninjurious limits. Actually, competitive play is structurally comparable to actions, which, if emitted under the influence of aggressive establishing operations and contexts, could result in severe injury or even death to the players. For dogs, play is an essential element in the development of healthy social attitudes and essential interactive repertoires with other dogs and people (Fagen, 1981).

Metacommunication and Play

Play depends on the exchange of various auditory, facial, and bodily expressions (e.g., play bow and play face) defining an intent to play. These play invitations are highly ritualized patterns of mutual identification, feigned diminutiveness, and neotenic care-seeking and active-submission behaviors. Bateson (1976) characterizes these various preliminary messages as a form of metacommunication, that is, expressive signals forming a communicative context by which the participants can properly interpret the behavioral events that follow. During an invitation to play, these various messages are communicated to reassure the other (and perhaps the sender) that the activity is, in fact, just play. According to Bateson, these various signals state, "These actions in which we now engage do not denote what those actions for which they stand would denote [otherwise]. . . . The playful nip denotes the bite, but it does not denote what would be denoted by the bite" (121). In other words, the preliminary signals communicate about the forthcoming events in terms that reach *beyond* the obvious denotations. He argues that the mammalian evolution of play signals may represent an important evolutionary step in the development of communication. Buytendijk (1936) argues that a dog's ability to communicate symbolically through gesture, body language, and vocalization has played a vital role in its successful domestic adaptation:

> Taking one thing with another, there is indeed no other animal in our environment that has so many means at its disposal for rendering the intensity of its actions symbolic. This explains (1) why man has ascribed to the dog as intense a faculty of feeling as he himself possesses; (2) why man believes he understands the dog; (3) why the dog is so exceptionally capable of accompanying man, and of being spoken to and treated as a house-mate, a friend, and brother. (65)

A common example of metacommunication related to play is the play smile or canine grin. Many dogs exhibit a "smile" during greetings and other times of excitement. The grin is superficially similar to the baring of teeth exhibited during agonistic displays. Both the grin and the snarl are formed by retracting the upper lip back and exposing the incisors and canines. Although a grin is sometimes confused with a snarl, many facial and bodily indicators confirm a nonaggressive and prosocial intention. Instead of communicating a threat, the play smile clearly invites playful social interaction. Darwin (1872/1965) long ago gave a very plausible account for the development of this canine social custom:

> Some persons speak of the grin as a smile, but if it had been really a smile, we should see a similar, though more pronounced, movement of the lips and ears, when dogs utter their bark of joy; but this is not the case, although a bark of joy often follows a grin. On the other hand, dogs, when playing with their comrades or masters, almost always pretend to bite each other; and they retract, though not energetically, their lips and ears. Hence I suspect that there is a tendency in some dogs, whenever they feel lively pleasure combined with affection, to act through habit and association on the same muscles, as in playfully biting each other, or their masters' hands. (120)

In another insightful passage, he keenly describes another common example of metacommunication at work:

> When my terrier bites my hand in play, often snarling at the same time, if he bites too hard and I say *gently, gently,* he goes on biting, but answers me by a few wags of the tail, which seems to say "Never mind, it is all fun." (120)

It should be noted that the canine grin may function in a variety of ways, some of which may be ambiguous and not indicative of an intention to play. Some dogs under the influence of conflicted or nervous intentions may grin in an effort to cut off interaction. Cutoff signals appear to be offered as gestures of compromise in situations involving social conflict (see *Cutoff Signals* in Volume 1, Chapter 10). The cutoff or compromise signal is not a submissive gesture but an opportunity for the contestants to call a draw and disengage without loss or gain. Generally, the cutoff signal appears to have a mutually pacifying effect that curtails tensions before they escalate into more serious conflict. Cutoff signals are often presented during playful activity, especially when things get too competitive or threatening for one of the players.

A common form of metacommunication exchanged by playing dogs is the play bow. Bekoff (1977) studied the function of play signals in both domestic and wild canids and observed that the play bow serves two primary functions: (1) the signal communicates an animal's intention to play in the first place, and (2) the signal confirms the continuance of a playful mood, thus preventing play from escalating into more serious fighting. Bekoff observed that play bows occur more frequently after certain agonistic actions (e.g., biting and

side-to-side head shaking) that might be misinterpreted by a playful opponent as a threat
(Bekoff, 1995). He argues that play bows
under such circumstances may serve to disambiguate the meaning and playful intention of
such behavior:

> In addition to sending the message "I want to
> play" when they are performed at the beginning
> of play, bows performed in a different context,
> namely during social play, might also carry the
> message "I want to play despite what I am
> going to do or just did—I still want to play"
> when there might be a problem in the sharing
> of this information between the interacting ani-
> mals. (426)

In the case of play between adult dogs and
puppies, the former might lie down on its
side or back and engage the latter in jaw
wrestling and gentle pawing. Figuratively
speaking, each player must temporarily dis-
card its social armor and weapons in order to
play. Play may evoke a shared sense of relief
from the various accustomed expectations and
roles ordinarily required from each of the participants. Between familiar dogs, dominant-
subordinate roles change fluidly during play,
but such transitions may be more stiff and
tenuous in the case of unfamiliar dogs playing
for the first time. In such cases, there is a significant risk that play may inadvertently escalate into overt fighting. Play may also turn
aggressive when one of the participants
abruptly decides to quit before the other is
ready. Usually, however, play is peaceful and
socially constructive, functioning to promote
harmonious interaction and mutual tolerance
between play partners.

Social Learning and Play

The ability to play is contingent on a balance
of health and emotional stability. Overly
aggressive, fearful, depressed, or sick dogs do
not show significant interest in play. Play
exudes a sense of security and well-being
together with an open willingness to accept
come-what-may during the course of playful
interaction and exploration. Play encourages
an empathic sensitivity involving gentleness
and tolerance while expressing oneself in
aggressive and sexual forms. Eibl-Eibesfeldt

(1971) reports that animals that fight among
themselves as adults practice agonistic skills as
young, learning appropriate restraints and bite
inhibition. If one partner in play bites too
hard, the "injured" play partner yelps, quits
playing, and may retaliate in earnest, thus
teaching the aggressor better bite inhibition in
the future. It is very likely that play is the
means by which dogs learn appropriate
restraint and inhibition over aggressive and
other socially disruptive behavior patterns
(Bekoff, 1972). In many respects, play is a
socially unifying activity that stands in direct
opposition to the socially dispersing influence
of agonistic behavior. Bekoff (1974) concluded from a comparative study of coyotes,
dogs, and wolves that "canids which play
together tend to stay together" (227). He
found that the relative amount of play exhibited versus agonistic behavior in early life is a
reliable indicator of the degree of sociability
exhibited by the animal as an adult. Play
appears to serve an important role in the facilitation of long-term affiliative behavior
among wolves and dogs—a tendency that is
notably lacking in the more socially aggressive
and *lonely* coyote.

Among wolf pups, aggressive behavior and
biting peak between weeks 8 and 12. During
play, participants learn "the fact that hard biting results in *aggressive reaction* (italics added)
by the wolf who has been bitten" (Zimen,
1981:186). As the result of aggressive retaliation and submission, play becomes more
friendly and social interaction progressively
more orderly and peaceful as bite inhibition
develops and the puppy learns to benefit from
social signals. In combination, social dominance and competitive success over the control
of food and other resources facilitate the emergence of more or less stable dominance relations between competing littermates. As a
result of such competition, a ranking order is
established to promote more peaceful and
cooperative interaction and the prevention of
disruptive fighting. As the result of playful
sparring and aggressive competition, the puppy
appears to internalize a lasting impression of its
relative status (that is, its general ability to control others in a competitive context). Although
highly aggressive puppies may secure and
maintain dominance from an early age, the

process of social definition is usually labile, with dominance relations becoming progressively stable between littermates between weeks 11 and 17 (Scott and Fuller, 1965).

Play facilitates social learning between dogs and between people and dogs. The presence of interactive tolerance and the exchange of affection during bouts of play provide an atmosphere of flexibility under which puppies and dogs can readily learn self-control and interactive restraint. This readiness coupled with a playful puppy's ability to switch back and forth quickly from behaviors belonging to unrelated functional systems gives play the ability to facilitate the formation of unique or new linkages, flexibility that is extremely useful for behavioral training efforts and the modification of various behavior problems. Play and exploratory curiosity are essential to learning both about the environment and about others—canine and otherwise:

> The animal collects experiences during play with conspecifics and learns the possible range of its own movements. Play always implies a dialogue with the environment, and this dialogue is always the result of an internal drive. One could even assume a separate drive for play, but I am inclined to believe that the drive to learn, which is the basis of all curiosity behavior coupled with an excess of motoric motivation, will suffice to account for the phenomenon of play. (Eibl-Eibesfeldt, 1970:240)

An important use of playful interaction among animals is the testing and probing of social relations, including social status. Pellis and Pellis (1996) note that the dominance-testing function of play is especially relevant in the case of postpubertal animals:

> We suggest that the primary function of postpubertal play fighting is that of social manipulation, either to recruit or maintain "friendships," or to improve one's status in the group. For the latter purpose, one animal has to test and probe its relationship with another. If such probing reveals weakness, the performer can increase the intensity or roughness of play or even switch to more explicitly agonistic behavior. In this way, the performer may intimidate the opponent, thus gaining access to current or future resources. But what if such rough play meets with strong resistance? The problem is then to back down, or de-escalate the encounter. An amicable signal that conveys the message "it was only play" would be invaluable. (260)

During playful interaction, aggressive behaviors are emitted at very low intensities and dogs are much more tolerant of provocative handling. Further, since dominant-subordinate roles are more fluid during play, a dominant dog or puppy can be more easily encouraged to adopt a subordinate role and learn the benefits of cooperation and submission by making various rewards available at such times. In an important sense, effective behavioral training is play with a structure and purpose. Structured play interaction provides an excellent tool for the modification of many emotionally debilitating problems besides dominance aggression. Play is commonly combined with other behavior-modification procedures in the management and control of fearful behavior, social excesses, and a variety of impulse-control problems.

Note: Initiating play with a dominant-aggressive dog with a history of serious attacks is potentially very dangerous. Such activities are only slowly and carefully introduced after significant behavior modification has taken place to reduce the risk. Dominant-aggressive dogs often exhibit a striking lack of interest in play and may resent playful initiatives and respond aggressively if prompted to play.

COGNITION AND AGGRESSION

Among highly evolved animals like dogs, executive cortical systems exercise significant regulatory control over the expression of emotional behavior. These cognitive appraisal and regulatory processes serve to excite or inhibit relevant motivational substrates selectively. Cognitive influences finely tune the dog's emotional state and prepare it for action according to the needs defined by the moment-to-moment circumstances confronting it, thus giving behavior a high degree of expressive accuracy and subtlety. Cortical and subcortical interactions are analogous to the relationship between a conductor and an orchestra. Although the orchestra is composed of many disparate musical instruments and sounds, it is given harmonious organization and direction under the executive command of the conductor's baton, thereby producing music instead of cacophony.

Unfortunately, executive cognitive control efforts often fail to regulate highly motivated behavior such as fear and rage. The afferent and efferent interconnections between the cortex and the subcortical areas responsible for the elaboration of fear, anger, and rage are asymmetrical, with stronger input going into the cortex than leaves it to modulate the activity of these influential areas of the brain (see *Cerebral Cortex* in Volume 1, Chapter 3). In other words, one cannot just command "Don't be afraid" or "Don't be angry" and expect the subcortical areas involved to be quieted. Executive control is not exerted like an on-off switch that activates or deactivates the selected arousal system; instead, such influences are mediated through the cortical activation of opposing motivational systems: *contraries cure contraries*. For example, an angry impulse may be offset by an opposing fearful impulse that is evoked by a *recognition* that aggression will probably not succeed and may actually fail and possibly cause the perpetrator harm. In this case, fear appears to restrain anger, whereas, in other cases, anger may reduce fear.

The central arousal of fear competes with anger and elevates behavioral thresholds for aggressive behavior, but only if such stimulation occurs before an attack is launched. Once an attack is under way, threats and efforts to physically punish aggressive behav-ior typically worsen the situation. Under the potentiating influence of rage, aggressive efforts become progressively immune to the restraining effects of fear. To inhibit aggression, fear must reach a sufficient threshold to generate an inhibitory response before a dog commits to an aggressive action. Once aggression occurs and rage is elicited, it is too late to attempt to restrain the behavior with fear-eliciting tactics. Finally, it appears that emotional impulses are hierarchically organized, with some being prepotent and inhibitory over the expression of less potent subordinate impulses (Izard, 1993). Although fear and anger tend to exert reciprocal inhibitory effects on each other, the relationship between rage and fear is not reciprocal: rage restrains fear, but fear does not appear to restrain rage.

ANXIETY, FRUSTRATION, AND AGGRESSION

Aggression (threat or attack) is driven by aversive affective states, prompted by natural or learned triggers, and guided by cognitive appraisal. Clearly, an increased likelihood of aggression occurs under conditions of heightened anxious or frustrative arousal (Figure 8.3). Both anxiety and frustration, occurring as the result of loss or threat, may trigger preparatory arousal (vigilance and behavioral invigoration) and lower aggression thresholds (Figure 8.4). Just as anxious arousal appears to reflect a mild stimulation of the fear system, frustrative

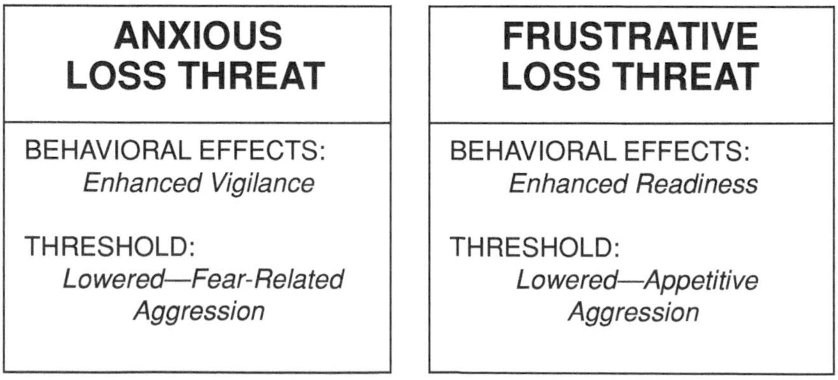

ANXIOUS LOSS THREAT	FRUSTRATIVE LOSS THREAT
BEHAVIORAL EFFECTS: *Enhanced Vigilance* THRESHOLD: *Lowered—Fear-Related Aggression*	BEHAVIORAL EFFECTS: *Enhanced Readiness* THRESHOLD: *Lowered—Appetitive Aggression*

FIG. 8.3. Control-related aggression thresholds are lowered by the presence of anxiety (enhanced vigilance) and frustration (enhanced readiness).

arousal may reflect mild activation of the aggression-rage system (Panksepp, 1998). In addition to the threshold-modulating influences of anxiety and frustration, a dog's disposition to behave aggressively depends on a past history of agonistic successes and failures. For example, under conditions of forceful restraint, both anxiety and frustration may be evoked, triggering autonomic arousal and behavioral invigoration that may result in aggressive efforts to escape. If the aggressive effort is successful, both anxious and frustrative arousal are immediately reduced and replaced by opponent relief and elation, potentially providing significant reinforcement for the behavior. Under similar circumstances in the future, stimuli associated with the situation may elicit preparatory anxious arousal in advance of impending restraint, thereby causing the dog to threaten or attack even before it is touched; that is, the dog may learn to respond preemptively to situations portending loss or threat. The decision to threaten or attack appears to be regulated by a cost-benefit assessment of the situation. Aggression is most likely to occur under circumstances in which the likelihood of success is high and the potential costs are low if aggression fails. Conversely, aggression is least likely to occur under circumstances in which the likelihood of success is low, and where a significant cost is at risk if aggression fails. Aggressive behavior is most likely to conform to a cost-benefit analysis under social circumstances that are both highly predictable and controllable. However, under the influence of uncontrollable and unpredictable circumstances involving high levels of anxiety and frustration, aggression may occur in a much more erratic and impulsive way (Figure 8.5).

To a significant extent, the behavioral treatment of aggression problems involves altering behavioral thresholds by appropriately modifying anxiety and frustration levels. Conditioned anxiety is addressed by means of various classical conditioning procedures, whereas conditioned frustration is modified by instrumental training efforts that give dogs constructive alternatives with which to control or cope with frustrating or threatening situations. In combination, these various behavior-modification procedures help to systematically disconfirm anxious-frustrative expectancies mediating aggressive behavior by fostering incompatible expectancies based on security and confidence, that is, heightened trust. Systematic training activities provide dogs with a highly predictable and controllable framework for experiencing and coping with motivational adversity.

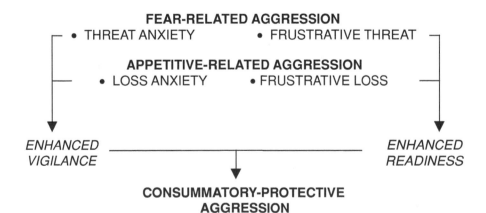

FIG. 8.4. Anxiety and frustration serve to prepare dogs for aggression by enhancing vigilance and motivational readiness.

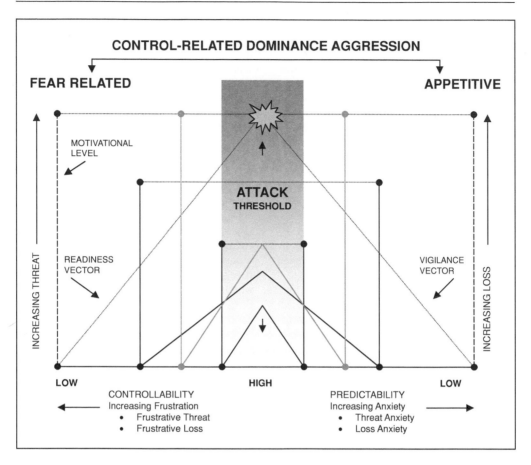

FIG. 8.5. Various contributory cognitive and motivational factors interact to influence the attack threshold. The perceived controllability and predictability of the situation exercise a pronounced influence. Under enhanced motivational conditions of impending threat or loss, vigilance and readiness vectors angle steeply in relation to the degree of control or predictability present, with an attack most likely under conditions where the event is both unpredictable and uncontrollable. Note that the likelihood of attack is correspondingly reduced as the size of the threat or loss is reduced and the event's controllability/predictability is increased.

BEHAVIORAL THRESHOLDS AND AGGRESSION

The vast majority of dogs go through life without ever exhibiting dominance-related aggression problems. Many dogs are exposed to similar rearing and training practices, but relatively few of them develop serious aggression problems. Presumably, permissive and unassertive owners would be more likely to foster dogs exhibiting dominance-related problems. Although some putative differences between owners of aggressors and nonaggressors have been suggested from time to time, nothing robust or explanatory has been iden-

tified. In fact, most studies to date have found little or no correlation between owner personality traits, anthropomorphic attitudes, or spoiling activities and the incidence of dominance-related aggression problems (Dodman, 1996; Goodloe and Borchelt, 1998; Voith et al., 1992) The relative independence of aggressive behavior and owner rearing or training practices reduces the likelihood that dominance-related aggression problems are caused primarily by status conflicts.

The control theory of aggression escapes similar criticism by emphasizing motivational considerations, such as anger, frustration, and irritability. These aggression-promoting establishing operations are offset or modulated by incompatible or affiliative establishing operations, such as affection and trust. The essential difference between control- and status-related dominance aggression is that control-related aggression is emitted in order to dominate some situation without reference to the relative status of aggressor and victim, whereas status-related aggression is emitted under circumstances in which a subordinate (past loser) fails to recognize and appropriately defer to an opponent's dominant status. Although status may be a significant factor in some cases of interspecific dominance aggression, unless the *status* concept is carefully delimited in functional terms, it may only confuse matters and impede training efforts. The status of social competitors is an emergent attribute defined by their relative successes or failures resulting from past conflicts and contests: winners are dominate and losers are subordinate. A potentially useful way to understand status in functional terms is provided by the control-vector analysis discussed in Chapter 7. In essence, status signals power and a history of aggressive success.

Many biological factors disposing dogs toward competitive success are inherited, for example, its size and physical health. In addition, various behavioral thresholds conducive to combative success appear to be inherited. Price (1998) argues that the primary effect of domestication on behavior has been to alter behavioral thresholds. Of particular interest is the alteration of behavioral thresholds controlling the freeze (mild fear), flight (strong fear), and fight reactions. Obviously, not all dogs show the same response to aversive stimulation; these differences of behavior are primarily due to emotional and behavioral thresholds. For example, some dogs exhibit a very low fear threshold and may freeze or flee in response to minimal fearful stimulation [e.g., fearful pointers (see *Nervous Pointer Dogs* in Volume 1, Chapter 5)], whereas other dogs may exhibit a very high fear threshold and exhibit extraordinary tolerance for such stimulation (Krushinskii, 1960). On the other hand, some dogs exhibit a low aggression threshold to provocative stimulation and are quick to *fight* in response to minimal annoy-

ance, whereas other dogs, possessing a high aggression threshold, may become aggressive only under the most extreme and provocative stimulation. Combining these opposing behavioral thresholds results in four sets of characteristics, latencies, and predictions (Figure 8.6). During competitive contests, dogs combining a low aggression threshold and a high fear threshold (quadrant 2) enjoy an advantage over opponents exhibiting a high aggression threshold and a low fear threshold (quadrant 3). For example, a dog that attacks with minimal provocation is likely to dominate a more inhibited counterpart who submits or runs away when minimally threatened (Pawlowski and Scott, 1956). Also, the tendency of male puppies to dominate female puppies may be due to the threshold-lowering effects of perinatal androgenization on neural substrates mediating the expression of aggressive behavior. Although these various thresholds are significantly influenced by biological factors, they are also subject to the actualizing influence of experience and learning (Krushinskii, 1960). Typically, dogs exhibiting control-related dominance aggression problems fall into quadrants 1 and 2. An important aspect of treating such problems involves systematically altering behavioral thresholds in the direction of quadrant 4. In the case of dogs exhibiting characteristics belonging to quadrant 1, behavior-modification efforts should aim at simultaneously elevating aggression and fear thresholds, whereas, in the case of dogs showing characteristics belonging to quadrant 2, training efforts should be primarily focused on elevating the aggression threshold. Note that attempting to increase control by lowering fear thresholds (flight) in dogs belonging to quadrant 2 may inadvertently push them in the direction of quadrant 1, with an increased risk of aggression and rage—an unfortunate and common iatrogenic outcome of training in cases in which overt aggression is physically punished.

This general scheme nicely explains how a dog possessing a high aggression threshold and a low fear threshold (quadrant 3) might be induced to attack. Under circumstances in which such dogs are strongly aroused with fear but prevented from escaping, the fight threshold may be finally reached, causing the

	LOW-FLIGHT	**HIGH-FLIGHT**
LOW-FIGHT	**1** LOW-FIGHT/LOW-FLIGHT *LATENCY:* Quick to aggression- Quick to fear *PREDICTION:* High probability to exhibit aggression with significant rage potential	**2** LOW-FIGHT/HIGH-FLIGHT *LATENCY:* Quick to aggression- Slow to fear *PREDICTION:* High probability to exhibit control-related dominance aggression
HIGH-FIGHT	**3** HIGH-FIGHT/LOW-FLIGHT *LATENCY:* Slow to aggression- Quick to fear *PREDICTION:* High probability to flee--low probability of aggression, unless flight is blocked	**4** HIGH-FIGHT/HIGH-FLIGHT *LATENCY:* Slow to aggression- Slow to fear *PREDICTION:* Low probability for aggression or fleeing, except under the most extreme duress or threat

FIG. 8.6. Matrix of behavioral thresholds controlling flight (fear) and fight (aggression).

dogs to attack the source of stimulation. If the attack is successful, such dogs may form a highly undesirable inference about how to control fearful stimulation or threats in the future, thereby lowering the controlling threshold for aggression. When threatened in future, a quadrant-3 dog may threaten or attack preemptively instead of waiting and possibly being hurt again. This *learned trigger* overrides or bypasses low-threshold fear inhibitions (freeze or flee) and directs the dog to attack. In this case, the dog attacks—not because of fear but in spite of fear. Under such influences, aggressive behavior may be liberated from modulatory threshold influences and natural triggers, gradually being elicited by a variety of stimuli and in minimally provocative and inappropriate contexts.

Under the assault of aversive stimulation, escape appears to be prepotent over attack, but attack is easily learned as an escape/avoidance response if it serves to terminate aversive stimulation (Azrin et al., 1967). The inhibitory effects of fear are especially compromised in situations where aggression has proven more successful than submitting or running away in the past. This particular form of aggression is especially responsive to behavior modification, since the *learned trigger* can be counterconditioned, causing the aggression threshold to gravitate gradually back to its *natural* level. In addition, such dogs are often very inhibited aggressors that seem to want to find a way out of conflict situations without resorting to aggression.

Theoretically, puppies exhibiting quadrant-1 traits would be at a higher risk of developing aggression problems as adults, regardless of owner rearing and training practices. When exposed to aversive stimulation, such puppies may respond to the punishing agent (e.g., the owner) with both fear and anger—a highly undesirable state of affairs. As a result of such motivational collision, fear may become progressively linked with anger and aggression. Instead of inhibiting attack (submission) or causing such puppies to submit, the elicitation of fear may stimulate aggression through its linkage with anger and rage circuits. Punishment in such cases may only stimulate more anger and aggression. The result is a spiraling escalation of rage, continuing until aversive stimulation is stopped. Conceivably, if such motivational cross-linkages are formed early enough in a dog's development, especially before fear and anger/rage neural circuits are fully differentiated and segregated, a very serious and explosive form of aggression might be incubated and finally expressed in adulthood (Panksepp, 1998).

AVERSIVE TRAUMA, SOCIAL LOSS, AND AGGRESSION

Although abusive treatment should be avoided in the rearing of dogs, punishment per se (even when highly aversive and non-contingent) may not always result in a predisposition for aggression or fearfulness in puppies with sufficiently high behavioral thresholds for aggression and fear. Although a history of abuse and trauma may represent a necessary cause, these experiences alone are not sufficient for the development of adult social behavior problems involving excessive fear or aggression. In fact, as shown by Fisher (1955), many puppies appear to be surprisingly resilient to the effects of traumatic treatment (see *Early Trauma and the Development of Behavior Problems* in Chapter 4). Fisher's findings draw into question the role of adverse and traumatic conditions in the development of maladaptive behavior in dogs. The modulating effects of behavioral thresholds provide a key to understanding why some dogs can undergo detrimental experiences but not exhibit lasting signs of disturbance,

whereas others appear to be profoundly and permanently debilitated by such experiences. Pavlov (1927/1960) was the first to recognize that certain temperament types are more susceptible to the elaboration of neurotic disturbances; especially vulnerable are those dogs prone to excessive excitation (choleric) or inhibition (melancholic) (see *Experimental Neurosis* in Volume 1, Chapter 9). Detrimental environmental conditions are most likely to exert lasting disturbances in dogs possessing excessively low thresholds to aversive stimulation. According to this analysis, a genetic predisposition affords conditions under which exposure to traumatic events may provide the conditions (distal setting events) under which influence adversity (proximal establishing operations) may result in persistent aggressive or fearful behavioral disturbances. Normally, aggression is physiologically and psychologically self-limiting and used only under adverse motivational conditions (e.g., frustration, irritability, and threat). Aggression occurring outside of this basic pattern is often the result of neurotic elaborations or an underlying physiological pathology.

Depending on individual temperament variations, stressful separation and loss may exert a pronounced effect on a dog's behavior by increasing social avoidance and aggression—changes that may persist even after contact with the attachment object is restored. E. C. Senay (1966) studied behavioral changes occurring in dogs following an abrupt cessation of social contact (abandonment) and subsequent reunion after 2 months of separation. Beginning at week 3 and continuing until 9½ months of age, the researcher established close contact with six German shepherd littermates. The behavior of the puppies was carefully monitored and evaluated prior to separation, after separation, and after reunion. During the 2-month period of separation (from 9½ to 11½ months), a noninteractive caretaker cleaned their pens and fed them.

From the onset and over the course of the study, the puppies exhibited consistent behavioral tendencies in terms of social affiliation and approach scores versus avoidance and aggression scores. Three of the puppies were highly cooperative and socially attracted to the experimenter and actively sought to maintain close contact with him (*approach temperament*), whereas the other three exhibited varying degrees of avoidance and aggression (*avoidance temperament*). Puppies exhibiting affiliative-approach tendencies received the highest scores with respect to responsiveness to discipline and trainability. These puppies showed a minimum amount of social avoidance when disciplined and a high degree of responsiveness to training. In contrast, socially avoidant and aggressive puppies received the lowest discipline and trainability scores, exhibiting a high degree of avoidance and resistance to training efforts.

Puppies exhibiting the highest preseparation approach scores showed increased social interest and attraction toward rater-observers entering the holding pen during the period. On the other hand, puppies exhibiting high avoidance and aggression scores prior to separation became even more avoidant and aggressive during the 2-month separation period. Interestingly, puppies with *avoidance temperaments* showed a significant decrease of activity during the separation period. Upon reunion with the experimenter, the trends toward increased attraction and affiliation, on the one hand, and increased avoidance and aggression, on the other, continued to increase during the first 2 weeks after reunion, before returning to preseparation levels after another 2 weeks of restored contact with the experimenter.

Senay observed a strong correlation between arousal levels and temperament type. Avoidant-aggressive puppies tended to exhibit a high level of general arousal and excitability, with tachycardia and excitable urination being exhibited by the most avoidant and aggressive puppies in the group, whereas puppies exhibiting less excitability and reduced arousal levels showed more approach behavior and *no* aggression:

> Early in life the animals seemed to possess differences in their neurophysiologic arousal systems. These differences seemed to determine whether object presentation [presence of the experimenter] would have organizing (approach temperament) or disorganizing (avoidance temperament) effects on the behavioral patterns of the animals. . .. The observations made here

suggest that with stimulation from the object held constant, animals possess individual differences in their arousal mechanisms and furthermore, that these differences are crucially involved in separation phenomenon. (70–71)

These findings underscore the importance of affectionate affiliation for the control and prevention of aggression problems, and emphasize the role of behavioral thresholds in their etiology and development. Separation from an attachment object may produce significant stress and alter avoidance and aggression thresholds in predisposed dogs possessing an *avoidance temperament,* while enhancing affiliative bonding and cooperation in dogs influenced by an *approach temperament.* Interpreted from a behavioral perspective, separation represents a setting event (distal influence) that motivationally alters a puppy's later responsiveness to establishing operations (proximal influence) associated with avoidance and aggression. Early traumatic experiences can be interpreted in similar ways. Predisposed puppies exposed to an excessively frightening experience (setting event) may be more responsive to similar conditioned and unconditioned experiences (establishing operations) occurring later in life. The early traumatic setting event may consequently cause such dogs to acquire related avoidance or aggressive behavior more rapidly and efficiently.

Learning and Dominance

As has already been repeatedly emphasized, dominance is synonymous with control. Dominance contests occur when a dog is prompted to do something it would prefer not to do, constrained to forego some preferred activity, or required to relinquish some possession it would prefer to keep. Consider, for example, a competitive contest by two dogs over a location or resource (Figure 8.7). During the contest, the more dominant of the two opponents will *prompt* the subordinate with a direct threat (e.g., stiff posture, stare, and snarl) to withdraw from the situation. If the subordinate fails to defer, the dominant animal may escalate its threats, or attack if its threats continue to be ignored. Assuming that the dominant dog's efforts are

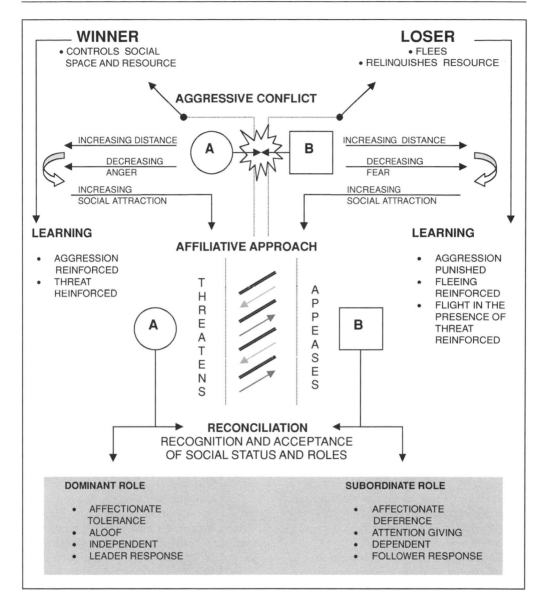

FIG. 8.7. Various outcomes resulting from agonistic interaction. Immediately following an aggressive encounter, anger and fear enhance social distance between combatants. Over time, anger and fear wane and are replaced by increasing levels of social attraction and affiliative interest. As contact is restored, threat and appeasement displays facilitate reconciliation, with opponents recognizing each other's social status and respective roles. Note the various effects that learning has on aggressive interaction.

successful, both the assertive behavior of the winner and the flight/submission of the loser are reinforced, but the reinforcement experienced by the two contestants is based on opposite reinforcing effects. The dominant dog's assertive behavior is positively reinforced twofold, since it successfully displaced the rival, as well as served to secure the resource (e.g., a bone). The subordinate's behavior is both punished and negatively reinforced. On the one hand, the subordinate's competitive adventure failed to control the resource (punishment), whereas, on the other, it succeeded in escaping the dominant dog's attack. As a result, during future competitive interaction between the two dogs, the dominant animal will be more likely to successfully assert rank, whereas the subordinate will be more likely to submit or flee. In addition, the subordinate will likely learn to avoid future contests with the winner. By exhibiting submissive behavior toward the threatening rival, the subordinate avoids attack and its submissive behavior is reinforced. Likewise, the subordinate's deferential response to threat or attack reinforces such displays in the dominant dog. In the future, contests between the two rivals are resolved largely through the exchange of ritualized threat and appeasement behaviors—displays that are highly *prepared* (species typical) and quickly learned.

Threat and appeasement displays may be conceptualized as triggers producing opposite establishing operations in the competitors. In the case of dominant animals, appeasement signals evoke motivational changes conducive to reducing aggressive behavior (reduces anger), whereas, in the case of subordinates, threats evoke motivation changes conducive to the emission of submissive behavior and withdrawal (increases fear). In both cases, under the influence of relevant establishing operations and motivational states, corresponding dominant-role and submissive-role *playing* is reinforced.

Following an assertion of dominance, the subordinate may run to a safe distance from the dominant alpha, but, as time wears on, affiliative pressures for social contact will cause it to gravitate back into closer proximity with the alpha. With contact restored, its social separation distress is reduced, thereby reinforcing affiliative behavior and increasing affection for the *magnanimous* alpha. Although the alpha may experience feelings of social loss as well, its distress may be felt much less keenly, since it is compensated with the elation and spoils of victory. Further, the alpha may view the social distance set between itself and its rival as part of its overall success. Dominant dogs possess a certain comfort with social distance, not appearing to need the reassuring social contact sought by submissive subordinates or at least not needing it in the same way or degree. Dominant dogs are more likely to receive affection rather than to give it out.

The direction of affectionate exchange supports the development of dominance-enhancing social polarity between the competitors, making the subordinate less likely to attack the alpha and making the alpha more tolerant of the subordinate's presence. Social polarity is a strong inhibitory and stabilizing influence on the dominant-subordinate relationship. Along similar lines, the alpha is more likely to emit distance-increasing (dispersal) behavior, whereas the subordinate is more inclined to emit distance-reducing (attraction) behavior. If the subordinate is to remain in close contact, however, it must accept a submissive role relative to the alpha's dominant status and prerogatives. Submission-enhancing interaction occurs among all group members until a hierarchy (not necessarily linear) of dominant-subordinate relations and dominance-supporting allegiances is formed.

Following a successful contest, future competitive interaction between the victor and the loser will probably take the form of threat and appeasement displays, indicating the importance of avoidance learning to the process of establishing social dominance. The threat or mere glance alone is now sufficient to evoke submission without needing to resort to an attack, although an occasional aggressive assertion of control may still occur from time to time. This appears to be a desirable arrangement for both the alpha and the subordinate. A possible factor restraining the alpha's use of overt aggression is that such behavior may be intrinsically aversive for it to perform—reminiscent of the reluctance of many owners to punish unruly dogs. Aggression may be *reinforced* insofar as it secures control but is probably not *reinforcing* for its own sake, at least not under normal circumstances. In fact, brain studies involving microstimulation of limbic system areas dedicated to the expression of aggression have shown that affective aggression is physiologically aversive for the stimulated animal (Adams and Flynn, 1966). Consequently, the alpha is not likely to attack subordinates casually or as a way to obtain *pleasure* at the subordinate's expense. For the subordinate, aggression is doubly aversive, because its own aggressive efforts are both intrinsically aversive and unsuccessful; that is, they result in punishment. Finally, there is always some risk of injury to the alpha as the result of fighting, so avoiding unnecessary combative contests would make sense on the level of self-preservation and safety, as well. Ultimately, the exchange of threat and appeasement display establishes a foundation for social organization and purposeful coordinated activity.

Submission behaviors appear to consist of exaggerated species-typical canine infant behaviors. Among many mammalian species, a strong inhibition prevents adults from attacking their young. Submission displays appear to take advantage of these innate inhibitions and taboos. Such displays are highly prepared responses learned without much experience and triggered by an alpha's threats. In turn, these submissive or appeasement gestures and postures trigger inhibitory control over the alpha's aggressive threats, preventing them from escalating into a full-fledged attack. In the presence of the alpha leader, the subordinate appears to act somewhat like an obsequious infant. These caricature infantlike behaviors appear to evoke paternal (or maternal) caregiving and protective responses toward the subordinate.

Although the subordinate may initially flee and stay away from the dominant victor, in time a growing need for social contact asserts itself. Submissive behavior emerges under the combined influence of fear and social attraction. In an important sense, social attraction overshadows fear and restrains the impulse to flee too far or stay away too long. Much like a rubber band stretched between the alpha and the subordinate, social attraction grows as a motivational tension in proportion to the distance and time spent fleeing. Gradually, needs for social contact attract the subordinate back into closer proximity with the alpha. The subordinate's approach takes place against a

building fear gradient but is facilitated under the counterconditioning influence of *affection*. The combination of fear and affection evokes the expression of submissive behavior. In short, *submission* is a motivational composite of *fear and affection*.

Gradually, the subordinate may learn that submissive displays *work* and can be used to manipulate the alpha. This *knowledge is power*, and the clever subordinate may even mock or tease the alpha, thereby narrowing the social distance and disturbing social stability between the two potential rivals. In addition, social polarity is shifted by the amount of attention and effort that the alpha must divert in the direction of the enterprising subordinate. The subordinate may also learn that the alpha does not really like being aggressive. At this point, the subordinate may become overtly obnoxious at times but immediately present a submissive token, if necessary, to placate the aroused and irritated superior. This transition involves a great deal of dominance testing, attention-seeking behavior (active submission), and playful competitive excesses. The alpha may rebuff these excesses but be gradually worn down by the subordinate's relentless and shrewd efforts. As time goes on, a critical point may be reached (especially in socially mature animals) where the provocative subordinate may lose its fear and respect for the alpha altogether and step over the line. If the alpha neglects to act decisively to the challenge, the subordinate may simply take over without a fight. Most often, however, such behavior is met with an immediate and assertive rejoinder, thereby subordinating the challenger (at least for a while). Unless resolved, the two rivals may eventually engage in earnest combat until one is injured, killed, or expelled from the group. These sorts of damaging dominance fights are relatively uncommon in nature but do occur. Serious dominance fights may play a genetic and ecological role in forcing the dispersion of *fit* second-ranking males and females into contact with other similarly expelled counterparts needing mates of their own, thereby encouraging outbreeding and avoiding the dangers of excessive inbreeding between close relatives.

SOCIAL COMPETITION, DEVELOPMENT, AND AGGRESSION

Serious dog aggression problems occur infrequently before the end of the first year and rarely in young puppies. Scott and Fuller (1965) *never* observed any serious attacks or threats in puppies toward humans administering handling tests designed to measure aggressive behavior. Most puppy agonistic behavior is playful, consisting of pawing and inhibited biting actions on hands and clothing. They concluded that "playful aggressiveness and serious aggressiveness are not necessarily correlated" (1965:137)—a finding recently reiterated by Goodloe and Borchelt (1998). Krushinskii (1960), however, has noted research suggesting that some forms of reflexive overt aggression *do* occur in young puppies. In one study, for example, researchers found that a 19-day-old puppy may exhibit an intense aggressive response to being suddenly awakened—a finding that may have relevance for understanding the etiology of this form of aggression in some adult dogs. Although reflexive aggression may be present at an early age, Krushinkii emphasized that "real" aggression toward humans infrequently occurred and not before the end of week 12. Although relatively uncommon, puppies do occasionally present inchoate aggressive tendencies and oppositional behavior that may portend more serious problems in adulthood. It is of great importance, therefore, to identify puppies at risk and to provide them with appropriate socialization and training.

Early Social Learning and Oppositional Behavior

As the result of genetic predisposition and early social learning involving competition with littermates and the mother, a puppy comes into the home *prepared* to accept an affectionate and cooperative (subordinate) place in the family structure, or may bring an enhanced readiness to resist control and assert a real challenge to the family's patience and training abilities. The cooperative and oppositional tendencies of most puppies fall somewhere in between these two extremes. In general, a subordinate or cooperative puppy more readily accepts social control, actively defers when challenged to submit, and exhibits strong bite inhibition, whereas a dominant or oppositional puppy is more likely to defy social control and, when challenged, may resort to aggression, perhaps neglecting to exercise appropriate bite inhibition. Such dominant or oppositional puppies may threaten or snap at family members who attempt to control them, especially around highly motivating activities and resources. The process of establishing control over oppositional puppies can be extremely frustrating and worrisome for novice puppy owners, who may not fully appreciate the potential resistance and persistence of such puppies. This situation is compounded by the owner's sincere desire to affectionately invite the puppy into the home as an equal family member. Unfortunately, affectionate efforts may only lead to unwanted aggressive play and disinhibited mouthing with sharp teeth.

Until the oppositional puppy learns to accept the owner's control and leadership initiatives, it is incapable of forming an affectionate and cooperative relationship. Oppositional puppies may resist instructional efforts to establish household manners, show an unwillingness to accept routine handling and petting, or exhibit intolerance for minimal frustration. In advance of an established leader-follower bond, the oppositional puppy may misinterpret the owner's affectionate efforts, thereby stimulating more social tension and conflict. Finally, early successes involving threats and biting directed against an ineffectual owner may set the precedence for similar behavior in the adult dog. Although it is difficult to make specific predictive statements about the influence of early experience on adult behavior, in comparison to more submissive and cooperative counterparts, puppies exhibiting intolerance for control are likely to continue exhibiting oppositional or aggressive behavior into adulthood unless the problem is addressed with appropriate training. Excessive competition between an oppositional puppy and family members may produce a number of adverse effects:

1. Social aggressive tensions and increased frustration may develop as the result of ineffectual owner efforts to assert control over the puppy.
2. The puppy's perception of social rank may be adversely affected by successfully evading owner control efforts.
3. Evasive chase-and-catch competition over *stolen* objects may be particularly problematical and conducive for the development of aggressive tensions.
4. Abusive punishment occurring out of anger may facilitate the development of defensive aggression.

Although such problems should be addressed and resolved through training, the excessive use of interactive physical punishment should be avoided in favor of positive reinforcement techniques, response prevention, response substitution-redirection, and time-out procedures.

Social versus Competitive (Possessive) Aggression

Competition is a normal aspect of canine social development (see *Social Dominance* in Volume 1, Chapter 2). Competitive success has often been evaluated in terms of a puppy's ability to secure and defend an attractive resource. For example, a common experimental procedure involves giving two hungry puppies a bone or a bowl of food big enough for only one of them to eat at a time. Under such circumstances, one of the puppies will likely displace the other by displaying various aggressive threats or by launching an actual attack, if necessary, to secure control of the bone or food bowl. Under similar circumstances in the future, the loser will tend to exhibit a more deferential pattern of social behavior toward the winner. The value of this procedure for assessing social dominance has been questioned, and some authors (see *Assessment and Identification*) have suggested that social dominance and competitive aggression may actually develop independently and segregate in adult dogs; that is, the dominance aggressor may exhibit competitive (possessive) aggression, but the possessive aggres-

sor is not necessarily dominant and may, in fact, be subordinate in all other situations (Borchelt, 1983). Wright (1980) performed a study designed to evaluate the relation between development, exploratory behavior, social dominance, and competitive (possessive) dominance. In his study, a group of five puppies were tested at three different ages (5½, 8½, and 11½ weeks). The German shepherd puppies showed considerable individual and developmental variations with respect to the expression of social and competitive aggression. Of particular interest was the behavior of the most socially dominant and controlling puppy [no. 2 (male)] when placed into an unfamiliar situation with a littermate and bone. Although otherwise highly aggressive toward littermates, when tested for its ability to control a bone in the novel environment, it scored much lower than less socially aggressive counterparts [e.g., no. 4 (male) and no. 5 (female)], at least during testing done at weeks 5½ and 8½. The two puppies that were most successful in controlling the bone (puppies 4 and 5) in the novel situation were more submissive than puppy 2 when interacting with littermates in familiar surroundings, at least initially. By 11½ weeks of age, however, puppy 2 had become significantly more successful in controlling the bone in the pen situation, superseding the competitive scores of puppy 5 and closing in on puppy 4. Interestingly, puppy 2 also exhibited significant changes in stimulus reactivity and exploration scores at 11½ weeks of age, suggesting the possibility that the puppy's increased competitive success may have been due to a reduction of fear in the novel situation.

The foregoing study does not necessarily support the notion that social dominance and competitive aggression function independently of each other (Reisner (1997). This view represents only one possible way to interpret Wright's findings, but not, perhaps, the most likely one, as Wright points out:

> The relationship between stimulus reactivity and competitive dominance indicates that those puppies that were the least neophobic were also the ones that were best able to control a desirable object in a competitive situation. . . . In other words, the most exploratory and less

timid puppies were not penalized during the bone-in-pen test by the strange setting, and thus were perhaps better able to control the bone than their more fearful, less exploratory littermates. (1980:23)

The lack of competitive effort exhibited by puppy 2 in the novel setting probably reflects a more general adverse motivational influence rather than the expression of different forms of aggressive behavior. In particular, fear and anxiety (neophobia) associated with the novel setting may be assumed to exert a dampening effect on both appetitive arousal and exploratory activity. In addition, since fear is motivationally antagonistic with aggression, the combined motivational influences associated with the novel setting may have simply suppressed interest in competing over the bone. With regard to the possibility of two forms of dominance (social versus competitive), the study provides no data with which to decide the matter, since appropriate controls were not present to isolate and track such agonistic differentiation independently of the suppressive effects of fear. Fear (neophobia) may generally diminish a puppy's motivation to compete and, in fact, dogs are often more competitive under the influence of familiar surroundings. If puppies had been tested with a bone placed into the home pen, perhaps the apparent differentiation of social dominance and possessive aggression would not have been observed at all. In summary, puppy 2's failure to control the bone in the novel setting at an earlier age may have been due to the inhibitory environmental effects of neophobia over appetitive and aggressive arousal, rather than the expression of different forms of aggressive behavior. Puppy 2's belated success in controlling the bone appears to have been the combined result of maturation and the repeated exposure (habituation) to the novel setting, thus causing a gradual diminution of fear and the simultaneous enhancement of appetitive and aggressive motivation to control the bone.

TEMPERAMENT TESTS AND AGGRESSION

Dominant-subordinate relations are formed under the constraints of genetics, maturation, and learning, with competitive relations and incentives changing as a puppy matures. Clearly, the playful competitive sparring between littermates is something quite different from the aggressive contests exhibited by socially mature dogs and wolves. Among adult dogs, for example, competition between adult conspecific males may occur over the possession of an estrus female, something that does not occur among puppies. Although a few constant themes or *individual differences* can be traced out over the course of social development (MacDonald, 1983), the meaning and purpose of competition undergo significant elaboration as an animal matures. The nature of these changes of intention and purpose are defined by biological and social demands placed upon the animal by the interaction of genes, ontogenesis, and environmental pressures. From puppyhood to old age, the direction of these changes is guided by epigenetic processes, incorporating and integrating the aforementioned factors under the selective influence of learning. Developmentally, agonistic behavioral thresholds and corresponding species-typical behavior patterns are strongly influenced by the variable and coordinated expression of genes. The expression of genes appropriate for adaptive success changes as the animal matures. In other words, behavioral traits and abilities appear and become functional according to a genetically orchestrated timetable. The functional influence of genes expressed during the early socialization period is not the same as those influences operating and affecting behavior at puberty or at social maturity. Even cognitive abilities such as *object permanence* are not fully functional in dogs until 11 months of age (Gagnon and Dore, 1994). Genes give structure and order to developmental processes via structural proteins and functional enzymes— enzymes that catalyze biochemical reactions. Enzymes both initiate and regulate the rate of biological activity in every bodily system, including the nervous system, where a precise system of pathways exists between genes, brain structure, neurochemical activity, and behavior (Dewsbury, 1978).

Although an element of continuity certainly exists from conception to senescence, functional elaborations take place throughout the course of a dog's life. These biological considerations present tremendous challenges for predicting adult behavior based on behavioral tendencies present at earlier stages of development. Over the course of development, genes are variably turned on and off or up- and downregulated under the influence of genes specialized for such purposes. These changes occur in a coordinated manner during a puppy's development. These genetic and experiential influences have important implications for puppy temperament tests and training activities. During early puppyhood, the infant dog's brain and body undergo rapid structural and functional change, reflecting underlying genetic changes controlled by operator genes (turning on or off genes) and regulator genes (increasing or decreasing the activity of genes). Not surprisingly, behavior also undergoes rapid change, and earlier stages of development may not be accurately reflected in later stages of development (see *Temperament Testing* in Volume 1, Chapter 5).

The labile character of aggressive behavior in young puppies makes it difficult to extract any hard and fast predictions about later behavior based on early agonistic indicators. For example, employing a social temperament test believed to perform such a predictive function by some breeders and trainers (Campbell, 1972), Beaudet and associates (1994) were unable to detect a predictive continuity with respect to dominance behavior in young dogs when tested at week 7 and again at week 16. The study involving 39 puppies found that dominance scores at week 7 were not predictive of dominance scores at week 16. The authors conclude that Campbell's test has "no predictive value regarding future social tendencies. In fact, the total value of the behavioral scores for social tendencies between the two age groups showed a trend toward regression from dominance to submission" (1994:273). The authors report that more significant predictive values were obtained by including a measure of activity levels but only in the case of female puppies. Similar predictive difficulties have been reported concerning the value of puppy tests used to help select working dogs (Dietrich, 1984; Wilsson and Sundgren, 1998). Recently, however, Slabbert and Odendaal (1999) reported significant predictive correlations by

testing dogs at different ages. In particular, retrieve test scores performed at 8 weeks and the scores of aggression tests performed at 6 and 9 months yielded highly significant predictive values. In combination, the three tests accounted for the prediction of 81.7% of unsuccessful police-dog candidates and 91.7% of those dogs successfully trained for police-dog service.

Perhaps, assessing approach-withdrawal tendencies, emotional arousal (especially fear) and reactivity levels, behavior thresholds, and recovery rates following fear- or aggression-eliciting stimulation at different ages might provide more predictive information about future agonistic tendencies [see Krushinskii (1960), Schneirla (1965), Martinek and Hartl (1975), and Goddard and Beilharz (1986)]. Sympathetic arousal and recovery as measured by changes of heart rate may provide a predictive indicator of temperament, especially with regard to the fear-withdrawal dimension (Fox, 1978). However, even these possibly more stable and heritable indicators undergo significant change over time as the result of developmental consolidation, biological alterations (e.g., hormonal changes), and learning. Nonetheless, assessing behavioral thresholds controlling fear/flight tendencies (passive defensive reactions) and anger/aggression tendencies (active defensive reactions) may provide an objective means for describing and predicting social aggressive behavior in dogs. As discussed in a previous section (see *Behavioral Thresholds and Aggression*), dogs at risk of developing an aggression problem may exhibit at an early age a relatively high response threshold to fear-eliciting stimulation (slow to flight), while showing a relatively low threshold for anger arousal and aggression (quick to fight). As a result, when faced with provocative stimulation, the *excitatory* or active defensive threshold may be triggered before the *inhibitory* or passive defensive threshold is reached. Puppies exhibiting lowered response thresholds for both fear (quick to flight) and anger (quick to fight) are probably at a significant risk of developing serious adult aggression problems involving rage. This risk may be particularly strong in cases in which both fear and anger are evoked at the same time, with the one motivationally cross-associating and fusing with the other. Under the simultaneous evocation of intense fear and anger, predisposed puppies may exhibit rage (a composite response of escalating fear and anger). As a result of the repeated or traumatic collision of fear and anger, abnormal aggressive behavior may develop (see *Experimental Neurosis* in Volume 1, Chapter 9). As adults, the conditioned or unconditioned elicitation of fear may serve to trigger (rather than inhibit) aggression, thereby releasing a cascade of escalating events in which fear and anger converge motivationally in the expression of uncontrollable rage. In support of this functional etiological analysis, many owners of adult dominance aggressors report a considerable admixture of fear and aggression in the behavioral histories of their dogs.

In addition to puppy tests, temperament evaluation procedures of various kinds have been devised to assess behavioral tendencies in adult dogs. Although the value of puppy temperament tests for predicting adult dog behavior has been challenged, temperament tests for assessing behavioral tendencies of adult dogs are still widely employed and used to help assess and predict future behavior. For example, these tests are often performed to evaluate and certify dogs used in nursing homes to comfort residents and to perform animal-assisted therapy (Fredrickson and Howie, 2000). Unfortunately, most temperament assessment procedures and tests have not been statistically validated for reliability or predictive value (Goodloe, 1996). In a study involving shelter dogs (N = 9) being selected for service work, Weiss and Greenberg (1997) were unable to find a correlation between their performance on an 11-part selection test and subsequent trainability for a service-related task (retrieving). Among tested parameters, they found that fearful submissive tendencies persisted from the initial testing phase into the training and evaluation phases of the study. Interestingly, in one case, a dog passed all test items and was ranked *excellent* but was unable to complete the training phase as the result of excessive excitability and "dominance" behavior. This latter finding underscores the unreliability of inferences about the future absence of some behavior or tendency based on its nonoccurrence during testing, especially in the case of tests not designed to specifically identify and measure its occurrence. In principle, the mere *absence* of some behavior is not a valid indicator of reliability for tests designed to predict behavior, at least insofar as one wishes to avoid running afoul of the *dead-dog rule* (see Chapter 2). Just because some behavior has not been observed to occur in the test or working situation does not rule out its possible occurrence in the future. At best, temperament tests can only reliably predict behavior or analogs belonging to the same general class of behavior observed and assessed during the test. Presumably these identified behaviors are statistically correlated with success in the performance of activities for which the test is applied (e.g., companion dog, therapy dog, or service dog), but even these important data are generally still lacking.

Exploratory efforts have been carried out to validate some behavior tests for identifying tendencies associated with aggression problems. For example, Netto and Planta (1997) have devised a temperament test involving 43 subtests used to identify and assess aggressive behavior in dogs. They report that the test yields significant validation (when compared with the results of owner questionnaires) and a high degree of reliability between test and retest scores involving interspecific attack and snapping directed toward human targets. However, some significant variations were identified between test and retest scores in the case of dog fighting. Intraspecific aggression appears to increase after retesting, suggesting that the dogs may have become less inhibited as the result of increased familiarity with the test area—a finding that has obvious parallels with Wright's study discussed previously. Van der Borg and coworkers (1991) devised and evaluated a series of tests for identifying dogs prone to exhibit a variety of common behavior problems, including aggression. The researchers found that the behavioral tests provided a better means for detecting potential problem behaviors than did the opinions of shelter staff. The opinions of shelter staff were 33% successful in predicting potential problem behaviors, whereas the tests proved to be 74.7% successful in predicting potential problems in adopted dogs.

PREVENTION

Puppies exhibiting incipient signs of aggression should be identified and referred for appropriate training and behavior modification. Behavior problems caught early enough are often highly responsive to training and therapy; however, as time goes on and they become established, significant change may become progressively harder to achieve: *organization impedes reorganization.* Puppies at high risk are those described by their owners to be difficult, testy, or reactive (quick to show fear or aggression); they are commonly hyperactive, possessive (growl and snarl) over food and toys, competitive and reactive to punishment, engage in habitual *stealing* of forbidden objects that they may then protect or stiffen over, aggressively resist routine grooming or handling efforts, engage in excessive or hard mouthing when touched, and resist basic training efforts. Members of a group at particular risk are those that resent touch and handling (e.g., being picked up) and exhibit other signs of contact aversion. Such puppies may resent even the most gentle petting and handling. While the aforementioned oppositional tendencies should prompt concern, not all puppies exhibiting reactive or competitive behavior necessarily grow up to become aggressive adults; nonetheless, it is important that owners presenting such behavior complaints be encouraged to seek appropriate professional training and counseling for their puppy.

First and foremost, behavior problems are prevented by establishing a human-dog bond informed by a high degree of affection, communication, and trust, that is, interactive harmony. Ultimately, though, preventing aggression problems can be realistically achieved only by genetically improving dogs for close association with people. Genetic improvement depends on selecting and breeding dogs that are less likely to produce overly aggressive offspring. In addition to improved genes, however, dogs need effective training, socialization, and the satisfaction of their basic social and biological needs. All of these considerations are indispensable for ensuring a dog's successful adaptation and the avoidance of adjustment problems—insofar as they are avoidable. Again, in terms of preventing or managing serious aggression problems in vulnerable dogs, considerable benefit can be achieved by initiating early and sustained integrated compliance training and incorporating various behavior modification efforts as needed over the course of the dog's life. Such training helps to modulate behavioral thresholds, reduces interactive frustration and irritability, enhances communication and affiliative cooperation, and promotes affection and relaxation. Finally, such training and socialization significantly improve a dog's overall quality of life, while enhancing the relationship between the owner and dog—the ultimate goals of cynopraxic therapy.

REFERENCES

Adams D and Flynn JP (1966). Transfer of an escape response from tail shock to brain stimulated attack behavior. *J Exp Anal Behav,* 8:401–408.

Aronson LP (1998). Systemic causes of aggression and their treatment. In N Dodman and L Shuster (Eds), *Psychopharmacology of Animal Behavior Disorders.* Malden, MA: Blackwell Science.

Azrin NH, Hutchinson RR, and Hake DF (1967). Attack, avoidance, and escape reactions to aversive shock. *J Exp Anal Behav,* 10:131–148.

Barrette C (1993). The "inheritance of dominance," or of an aptitude to dominate? *Anim Behav,* 46:591–593.

Bateson G (1976). A theory of play and fantasy (1955). In JS Bruner, A Jolly, and K Sylva (Eds), *Play: Its Role in Development and Evolution.* New York: Basic.

Beaudet R, Chalifoux A, and Dallaire A (1994). Predictive value of activity level and behavioral evaluation on future dominance in puppies. *Appl Anim Behav Sci,* 40:273–284.

Bekoff M (1972). The development of social interaction, play, and metacommunication in mammals: An ethological perspective. *Q Rev Biol,* 47:412–434.

Bekoff M (1974). Social play in coyotes, wolves, and dogs. *BioScience,* 24:225–230.

Bekoff M (1995). Play signals as punctuation: The structure of social play in canids. *Behaviour,* 132:419–429.

Borchelt PL (1983). Aggressive behavior of dogs kept as companion animals: Classification and influence of sex, reproductive status, and breed. *Appl Anim Ethol* 10:45–61.

Borchelt PL and Voith VL (1985). Aggressive behavior in dogs and cats. *Compend Contin Educ Pract Vet,* 7:949–957.

Borchelt PL and Voith VL (1986). Dominance aggression in dogs. *Compend Continuing Educ Pract Vet,* 8:36–44.

Borchelt PL and Voith VL (1996). Dominance aggression in dogs. In VL Voith and PL Borchelt (Eds), *Readings in Companion Animal Behavior.* Trenton, NJ: Veterinary Learning Systems.

Buytendijk FJJ (1936). *The Mind of the Dog.* Boston: Houghton Mifflin.

Campbell WE (1972). A behavior test for puppy selection. *Mod Vet Pract,* 12:29–33.

Campbell WE (1992). *Behavior Problems in Dogs.* Goleta, CA: American Veterinary Publications.

Chance MRA (1967). Attention structure as the basis of primate rank orders. *Man,* 2:503–518.

Darwin C (1872/1965). *The Expression of the Emotions in Man and Animals.* Chicago: University of Chicago Press (reprint).

Dewsbury DA (1978). *Comparative Animal Behavior.* New York: McGraw-Hill.

Dietrich C (1984). Temperament evaluation of puppies: Use in guide dog selection. In RK Anderson, BL Hart, and LA Hart (Eds), *The Pet Connection: Its Influence on Our Health and Quality of Life.* Minneapolis: University of Minnesota.

Dodman NH, Miczek KA, Knowles K, et al. (1992). Phenobarbital-responsive episodic dyscontrol (rage) in dogs. *JAVMA,* 201:1580–1583.

Dodman NH, Moon R, and Zelin M (1996). Influence of owner personality type on expression and treatment outcome of dominance aggression in dogs. *JAVMA,* 209:1107–1109.

Dollard J, Miller, NE, Doob LW, et al. (1939). *Frustration and Aggression.* New Haven: Yale University Press.

Drews C (1993). The concept and definition of dominance in animal behaviour. *Behaviour,* 125:283–313.

Eibl-Eibesfeldt I (1970). *Ethology: The Biology of Behavior.* New York: Holt, Rinehart and Winston.

Eibl-Eibesfeldt I (1971). *Love and Hate: The Natural History of Behavior Patterns.* New York: Holt, Rinehart and Winston.

Eibl-Eibesfeldt I (1979). *The Biology of Peace and War: Men, Animals, and Aggression.* New York: Viking.

Fagen R (1981). *Animal Play Behavior.* New York: Oxford University Press.

Fisher AE (1955). The effects of early differential treatment on the social and exploratory behavior of puppies [Unpublished doctoral dissertation]. State College: Pennsylvania State University.

Fonberg E (1988). Dominance and aggression. *Int J Neurosci,* 41:201–213.

Fox MW (1971). *Integrative Development of Brain and Behavior in the Dog.* Chicago: University of Chicago Press.

Fox MW (1973). Social dynamics of three captive wolf packs. *Behaviour,* 47:290–301.

Fox MW (1978). *The Dog: Its Domestication and Behavior.* Malabar, FL: Krieger.

Frank H and Frank MG (1982). On the effects of domestication on canine social development and behavior. *Appl Anim Ethol,* 8:507–525.

Fredrickson M and Howie AR (2000). Methods, standards, guidelines, and considerations in selecting animals for animal-assisted therapy. Part B: Guidelines and standards for animal selection in animal-assisted activity and therapy programs. In A Fine (Ed), *Handbook on Animal-Assisted Therapy.* New York: Academic.

Gagnon S and Dore FY (1994). Cross-sectional study of object permanence in domestic puppies (*Canis familiaris*). *J Comp Psychol,* 108:220–232.

Goddard ME and Beilharz RG (1986). Early prediction of adult behaviour in potential guide dogs. *Appl Anim Behav Sci,* 15:247–260.

Goodloe LP (1996). Issues in description and measurement of temperament in companion dogs. In VL Voith and PL Borchelt (Eds), *Readings in Companion Animal Behavior.* Philadelphia: Veterinary Learning Systems.

Goodloe LP and Borchelt PL (1998). Companion dog temperament traits. *J Appl Anim Welfare Sci,* 1:303–338.

Hart BL and Hart LA (1985). *Canine and Feline Behavioral Therapy.* Philadelphia: Lea and Febiger.

Immelmann K (1980). *Introduction to Ethology.* New York: Plenum.

Izard CE (1993). Four systems for emotion activation: Cognitive and noncognitive processes. *Psychol Rev,* 100:68–90.

James W (1896/1956). Is life worth living? In *The Will to Believe.* New York: Dover (reprint).

Konorski J (1967). *Integrative Activity of the Brain: An Interdisciplinary Approach.* Chicago: University of Chicago Press.

Krushinskii LV (1960). *Animal Behavior: Its Normal and Abnormal Development.* New York: Consultants Bureau.

Landsberg GM (1991). The distribution of canine behavior cases at three behavior referral practices. *Vet Med,* 86:1011–1018.

Line S and Voith VL (1986). Dominance aggression of dogs towards people: Behavior profile and response to treatment. *Appl Anim Behav Sci,* 16:77–83.

Lockwood R (1979). Dominance in wolves: Useful construct or bad habit? In E Klinghammer (Ed), *The Behavior and Ecology of Wolves.* New York: Garland STPM.

Lorenz K (1964). Ritualized fighting. In JD Carthy and FJ Ebling (Eds), *The Natural History of Aggression.* New York: Academic.

Lorenz K (1966). *On Aggression.* New York: Harcourt Brace Jovanovich.

MacDonald K (1983). Stability of individual differences in behavior in a litter of wolf cubs (*Canis lupus*). *J Comp Psychol,* 97:99–106.

Martinek Z and Hartl K (1975). About the possibility of predicting the performance of adult guard dogs from early behavior: II. *Act Nerv Super (Praha)* 17:76–77.

Mech LD (1970). *The Wolf: The Ecology and Behavior of an Endangered Species.* Minneapolis: University of Minnesota Press.

Most K (1910/1955). *Training Dogs.* New York: Coward-McCann (reprint).

Netto WJ and Planta DJU (1997). Behavioural testing for aggression in the domestic dog. *Appl Anim Behav Sci,* 52:243–263.

Netto WJ, Van der Borg JA, and Sleger JF (1992). The establishment of dominance relationships in a dog pack and its relevance for the man-dog relationship. *Tijdschrift voor Diergeneeeskunde,* 117(Suppl 1):51S–53S.

Panksepp J (1998). *Affective Neuroscience: The Foundations of Human and Animal Emotions.* New York: Oxford University Press.

Papero DV (1990). *Bowen Family System Theory.* Boston: Allyn and Bacon.

Pavlov IP (1927/1960). *Conditioned Reflexes: An Investigation of the Physiological Activity of the Cerebral Cortex,* GV Anrep (Trans) New York: Dover (reprint).

Pawlowski AA and Scott JP (1956). Hereditary differences in the development of dominance in litters of puppies. *J Comp Physiol Psychol,* 49:353–358.

Pellis SM and Pellis VC (1996). On knowing it's only play: The role of play signals in play fighting. *Aggressive Violent Behav,* 1:249–268.

Polsky RH (1993). Does thyroid dysfunction cause behavioral problems? *Canine Pract,* 18:6–8.

Preti G, Muetterties EL, Furman JM, et al. (1976). Volatile constituents of dog (*Canis familiaris*) and coyote (*Canis latrans*) anal sacs. *J Chem Ecol,* 2:177–186.

Price EO (1998). Behavioral genetics and the process of animal domestication. In T Grandin (Ed), *Genetics and the Behavior of Domestic Animals.* New York: Academic.

Rabb GB (1967). Social relationships in a group of captive wolves. *Am Zool,* 7:305–311.

Reinhard D (1978). Aggressive behavior associated with hypothyroidism. *Canine Pract,* 5:69–70.

Reisner IR (1997). Assessment, management, and prognosis of canine dominance-related aggression. *Vet Clin North Am Prog Companion Anim Behav,* 27:479–495.

Reisner IR, Erb HN, and Houpt KA (1994). Risk factors for behavior-related euthanasia among dominant-aggressive dogs: 110 cases (1989–1992). *JAVMA,* 205:855–863.

Romanes GJ (1888). *Animal Intelligence.* New York: D Appleton.

Rowell TE (1974). The concept of social dominance. *Behav Biol,* 11:131–154.

Schenkel R (1967). Submission: Its features and function in the wolf and dog. *Am Zool,* 7:319–329.

Schjelderup-Ebbe (1935). Social behavior of birds: In A Murchinson (Ed), *A Handbook of Social Psychology.* Worcester, MA: Clark University Press.

Schneirla TC (1965) Aspects of stimulation and organization in approach-withdrawal process underlying vertebrate behavioral development. *Adv Study Anim Behav,* 7:1–74.

Scott JP (1991). The phenomenon of attachment in human-nonhuman relationships. In H Davis and D Balfour (Eds), *The Inevitable Bond: Examining Scientist-Animal Interactions.* Cambridge: Cambridge University Press.

Scott JP and Fuller JL (1965). *Genetics and the Social Behavior of the Dog.* Chicago: University of Chicago Press.

Slabbert JM and Odendaal JSJ (1999). Early prediction of adult police dog efficiency: A longitudinal study. *Appl Anim Behav Sci,* 64:269–288.

Senay EC (1966). Toward an animal model of depression: A study of separation behavior in dogs. *J Psychiatr Res,* 4:65–71.

Sommerville BA and Broom DM (1998) Olfactory awareness. *Appl Anim Behav Sci,* 57:269–286.

Trumler E (1973) *Your Dog and You.* New York: Seabury.

Uchida Y, Dodman N, DeNapoli J, and Aronson L (1997). Characterization and treatment of 20 canine dominance aggression cases. *J Vet Med Sci,* 59:397–399.

Van der Borg JAM, Netto WJ, and Planta DJU (1991). Behavioural testing of dogs in animal shelters to predict problem behaviour. *Appl Anim Behav Sci,* 32:237–251.

Van Hoof JARAM and Wensing J (1987). Dominance and its behavioral measures in a captive wolf pack. In H Frank (Ed), *Man and Wolf.* Dordrecht, The Netherlands: Dr W Junk.

Voith VL (1980a). Play: A form of hyperactivity and aggression. *Mod Vet Pract,* 61:631–632.

Voith VL (1980b). Play behavior interpreted as aggression or hyperactivity: Case histories. *Mod Vet Pract,* 61:707–709.

Voith VL (1989). Behavioral Disorders. In JS Ettinger (Ed), *Textbook of Veterinary Internal Medicine.* Philadelphia: WB Saunders.

Voith VL and Borchelt PL (1982). Diagnosis and treatment of dominance aggression in dogs. *Clin North Am Small Anim Pract,* 12:655–663.

Voith VL, Wright JC, Danneman PJ, et al. (1992). Is there a relationship between canine behavior problems and spoiling activities, anthropomorphism, and obedience training? *Appl Anim Behav Sci,* 34:263–272.

Weiss E and Greenberg G (1997). Service dog selection tests: Effectiveness for dogs from animal shelters. *Appl Anim Behav Sci,* 53:297–308.

Wilson EO (1975). *Sociobiology: The New Synthesis.* Cambridge: Belknap Press of Harvard University Press.

Wilsson E and Sundgren PE (1998). Behavioral test for eight-week old puppies—heritabilities of tested behaviour traits and its correspondence to later behaviour. *Appl Anim Behav Sci,* 58:151-162.

Wright JC (1980). The development of social structure during the primary socialization period in German shepherds. *Dev Psychobiol,* 13:17–24.

Zimen E (1981). *The Wolf: His Place in the Natural World.* London: Souvenir.

9

Appetitive and Elimination Problems

For a dog, when he comes to a rosebush or some other shrub, though he cannot urinate, yet he will lift up his leg and make a pretense of doing so.

GEOFFREY CHAUCER, *Canterbury Tales* (1394/1929)

PART 1: APPETITIVE PROBLEMS

EXCESSIVE EATING AND OBESITY

Malnutrition resulting in excessive weight gain or loss occurs when dogs either ingest too much or too little food for their biological needs. If dogs ingest more calories than they need to support biological functions, the excess is converted and stored as fat. As the result of habitually eating more food than is required, the dog's body weight will gradually increase over time. On the other hand, if dogs eat too little food for their needs, fat reserves are gradually depleted and their body weight will decrease.

Definition and Incidence

As in humans, obesity is a common problem among dogs. Obesity can be defined as a condition in which fat reserves accumulate to a point such that the dog's health may be adversely impacted. The extent of the problem has been estimated to affect between 24% and 34% of the dog population (Markwell, 1990), although one practitioner reported that as many as 44% of the dogs visiting an Austrian small animal clinic were overweight [see Edney and Smith (1986)]—an estimate echoed by Morris and Beaver (1993), who indicate that 44% of the overall companion animal population may be overweight. A dog is considered obese when its body weight exceeds its ideal weight by 15% to 20%, but even excess weight 10% above a dog's ideal weight can have significant health and quality-of-life implications. A simple way to judge roughly whether a dog is underweight or overweight is to observe and palpate its ribs (Sibley, 1984). If a dog's ribs are visible, this is a sign of malnutrition in the direction of inadequate caloric intake, whereas, if the ribs cannot be felt, the thick layer of fat indicates that the dog may be eating too much for its energy needs. Significant evidence suggests that excessive weight gain early in life adversely influences osteoarthritis associated with hip dysplasia. Keeping a dog's weight at optimal levels appears to reduce the severity of radiographic signs of hip osteoarthritis in adult dogs (Kealy et al., 1997). Recently, Impellizeri and colleagues (2000) reported promising evidence suggesting that weight control in adult dogs can significantly reduce observed signs of lameness associated with hip osteoarthritis. The nine dogs, estimated to be 11% to 12% over their ideal weight, lost 11% to 18% of their initial weight while fed a reduced-calorie diet for 10 to 19 weeks. As a group, they showed a steady reduction in lameness over the course of the dieting period.

Feeding and Obesity

Dogs gain weight because they eat more food than they need to satisfy their biological and energy requirements. Of course, this is largely an avoidable problem, since owners control what dogs eat. The causes of overfeeding are varied. Puppy owners are often under the false opinion that a plump puppy is a more healthy puppy and more likely to attain its full size. Consequently, they may overfeed the puppy or supplement its diet in various ways to cause it to eat more than it needs. These efforts may include frequently changing diets, enhancing the ration's palatability by adding canned food or table scraps, and feeding between-meal treats. In some cases, owners may feed a premium diet containing highly digestible food in excessive amounts; however, even in cases where a dog is fed according to the manufacturer's instruction, the dog may still gain weight. Breed, sexual status (spayed or neutered), and health may affect metabolic efficiency or energy expenditure. In addition, food needs vary with activity levels (exercise) and seasonal influences on thermoregulation. Also, despite owner protests otherwise, a little detective work often reveals that a dog is getting additional sources of food besides what is provided in its bowl. For example, some owners may use biscuits to reward good behavior and inadvertently cause their food-trained dogs to become overweight. Small food rewards are usually adequate for training purposes. Further, problems can be avoided by subtracting the amount of food given during training activities from the dog's daily ration. In large families, dogs may receive additional food and treats by begging from different family members. Since only a very small amount of excessive food can result in significant weight gain over time, such incidental sources of food may represent a significant cause of obesity.

Overeating may also result from social facilitation when dogs are fed in close proximity of one another (James and Gilbert, 1955). In some cases, however, close feeding proximity may result in appetitive inhibition and weight loss, especially in the case of dogs that do not get along together on peaceful terms. Mugford (1977) found that feeding a group of dogs on an ad libitum basis (free feeding) significantly curtailed social facilitation, with dogs only infrequently eating together if they had food continuously available to them. In addition to social facilitation, eating excesses may also result from compulsive conflict. For example, Fox (1962) describes an unusual case involving a 12-year-old male Welsh terrier that developed a compulsive eating habit (polyphagia) after a cat was introduced into the household. When in the presence of the cat, the dog ate five times more food than normal. Within 6 weeks, he was grossly overweight and exhibited persistent flatulence. Fox theorized that the dog's excessive eating when near the cat was the result of a summation of appetitive and attention-seeking motivations; that is, in the presence of the owner, attention-seeking behavior and eating behavior became motivationally cross-connected in a compulsive manner.

Metabolic Considerations

In many ways, obesity appears to be more of a metabolic problem rather than an eating problem. Aside from the possibility of a systemic disorders (e.g., hypothyroidism), some dogs simply appear to possess a more efficient metabolic system. As a result, such dogs may be more prone to gain weight because they are better equipped to digest and assimilate more of what they eat while expending a minimal amount of energy doing so. Naturally, dogs with an efficient metabolism would tend to deposit, store, and conserve more fat than counterparts possessing a less efficient metabolism. Evolutionary pressures appear to favor the development of a highly efficient metabolism. A highly efficient digestive and metabolic system would make the most competent use of available food. The storage of fat reserves during times of plenty would help to ensure the animal's survival when faced with adverse conditions of food scarcity or starvation. Under natural conditions, this hypothetical protective mechanism is functional and very useful, since food is not easily and consistently obtained; however, under the superabundance and variety (cafeteria-diet effect) often associated with the domestic situation, dogs may ingest far more food than is necessary for their basic biological needs. The net result is excessive weight gain. In addition to depositing and storing fat, under adverse foraging conditions an animal's metabolism may undergo changes toward becoming more efficient. This adaptive mechanism appears to enhance metabolic efficiency under conditions of starvation [see Brownell et al. (1986)], perhaps helping to explain the tendency of animals and persons to gain weight on a lower-calorie diet or to regain lost weight and more when they go off the diet.

Energy is primarily expended in one of two ways: exercise and heat production. The majority of energy expended by the body is consumed by thermoregulation, with approximately 70% to 85% of caloric energy being used to maintain resting-state metabolism, and the digestion-assimilation of nutrients (Carlson, 1994). Durrer and Hannon (1962) reported a significant relationship between environmental temperature, food intake, and weight gain or loss among a group of Alaskan huskies. Despite eating nearly twice as much food during the winter than during the summer, the dogs tended to lose weight during the cold Alaskan winter months—weight they gained back again during the much warmer summer months. Even under the influence of more modest seasonal temperature changes (Florida), dogs tend to eat significantly less in the summer than in the winter (Rashotte et al., 1984). Although exercise is very beneficial in terms of promoting general health and a sense of well-being, physical activity appears to account for a relatively small number of calories burned. Consequently, weight-loss plans usually emphasize the input (food ingestion) side of the weight problem rather than the output (e.g., exercise) side, but both food restriction and exercise are necessary for effective weight control. In addition to quantity, the digestibility and nutritional density of the food also plays a significant role.

Neurobiological Control of Hunger and Satiety

Another potential cause of overeating is a physiological dysfunction or interference of hunger and satiety signals. Traditionally, opponent set points in the hypothalamus were believed to regulate food intake by inducing hunger (lateral area), on the one hand, and triggering satiety (ventromedial area), on the other (Johnson et al., 1962). Although the lateral hypothalamus (LH) appears to mediate hunger and appetitive preparatory activities via seeking-system circuits, the role of the ventromedial hypothalamus (VMH) in mediating satiety has been found to be more complex than previously believed. In fact, both hunger and short-term satiety signals instructing animals to stop eating probably originate within the LH (not the VMH), whereas the long-term *energy balance system* responsible for regulating food intake appears to originate within the VMH (Panksepp, 1998). Together, these areas of the brain modulate many aspects of the short- and long-term appetitive-seeking system, thereby keeping energy input and energy output in balance. Under certain conditions, dysregulation of hunger-satiety control may occur. For example, incentive motivation derived from the ingestion of novel or highly palatable food items may overshadow or confound satiety signals, thereby causing a dog to eat more than it needs. Bradshaw and Thorne (1992) suggest that overeating (and undereating), resulting from the ingestion of novel foods, may occur because dogs are unable to predict the nutritional value of the unfamiliar food and do not "know" when to stop eating:

> Most mammals stop eating long before the equilibrium state of the body has been restored, the delay being due to the digestion of many key nutrients, so meal-end must be controlled by some signal that sufficient food has been taken into the stomach. This can only be accurate if the end product of digestion can be predicted, which normally means that the food is a familiar one. Thus both cats and dogs may under- or over-eat if presented with a new food, particularly if it is of a new type; for example, semimoist food can induce this kind of temporary error when first introduced into the diet. (121)

Whatever the causes, the ingestion of novel food items is believed to facilitate obesity. In the laboratory, a common means to induce obesity is to provide animals with a "cafeteria diet" consisting of a variety of high-energy and palatable food items, thus causing hyperphagia and rapid weight gain (Rothwell et al., 1982).

Significant research has been focused on the role of the neurotropic hormone leptin in the etiology of obesity (Friedman and Halaas, 1998; Friedman, 2000). Leptin is produced by fat tissue and exerts an influence on appetite and fat reserves via leptin receptors located in the hypothalamus. Most of the leptin research has been carried out on mutant obese mice possessing a defective gene needed to produce leptin. When obese mice are injected with leptin, they rapidly lose fat reserves (30% in 2 weeks) by not eating as much and by increasing energy expenditure. In contrast to weight loss achieved by dietary restriction, where both fat reserves and muscle tissue are lost, losses produced by leptin injection specifically target eating behavior and

reduce weight by decreasing fat reserves only. Obviously a factor in the regulation of appetite and weight gain, leptin itself may not represent a cure for obesity, however. Obese people, for example, appear not to be lacking in leptin hormone production (in fact, they typically possess much higher levels than lean counterparts) or lack hypothalamic leptin receptors (Panksepp, 1998). The presence of high levels of leptin in obese people suggests that they may produce increased hormone in an effort to compensate for a defect somewhere in the satiety-signaling system (Friedman et al., 1995). The inability of leptin to signal satiety and inhibit eating may be mediated by another gene (SOCS-3), whose expression is turned on in the presence of high leptin levels and inhibits the action of leptin on satiety control centers (Bjorbaek et al., 1998). Finally, Friedman and colleagues have found that dieting results in lowered levels of leptin, perhaps helping to explain the increased appetite, slower metabolism, and weight regain associated with on-again, off-again dieting. Although not a likely cure for obesity, the researchers suggest that leptin may eventually prove beneficial as a means for reducing appetite and helping to maintain weight loss after dieting.

Drinking behavior appears to be under the influence of serum osmotic pressure and blood volume, with drinking being stimulated when serum osmotic pressure rises between 1% and 3% (Wolf, 1950). These changes in osmotic pressure are detected by osmoreceptors in the anterior hypothalamus. Drinking is stopped by a combination of signals, including stomach sensations, dilute blood, and the completion of drinking movements (Johnson et al., 1962).

Owner Attitudes

Kienzle and colleagues (1998) learned that obesity in dogs is affected by the owner's attitude toward the dog and food. They performed a study comparing the personal characteristics and rearing practices of owners of obese dogs with owners of normal dogs. The researchers found that obese dogs were often treated as *fellow humans* by their owners. Also, the owners of obese dogs were often overweight themselves because of the same lifestyle shortcomings that caused their dogs to become overweight:

> The results of this survey indicate that owners of obese dogs tend to interpret their dog's every need as a request for food. It appears that this is due, in part, to a transfer of their own health and eating habits, including a certain laziness and a lack of appreciation of the dog's nutritional and health requirements. In counseling these owners, they should be encouraged to respond to the dog's requests for attention not always with food, but more frequently with physical activities, such as brisk walks or regular play sessions. There will be benefit for both dog and owner. (2780S)

INAPPETENCE AND ANOREXIA

Dogs sometimes lose weight because of inappetence. Although appetite loss is often associated with medical problems, and should be brought to a veterinarian's attention, anorexia (cessation of eating) is frequently the result of psychogenic causes such as anxiety or separation distress. The suppression of appetite as the result of anxiety can represent a significant obstacle for counterconditioning and training efforts using food. As already mentioned, separation-anxious dogs exhibit a significant loss of appetite when separated from their owners. When left in a kennel for a long time, such dogs may suffer significant weight loss stemming from anorexia.

Dogs may become problem eaters as the result of improving the palatability of ordinary food in order to increase their willingness to eat it. Not only do enhanced diets encourage overeating and possessiveness around the food bowl, they may stimulate dogs to seek even more novel foods. Regardless of what they are given, such dogs may not remain satisfied for very long before they start holding out for something even better. Also, dogs fed savory or varied food items in order to improve appetite may inadvertently learn to manipulate the owner by begging or by abstaining from eating for progressively longer periods. Such dogs may become finicky and refuse to eat ordinary dog food when it is offered to them, especially if it is not mixed with a tasty incentive. A finicky

dog can learn to eat regular food again, but only if its owner stays firm and does not yield to the dog's importunate demands for something better. Another possible cause of anorexia in dogs is taste aversion (Houpt, 1982). Following a serious sickness involving nausea, a previously acceptable food associated with acute internal distress may be avoided after the dog recovers.

PICA AND DESTRUCTIVE BEHAVIOR

Destructive behavior is driven by diverse motivational considerations. A brief inventory of the pertinent factors, includes anxiety, boredom, frustration, attention seeking, nutritional deficiencies, insufficient exercise, hunger tensions, and inadequate training. In addition, destructive behavior is often associated with common diagnostic entities such as separation distress and hyperactivity. Obviously, it is important to assess each case carefully and to determine the likely causative factors involved before drawing premature conclusions and possibly implementing inappropriate or ineffective training. This caution is particularly important with regard to destructive behavior associated with hyperactivity and separation distress (boredom, frustration, and anxiety) and other reactive emotional states.

The term *pica* [after the Latin name for the magpie (*Pica pica*)—a bird reputed to eat a wide variety of things] is used to designate nonnutritive eating of things like cloth, wood, plastics, stones, dirt, or just about anything else a dog can seize with its mouth and swallow. A very common form of pica is grass eating. The causes of grass eating are still unknown but have attracted a range of opinions from a vegetable dietary supplementation, gastric pH regulation, natural purge for worms, and a learned way to induce vomiting when a dog feels nauseous (Beaver, 1981) to perhaps a natural remedy for gastrointestinal irritation (McKeown, 1996). Another common pica habit is chewing and eating stones—which may result in excessive dental wear and gastric obstruction (Fox, 1963). In some cases, this habit may exhibit a compulsive character, as the following anecdote reported by Unwin (1994) seems to indicate:

The patient was a young male basset hound. Diagnosis was not difficult—he rattled when he moved. After his third gastrotomy I took him out for a walk. Although wobbly from the anaesthetic, when we approached a gravel path he brightened up and attempted to prize a stone out of the ground. (511)

Like other forms of pica, it has been speculated that stone chewing may be related to a nutritional deficiency or malabsorption problem, but this connection has not been experimentally demonstrated. Some puppies and dogs are highly attracted to a variety of household items (e.g., clothing, tissues, paper, toys, carpet matting)—items that may be ingested and cause gastric impaction or bowel occlusion requiring veterinary surgical intervention. Such animals need to be carefully supervised or restrained to prevent such behavior until the underlying causes can be identified and appropriate behavior modification carried out.

Pica is sometimes associated with an underlying medical condition, and therefore its evaluation should include a veterinary examination, especially in cases that involve the ingestion of large of amounts of nonnutritive material. Commonly cited medical causes of pica include a variety of gastrointestinal disorders, including parasitic infestation. Other possible causes of pica include toxins, metabolic disorders, nutritional deficiencies, and neurogenic pathology. Lead toxicosis should be considered as a possible factor in cases where a history of chewing on wood painted with lead-based paint is evident. Lead may also be ingested by puppies that chew or eat newspapers and magazines (Hankin et al., 1974), although such sources of contamination are probably less significant today than they were in the past. Lead, which is a common source of poisoning, may be associated with hyperkinesis, especially in dogs known to have been exposed to lead at an early age. Other behavioral signs of lead poisoning include anorexia, hyperexcitability, compulsive barking, champing fits, convulsions, muscular spasms, and increased sensitivity to touch (Zook et al., 1969). Although pertinent statistics are not available for dogs, 70% to 90% of children testing positive for lead poisoning also have a history of pica (Feldman, 1986).

Some forms of compulsive pica may stem from a malfunction of the limbic system. Bilateral ablation of the temporal lobes in monkeys results in compulsive orality: "The hungry animal if confronted with a variety of objects will, for example, indiscriminately pick up a comb, a bakelite knob, a sunflower seed, a screw, a stick, a piece of apple, a live snake, a piece of banana, and a live rat. Each object is transferred to the mouth and then discarded if not edible" (Kluver and Bucy, 1937:353). The researchers characterized the condition as a "psychic blindness," leaving the animals unable to determine, in advance of placing the item in the mouth, whether it was edible or not.

Nutritional Deficiency

Various nutritional hypotheses have been proposed to explain destructive chewing and other forms of inappropriate appetitive interest or ingestion. Studies of children have found an apparent causal connection between pica and nutritional deficiencies, particularly involving trace metals like zinc and iron. The most frequently cited cause of pica in humans is iron deficiency. For example, among persons exhibiting mental retardation, the frequency and severity of pica are directly correlated with the degree of iron deficiency. In the case of laboratory rodents, iron-deficient rats exhibit 50% lower levels of dopamine (D2) receptors in various areas of the brain. Some authorities have speculated that reduced dopamine neurotransmission is an instrumental neural chemical substrate underlying increased levels of pica activity. Following this line of reasoning, Singh and colleagues (1994) tested the effect of two drugs that have opposing effects on dopamine, one depressing dopaminergic activity (thioridazine) and the other stimulating it (methylphenidate). When given methylphenidate, mentally retarded persons with pica exhibit a sharp decrease in the habit to negligible levels while showing a symmetrically dramatic increase in pica when treated with the D2-antagonist thioridazine. In cases where malabsorption of iron is suspected, vitamin-C supplementation may be beneficial, since ascorbic acid appears to facilitate the absorption of iron (Levine et al., 1999).

Reactive Emotional States and Destructiveness

Dogs appear to engage instinctively in chewing and digging when they are restrained, frustrated, or distressed in an effort to break free or otherwise resolve a stressful situation. For wild canids, chewing and digging are also valuable means for exploring the environment and achieving control over the natural resources needed for survival (e.g., burying and recovering caches of food, uncovering cool earth to enhance thermoregulation, den construction, and foraging on plant matter). Under domestic conditions, these tendencies to chew and dig may become destructive and problematic when they are directed toward personal belongings and carefully planted gardens. In addition, domestic dogs may fall under the influence of various stressors and emotional influences that trigger maladaptive chewing and digging activity. For example, separation anxiety is considered a leading cause of destructive behavior occurring in an owner's absence (Lindell, 1997). Separation anxiety should always be considered as a possible cause in cases were destructive behavior is directed toward door frames, nearby carpeting, and window casings. Such behavior may also be driven by barrier frustration evoked by the owner's departure or outdoor activities (e.g., passing dogs or other animals). Other sources of distress include fear and boredom. Thunder-phobic dogs are prone to scratch and bite on doors and walls when left alone during a storm. Some storm-thunder-phobic dogs routinely flee into closets only to scratch and chew through drywall, sometimes injuring themselves in the process. Finally, simple boredom has been frequently implicated in destructiveness (Voith, 1980; Turner, 1997).

In cases where a stress-related etiology is suspected, the various sources of stress must be identified and addressed with appropriate conditioning, training, and environmental change. Separation-anxious dogs, for example, need help learning to cope with loneliness and distress at separation, frustrated dogs must learn to accept constraining situations imposed upon them, fearful dogs must be systematically desensitized, and bored dogs need to be provided with alternative means for obtaining the stimulation that they crave. Once the underlying causes are alleviated, a dog's destructive tendencies often undergo spontaneous reduction without further training. In some cases, however, a dog may acquire a refractory appetite for destructive activity and consequently fail to stop engaging in the habit, even though the original causes have been removed. Destructive chewing, in particular, may easily develop into such a "vice." In such cases, the object continues to attract the dog's chewing activity and may require inhibitory training or aversive counterconditioning and the redirection of chewing activity into more acceptable outlets.

PICA AND SCAVENGING

Scavenging is a normal canine activity that has served dogs' survival in close habitation with humans for many thousands of years. Current theories of domestication underscore the significance of scavenging for the mediation of close contact between semiwild protodogs and early humans (see *Interspecific Cooperation: Mutualism* in Volume 1, Chapter 1). Most dogs show some degree of interest in scavenging, but some dogs may become virtually obsessed with finding and eating the most unappealing things, at least with respect to the human eye and palate. Scavenging dogs can be extremely frustrating for their owners, making walks a harrowing lunge and yank from one thing to another. Sticks and leaves, rocks, tissues, animal carrion, bits of garbage, everything seemingly draws the dog's fleeting attention. This habit is particularly common in excitable and hyperactive dogs, especially young sporting dogs like the golden, Labrador, and Chesapeake Bay retrievers. The habit should be carefully managed, since improper training could very easily cause a nuisance to escalate into a more serious problem. Such dogs may become progressively possessive and defensive about their prizes, perhaps culminating in embarrassing public affrays over scavenged objects. Many dog owners have been seriously bitten attempting to pry a tissue or piece of plastic wrap from the mouth of their scavenging dog. Possessive aggression problems are frequently traced to competitive interaction over scavenged or *stolen* items and the punitive removal of such things from the dog's mouth. The risk of aggression is increased by chasing after a dog that has managed to grab something, especially if it is cornered and forced to release the object. Such activities, while occasionally necessary for a dog's safety, should be avoided whenever possible. Instead of forcefully removing objects from a dog's mouth, the owner should train the dog to trade its prize for a reward.

COPROPHAGY

In many species, such as the rabbit, coprophagy (stool eating) is a normal ingestive behavior that provides a variety of vital nutrients, including B-complex vitamins (Soave and Brand, 1991). Denying rabbits, for example, access to fecal droppings produces nutritional deficiencies and health problems, and, in the case of young rabbits, retards normal growth and weight gain. In the case of rats, 5% to 50% of their fecal output is eaten, providing them with an important source of thiamine and vitamin K. Although dogs do not need to eat feces for good health, when they are fed a thiamine-deficient diet, dogs will engage in coprophagy to stave off physical symptoms and attenuate neurological signs of thiamine deficiency, at least temporarily (Reed and Harrington, 1981). In horses, foals under 20 weeks of age show a preference for their mother's feces, which they eat (Crowell-Davis and Houpt, 1985). A similar phenomenon exists in rats. Rat pups appear to be attracted to maternal feces in order to obtain deoxycholic acid, a chemical that protects them against enteritis and facilitates the digestion and absorption of fatty acids needed for the manufacture of myelin. Finally, equine coprophagy may provide foals with various nutrients (e.g., vitamins and protein) and beneficial bacterial flora needed for digestion (Crowell-Davis and Caudle, 1989). Perhaps similar pheromones and biological benefits are obtained by puppies when they eat feces—a hypothesis that remains to be tested.

Mother dogs instinctively elicit elimination and ingest their puppies' excrement from birth to approximately 3 weeks of age. Particularly fastidious mothers will sometimes continue to "clean up" after their puppies long after week 3, however. Adult males will also ingest feces produced by young puppies. Among wolves, mothers only ingest "milk scats" and refrain from eating fecal material after the puppies begin to eat meat at approximately 3 to 4 weeks of age (Allen, 1979). Although dogs of all ages may show the behavior, coprophagy is particularly prevalent among puppies and young dogs between 4 and 9 months of age. Besides eating their own feces (*autocoprophagy*), some dogs ingest the feces of other dogs and animals (*allocoprophagy*), especially cat and horse droppings. Most dogs actively explore the droppings of other dogs and animals, but, for some dogs, something in the feces is sufficiently compelling and attractive for them to go further and eat it. The texture and smell (taste) of the feces appear to be significant factors. Many coprophagous dogs are particularly attracted to frozen *poopsicles* or firm stools. Such dogs rarely eat soft or poorly formed stools and are less likely to ingest stools that have been rendered objectionable through dietary manipulation or tainted by various repellents.

Coprophagy is considered normal among puppies and represents a small health risk to the offending puppy eating its own feces (Hubbard, 1989), but eating the feces of other dogs may cause parasitic infections (e.g., coccidiosis) or increase a puppy's risk of coming into contact with viral pathogens (parvovirus) shed in the feces. Despite reassurances, owners are often disgusted with the habit and may be unwilling to tolerate it. Many persistent coprophagous dogs have been given up for adoption as a direct result of stool-eating behavior. The problem is especially intolerable in situations where a dog comes into close contact with children, who may be licked on the mouth by the dog. Sadly, some owners may even seek euthanasia in refractory cases—an outcome recommended by some authorities in cases in which the owner's "bond with their is dog irreparably damaged" (McKeown et al., 1988:850) by the habit. However, euthanizing a dog because of coprophagy seems to be a rather extreme and questionable practice.

PUTATIVE CAUSES OF COPROPHAGY

The exact causes of the habit are unknown, but several etiologies have been described. There appears to be some connection between excessive coprophagy and nutritional deficiencies, stress, boredom, unsanitary rearing conditions, and restrictive housing.

Environmental Stress

Overly restrictive or isolatory confinement has been correlated with a higher incidence of coprophagy in dogs. Houpt (1982), for example, has reported that dogs exposed to excessive isolation (kept in kennels or basements) are more likely to engage in the habit than dogs kept in close contact with people. Beerda and coworkers (1999) reported evidence suggesting that restrictive confinement may represent a significant factor in the etiology of coprophagy. In addition, they reported that pica (gnawing behavior) similarly increased among dogs housed under restrictive conditions, suggesting that both coprophagy and pica may be influenced by environmental stress. The dogs (beagles) in the study were first housed under unrestricted (outdoor) conditions before being moved to more restrictive (indoor) housing conditions. The procedure suggests that the causative variable may not be restrictive/isolatory confinement per se but rather points to the possibility that the stressful change and adaptation associated with the transition from outdoor to indoor housing conditions may play a role in precipitating coprophagous activity. In conclusion, at least in some cases, coprophagy may be part of a general pattern of behavioral adaptation to stressful housing conditions, especially those involving increased restriction and social isolation.

Anxiety Reduction and Attention Getting

Anecdotal correlations between coprophagy and various psychological states, such as anxiety reduction and attention seeking, have been suggested but not convincingly demonstrated. Campbell (1975), for example, argues that coprophagy is often exhibited as an anxiety-reducing response acquired as the result of inappropriate punishment during house training or in association with normal fecal interest and exploration. According to his theory, coprophagous dogs choose to eat their feces because it eliminates the *evidence* and the threat of punishment. However, instead of being successful, the act is followed by additional punishment, more anxiety in the presence of feces, and, consequently, more stool eating. Hart and Hart (1985) have speculated about a similar—but opposite—vicious circle. They have noted that some cases of coprophagy may be calculated to attract the owner's attention; that is, eating feces is interpreted as a form of attention-seeking behavior:

> Owners may react emotionally to the sight of their dogs going after feces, and a dog may pick up this reaction as a means to garner additional attention. (107)

Nutritional Causes

A common assumption holds that coprophagy is related to some sort of nutritional problem or deficiency. These theories generally emphasize one of two possibilities: (1) coprophagy is a search for nutrients lacking in a dog's diet or (2) the habit is motivated to consume undigested nutrients passed into the feces. Vitamin-B deficiencies have been frequently implicated. In this regard, Reed and Harrington (1981) note that canine fecal microbial activity synthesizes thiamine and other B vitamins, with coprophagy providing some relief to thiamine-deprived dogs. Landsberg and colleagues (1997) summarized the results of an unpublished study involving nine coprophagous dogs. All exhibited at least one laboratory abnormality that could explain the development of the problem. The majority of the dogs exhibited low to borderline levels of trypsinlike immunoreactivity. Some dogs exhibited abnormal folate or cobalamin levels but none exhibited abnormal fecal fat or trypsin levels. Finally, no evidence of intestinal parasites was revealed by fecal exams. One author claims rapid control of coprophagy by increasing the ration's protein and fat content, reducing the amount of carbohydrates, and supplementing with brewer's yeast (Cloche, 1991). Another obvious nutritional possibility to consider, and one perhaps more directly linked with a nutritional function, is that coprophagous dogs may simply be harvesting undigested food passed in the feces.

Enzyme Conservation

Besides undigested food and other nutrients, feces is a rich source of digestive enzymes and bacteria. Whether or not the ingestion of alimentary bacteria is of any benefit to dogs is not known, but some evidence suggests that digestive enzymes may play a role in the control of coprophagy. Many veterinarians and dog trainers report anecdotal success when a meat tenderizer containing papain (a proteolytic enzyme) is added to the coprophagous dog's diet. In the aforementioned report by Landsberg and colleagues (1997), the authors found that four of the nine dogs treated with a plant-based enzyme supplement responded favorably to the therapy. McCuistion (1966) argues that, as the result of living in close association with people, the dog's eating habits and sources of food have changed from a diet proportionately high in animal protein content to one high in carbohydrates and vegetable proteins. He believes these are changes that the canine digestive system has not fully accommodated.

A critical factor influencing a dog's digestive efficiency is the presence of adequate levels of various digestive enzymes specifically designed to metabolize proteins, carbohydrates, and lipids. McCuistion argues that coprophagous dogs eat feces to collect and conserve these critical enzymes, especially those involved in the digestion of carbohydrates and proteins. The theory makes some sense and, perhaps, enzyme deficiency is a relevant factor in some cases of coprophagy. After all, although dogs can survive on a vegetarian diet alone (Thorne, 1996), they are preferentially opportunistic carnivores adapted to eat and digest an omnivorous diet containing a significant proportion of animal protein. Under domestic conditions, dogs are made to eat relatively monotonous diets consisting of high levels of carbohy-

drate and protein content derived from plant sources. It is reasonable to suspect that some predisposed dogs may exhibit an insufficiency of digestive enzymes needed to digest such food thoroughly, enzymes that they conserve or harvest by eating their own or other animal's feces.

Wolves are particularly attracted to the viscera and contents of the gut, which they eat first—before the more protein-rich and muscled areas of their prey. The canid's predilection to eat gut contents first may have evolved as a means to obtain exogenous digestive enzymes needed to assist in the digestion of gorged flesh protein. Some dogs are particularly attracted to horse manure and apparently relish the opportunity to eat it—could they be seeking similar digestive components? According to McCuistion, some dogs appear to have suffered inadvertent physiological alterations as the result of selective breeding—changes that may reduce the production of proteolytic and other enzymes. Dogs are commonly attracted to cat feces—an interest, again, that may be related to harvesting digestive enzymes or partially digested food passed in the feces.

The enzyme theory is appealing, particularly when one considers that coprophagy is most often exhibited by young dogs. Puppies ingest large amounts of food (proportionately, about twice as much as adults) and might benefit from the supplemental ingestion of exogenous digestive enzymes and partially digested food. If nothing else, perhaps such enzymes and other active digestive aids and nutrients recycled from the stool facilitate the digestive process, making it more efficient and thorough. The central question remains, though: Does a nutritional or enzyme deficiency stimulate dogs to eat feces? Most dogs do not develop coprophagy, even when they are on a less than ideal diet or starved (Crowell-Davis et al., 1995). Also, dogs suffering from pancreatic insufficiency or malabsorption disorder may exhibit such behavior but only after becoming seriously ill and exhibiting other clinical signs of disease. These questions are enough to regard the enzyme theory with some skepticism, at least until additional research is carried out.

Counterconditioning Hypothesis

Associative learning and counterconditioning may gradually supplant an innate aversion and avoidance toward feces and replace it with an appetitive attraction. This process may be facilitated by the habitual association of feces with highly attractive sources of appetitive stimulation. For example, under unsanitary conditions in which excrement is left to lie about a nursery, puppies may be exposed to the odor of feces in combination with three potential sources of appetitive counterconditioning:

—Food: Eating in the close vicinity of feces may forge an associative link between its odor and food. This association may cause feces to later become inappropriately identified as a potential food item.

—Nursing mother: In situations where the mother is obligated to eat the feces of her young (especially after they begin to eat solid food), the puppies may smell the feces on her breath and identify the odor with food. This may be an especially potent influence in the case of hungry puppies that beg for food by sniffing and licking at the mother's mouth and muzzle. If, at such times, the mother happens to regurgitate food mixed with feces, an even stronger impression may be made—a kind of *appetitive inoculation* may occur that predisposes puppies for coprophagy. Puppies may also learn to eat feces by observing the mother eating it.

—Exploratory play: Finally, under filthy and environmentally barren conditions, puppies may play with and ingest feces.

EVOLUTIONARY RATIONALE

Some clues to the origin of coprophagy may be obtained by interpreting the habit in terms of evolutionary fitness and function. In advance of true domestication, early protodogs are believed to have followed nomadic hunting groups moving across Eurasia at the end of the Ice Age. These early dogs were probably scavengers that survived on whatever was left behind in the wake of these vast human migrations. Socially confident dogs had a distinct advantage over fearful counterparts when it came to exploiting dis-carded offal and garbage. Confident dogs would have been able to approach closer and stay longer near human encampments and, thereby, obtain the most nutritious portions of the refuse left behind. Eating human feces conceivably offered another advantage by providing supplementary enzymes and microbial nutrients supplementing the less than ideal omnivorous diet.

As a consequence of the vicissitudes of domestication, dogs surely fell upon hard times during their long historical journey in the shadow of early humans, at times, perhaps, having little more to survive on than garbage and feces. Eating feces and garbage during times of starvation may have been encoded over time as a genetic trait. Dogs that could subsist on such a diet would have had a distinct survival and reproductive advantage over dogs that refused to eat such things.

An old Crow story, quoted by Lopez (1978), describes habits consistent with those just outlined regarding the feeding behavior of early dogs, including the eating of refuse and human feces, when necessary. The story recounts a dialogue between a dog and a wolf debating the various advantages and disadvantages of domestic life:

> A Crow woman was out digging roots when a wolf came by. The woman's dog ran up to the wolf and said, "Hey, what are you doing here? Go away. You only come around because you want what I have."
>
> "What have you got?" asked the wolf. "Your owner beats you all the time. Kids kick you out of the way. Try to steal a piece of meat and they hit you over the head with a club."
>
> "At least I can steal the meat!" answered the dog. "You haven't anything to steal."
>
> "Huh! I eat whatever I want. No one bothers me."
>
> "What do you eat? You slink around while the men butcher the buffalo and get what's left over. You're afraid to get close. You sit there with your armpits stinking, pulling dirt balls out of your tail."
>
> "Look who's talking, with camp garbage smeared all over your face."
>
> "Hrumph. Whenever I come into camp, my owner throws me something good to eat."
>
> "When your owner goes out to ease himself at night you follow along to eat the droppings, that's how much you get to eat."

"That's okay! These people only eat the finest parts!"

"You're proud of it!"

"Listen, whenever they're cooking in the camp, you smell the grease, you come around and howl, and I feel sorry for you. I pity you. . ."

"When do they let you have a good time?" asked the wolf.

". . .I sleep warm, you sleep out there in the rain, they scratch my ears, you—"

Just then the woman shouldered a bundle of roots, whacked the dog on the back with a stick, and started back to camp. The dog followed along behind her, calling over his shoulder at the wolf, "You're just full of envy for a good life, that's all that's wrong with you."

Wolf went off the other way, not wanting any part of the life. (110–111)

Tolerance for Nausea and Taste Aversion

Of necessity, dogs feeding on refuse would have acquired a considerable tolerance for nausea and other sicknesses associated with the ingestion of spoiled or rotting food. Circumstantial support for this hypothesis comes from the difficulty of establishing taste aversions in dogs (see *Taste Aversion* in Volume 1, Chapter 6). Although some authorities have claimed to achieve positive results by using taste-aversion procedures to control coprophagy (Houpt, 1991; Landsberg et al., 1997), others have been disappointed by the procedure. Hart and Hart (1985), for example, reported "little success" (106) with taste aversion for controlling coprophagy in dogs. Similarly, Rathore (1984) was unable to obtain a lasting taste-aversion effect persisting longer than 24 to 48 hours. In Rathore's study, 10 dogs were given 6 to 10 grams of lithium chloride placed inside various kinds of meat. Not only did the technique fail to yield a lasting aversion, surprisingly, upon vomiting, the dogs actually ate the nauseant-tainted vomitus. Subsequently, untainted meat associated with lithium-chloride-induced nausea was avoided for 7½ hours—a very transient effect. Also, Hansen and coworkers (1997), utilizing a taste-aversion procedure, were unable to control dog attacks on sheep effectively. They did, however, report significant side effects, including increased aggression. Although taste aversion

has been reported in a number of species, including coyotes (Gustavson et al., 1974), many dogs appear to be biologically *immunized* against this sort of learning. Bradshaw and Thorne (1992) suggest that dogs may have undergone various changes as the result of domestication that militates against such learning. Perhaps the key alteration was the development of an increased tolerance for nausea. The dogs' historical dependence on less than optimal food sources, including spoiled or rotting food (a potential source of significant nausea), may have resulted in the gradual immunization of a subgroup of the dog population against nausea and the taste-aversion effect. According to this hypothesis, dogs exhibiting an increased tolerance for nausea (evolutionary immunization) may be more inclined to eat feces.

Pro and Con Evidence

Following this line of reasoning, one would expect to find a higher incidence of coprophagy among dogs on an insufficient diet or those showing a failure to digest or absorb food properly. It is noteworthy here that coprophagy is commonly observed in malabsorption disorders or starvation. Interestingly, in this regard, Serpell and Jagoe (1995) report that dogs exhibiting coprophagy are more often obtained off the street or from an animal shelter than from other sources, suggesting that some of them may have relied on feces as a source of nutrition while struggling to survive on their own. Not all the evidence supports this hypothesis, however. In an experiment reported by Crowell-Davis and coworkers (1993), several dogs were put on restricted diets and observed for behavioral changes. Given the aforementioned evolutionary hypothesis, one might expect to find increased coprophagy under conditions of reduced caloric intake. Although restricted feeding had significant effects on activity levels and some other behavioral parameters, there was no evidence of an increased tendency to eat feces by the dogs in the study.

The absence of coprophagy in dogs on restricted diets raises some doubt about the aforementioned hypothesis, but the findings do not necessarily invalidate it. First, the level of hunger induced by the Crowell-Davis experiment may not have been sufficient to evoke coprophagy. Second, the hypothesis does not assume that all dogs are prone to develop coprophagous habits under the influence of hunger. Third, the hypothesis does not maintain that all dogs show a tolerance for nausea but only suggests that dogs that exhibit coprophagy may possess an increased tolerance for nausea. Before any decisive conclusions can be arrived at concerning the role of domestic evolution on coprophagy, much yet remains to be learned about its etiology.

Encoded Survival Habits

Whatever the causes of the habit, the resistance of coprophagy to punitive training efforts suggests that a very compelling motivational substrate underlies its expression. Consistent with the evolutionary hypothesis already discussed, coprophagy may be one of several appetitive *survival behaviors* that have evolved to cope with the periodic adversity of starvation. Such behavior may be maintained by a very lean schedule of reinforcement, respond atypically to punishment, and exhibit relative immunity to taste-aversion procedures. Consequently, some dogs may persistently scavenge on refuse, bones, and various other nonnutritive items, despite the presence of high levels of punishment and the absence of credible reinforcement to explain the maintenance of the behavior. Perhaps, as the result of some generalized motivational state of agitation (e.g., stressful conflict, frustration, or anxiety) or social need, some vulnerable dogs may exhibit displacement survival behavior despite the absence of actual starvation. In other words, under the influence of chronic stress, scavenging may be emitted as a displacement or compulsive activity. Indeed, pica, in many cases, appears to be driven by a compulsive urge to eat feces or to find, seize, and protect the most inconsequential and nonnutritive items.

PART 2: ELIMINATION PROBLEMS

The first major training chore encountered by new dog owners is house training. Effective house training depends on watchful supervision and the provision of realistically scheduled opportunities for puppies to eliminate outdoors. Most young dogs naturally tend to concentrate the placement of elimination in places away from were they eat and sleep, and readily eliminate outdoors if access is provided to them. Ross (1950) found that puppies rarely eliminated in straw-covered sleeping areas from 5 weeks of age onward, suggesting that the habit of not eliminating in areas used for sleeping begins prior to week 5. By the time puppies are 7 to 8 weeks of age, they begin to exhibit location and substrate preferences (Scott and Fuller, 1965). Such evidence suggests that preliminary house-training efforts should be initiated by the breeder prior to placing the puppy into its new home.

PHYSIOLOGY, NEURAL CONTROL, AND LEARNING

Elimination is interesting from a behavioral point of view because it involves the coordinated operation of Pavlovian and instrumental mechanisms. Numerous conditioned and unconditioned digestive reflexes are triggered as soon as a bite of food is taken into the mouth. As food enters the stomach, a gastrocolic reflex is elicited that causes increased colonic motility or a *mass movement*. A mass movement is a sustained peristaltic contraction that pushes gut content through the colon toward the rectum, thereby setting the stage for defecation (Berne and Levy, 1996). The structures and mechanisms controlling elimination (defecation and urination) are composed of both striated and smooth muscle tissue. The peristaltic activity occurring on the inside of the rectum is produced by smooth muscle tissue that is regulated by the autonomic nervous system. These internal alimentary reflexes function under the influence of classical conditioning. The anal sphincter, however, is composed of striated muscle tissue that is under voluntary control and subject to instrumental conditioning. In the case of urination, urine moves from the kidneys through the ureters into the bladder. As the bladder distends, a micturition reflex is elicited, stimulating internal and external sphincter contractions and detrusor inhibition (Nickel and Venker-van Haggen, 1999). When the bladder needs to be emptied, the internal sphincter located within the neck of the bladder is reflexively stimulated to release urine into the urethra. However, the final decision to urinate is controlled by an external sphincter regulated by cortical inhibition (Berne and Levy, 1996). For urination to occur, the external sphincter must be voluntarily relaxed—a process that is strongly influenced by instrumental learning.

In addition to pressure-sensitive bladder reflexes, the dog's urinary activity is strongly influenced by olfactory stimulation. Shafik (1994) demonstrated the existence of an *olfactory micturition reflex*. Electrostimulation of the nasal mucosa results in reduced activity within the smooth muscle of the internal urethral sphincter while producing no response in the external urethral sphincter. The researcher speculates that sniffing urine marks stimulates a readiness to eliminate, despite the absence of a full bladder.

Classical and Instrumental Learning

Both classical and instrumental learning processes interact together in the acquisition and extinction of eliminatory habits. Although reflexive interoceptive stimuli do signal an internal readiness or need to eliminate (establishing operations), these preparatory reflexes are modulated by exteroceptive or external cues that define specifically when and where elimination will take place (discriminative stimuli). Ultimately, a dog's decision to eliminate is an instrumental (i.e., voluntary) act controlled at a cortical level of organization and coordinated by limbic modulatory influences and pontine urine storage and emptying centers (Nishizawa and Sugaya, 1994):

> The cerebral cortex, limbic lobe, basal ganglia, and hypothalamus in suprapontine levels and cerebellum all function in some way which modulates the lower urinary tract function with input-output relationships to the PMC [pontine micturition center]. In this connection, the frontal cerebral cortex initiates voluntary micturition with descending input to the PMC. (169)

O'Farrell (1986) argues that elimination is under the exclusive control of classical conditioning and associated reflexive mechanisms. According to her theory, elimination need not

be followed by an *external reward* to encourage the habit:

> Most owners are content if the responses are conditioned to out-of-doors stimuli and not to in-the-house stimuli, but it is possible to condition the responses to much more specific stimuli, such as the gutter or a piece of grass. The practical relevance of the fact that this learning is based on classical conditioning rather than on instrumental learning is that an external reward is not necessary. . . The owner does not need to reward successes or punish failures. (32)

Although it is true that one need not explicitly reinforce elimination habits in order to strengthen them, it does not follow that they are not undergoing instrumental reinforcement. What appears to have confused O'Farrell, causing her to confound reflexive and voluntary eliminative behavior, is a failure to recognize the role of intrinsic reinforcement in the process of acquiring house-training habits. Not all reinforcers controlling instrumental behavior are present as external rewards; in fact, many voluntary behaviors are controlled by intrinsic sources of reinforcement associated with the act itself. Elimination appears to be one of these self-reinforcing behaviors.

Punishment

O'Farrell's assessment appears to have led some behavior modifiers to the fallacious conclusion that inhibitory procedures ought not be used during house training, after all—you cannot punish a reflex. In fact, mild punishment is often very expedient for promoting house training and surely should be applied whenever a puppy or dog is caught in the act of eliminating in the house. Timing is very important when applying effective punishment. The first general rule of effective punishment is that it must occur contiguously with the act of elimination—not minutes or seconds afterward but immediately and overlapping the act itself.

Unfortunately, retroactive or noncontingent punishment is still defended by some dog trainers and is still widely practiced by dog owners (see *Noncontingent Punishment* in Volume 1, Chapter 8). Excessive and inappropriate punishment should also be avoided.

For example, the practice of rubbing a puppy's nose in its urine or feces is often carried out in conjunction with the delivery of a sharp smack to its rear end with a rolled-up newspaper. Such repulsive methods are entirely without behavioral justification, even if the puppy is caught in the act. A startling sound such as a sharp tone of voice or clap of the hands is often a sufficient deterrence.

A dog's cleanliness and responsiveness to house training represents a significant factor in its success as a domestic companion. If dogs were not able to learn to urinate and defecate outdoors on schedule, it is unlikely that they would have attained the close social proximity that they currently enjoy with people. Fortunately, the vast majority of dogs are easily and permanently house trained, often in spite of poorly organized and implemented house-training efforts. Notwithstanding the ease with which most dogs are house trained, some fail to acquire good habits in the first place or develop various behavior problems involving inappropriate elimination as they develop.

ELIMINATION BEHAVIOR

Urine Marking

Urine marking is familiar to anyone who has ever spent time around dogs. Intact male dogs are prone to show this activity, expending large amounts of energy on the investigation of attractive spots before urinating over them. Dogs exhibit various searching activities involving sniffing, licking, and sometimes gently scrapping the ground with the front paws, as though to turn up a fresher scent located below the surface. When satisfied with their olfactory inquiry, they appear duty-bound to add a splash of their own to the community *bulletin board*. Some may become rather compulsive about the habit, urinating dozens of times until the effort is reduced to dry *blanks*—a phenomenon that Bekoff (1979) interprets as a visual dominance display. As previously noted, the marking response appears to be mediated by an olfactory micturition reflex (Shafik, 1994). Dogs tend to urinate more often when off leash than when on leash, with both male and

female dogs being more likely to defecate when walked off leash (Reid et al., 1984). Interestingly, Reid and coworkers also found that purebred dogs tend to urinate more often than mixed-breed dogs.

Elimination Postures

Male and female elimination postures begin to differentiate along sexually dimorphic lines by 3 to 5 weeks of age, with some male puppies exhibiting a full leg-lift posture by 19 weeks of age (Berg, 1944). Beach (1974) found that urinary postures become sexually dimorphic by 5 to 7 weeks of age, with some male beagles using the leg-lift posture as early as week 16. The discrepancies between Berg's and Beach's observations concerning the onset of leg-lifting behavior suggest that some breed differences may exist with regard to the ontogenesis of the leg-lifting posture.

Another disagreement between Berg's earlier findings and later research is the degree of stereotypy evident in male and female elimination postures. Berg claims to have never observed a female dog elevate her leg during urination. Sprague and Anisko (1973), however describe a significantly different picture with regard to male and female elimination postures. Whereas male dogs were observed to use the elevated leg posture to eliminate almost exclusively (97% of the time), females squatted only 68% of the time, with the remaining 32% of female urinations involving some other variation, including leg lifting. The researchers identified a variety of distinct postures used by males and females to urine mark, including stand, lean, raise, elevate, flex, squat, lean-raise, flex-raise, handstand, arch, squat-raise, and arch-raise (Figure 9.1). Males tend to eliminate more frequently than females. One male dog was observed to eliminate or *pseudo-urinate* 60 to 80 times over a 3- to 4-hour period (Sprague and Anisko, 1973). Usually, females fully evacuated their bladders with one or two urinations. Another prominent difference between male and female urinary activity is its directionality. Among male dogs, urine is most often directed toward the scent of other male dogs, especially involving vertical objects, whereas female dogs tend to be less selective about the

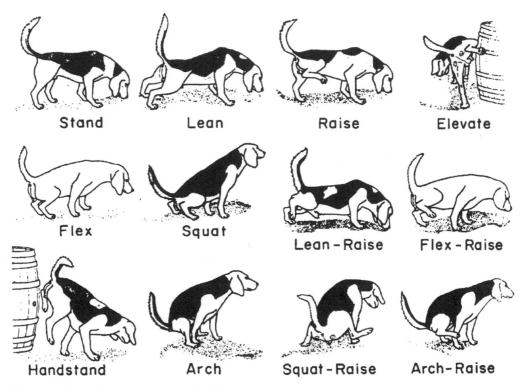

FIG. 9.1. In addition to squatting and leg lifting, dogs exhibit a variety of postures while urinating. After Sprague and Anisko (1973).

placement of urine, suggesting that urination for the female probably is restricted to a physiological function, at least during anestrus. Females were infrequently observed to sniff elimination areas before urinating. Male dogs show a definite preference toward sites frequented by females in estrus and urine-marked sites containing the scent of unfamiliar males (Dunbar and Carmichael, 1981). In addition, Dunbar and colleagues (1980) found that the stimulus value of urine to males was increased when females were injected with the estradiol and reduced when injected with testosterone.

Functions of Urine Marking

Urine marking appears to serve two primary communicative functions: (1) communication between male dogs, and (2) communication of reproductive status between males and females. These social and biological functions appear to be controlled by a hormonally modulated mechanism. Many studies have demonstrated a linkage between urine-marking behavior and the influence of endogenous hormonal activity, but this relationship is problematic. For example, Hart (1974) reported that, although castration reduced mating frequency and the duration of coital lock within 2 months after surgery, the latency and frequency of urinary marking was unaffected by castration after 5 months. Male dogs usually begin to urine mark as they reach puberty, perhaps in response to increasing concentrations of circulating testosterone (Hart, 1985). Although testosterone appears to exert an influence on urine-marking behavior, the behavior does appear to be dependent on the presence of circulating gonadal testosterone. Beach (1974) found that many dogs castrated just after birth (48 hours postpartum) or prepubertally (4 to 4½ months of age) go on to exhibit the leg-lifting posture as adults. Further, he found that castration performed on adult dogs (15 to 17 months) had no observable effect on urine-marking postures.

Despite the relative independence between urine marking and a dog's reproductive status, Hopkins and coworkers (1976) found that household urine marking was gradually or rapidly reduced as the result of castration in about 50% of the dogs surveyed. Consistent with aforementioned reports, they found that urine marking away from the home was relatively unchanged in the neutered dogs:

> Several owners in the present study indicated that urine marking in relatively novel areas (e.g., sidewalks and parks) was unchanged in their dogs, whereas urine marking in the house was eliminated. These differences in castration effects between urine marking in the home and away from the home are probably related to the fact that olfactory stimuli from the urine of other dogs (which are undoubtedly the most important stimuli for urine marking) are strongest outside the home. (1110)

One way that has been proposed to resolve some of these problematic aspects associated with the hormonal mediation of urine marking is to assume that the connection is formed at an earlier point in the animal's ontogenetic development than puberty. In fact, it is known that the fetus is exposed to a significant surge of in utero testosterone secreted just before birth or immediately afterward (Hart, 1985). These androgen secretions serve to masculinize the fetus by producing sexually dimorphic changes in the neonate's brain and various biobehavioral systems. Beach (1974) found that 50% of the females perinatally implanted with a pellet of testosterone tended to exhibit malelike elimination postures. These early hormonal influences may sensitize and promote the development of certain sensory and motor neural connections that are later activated with the onset of puberty. The aforementioned variable responses to neutering, especially the persistence of urine marking in spite of prepubertal castration, may be due, in part, to the formation of such early predispositions.

COMMON ELIMINATION PROBLEMS

House-training problems are a common reason that people seek behavioral advice and training regarding their dogs. Yeon and coworkers (1999) reported that 9% of the cases seen at the Cornell Animal Behavior Clinic between 1987 and 1996 (N = 1173) were house-soiling problems. Voith and Borchelt (1985) reported that approximately 20% of the overall cases presented for behavioral treatment involve elimination problems. Similar statistics concerning the relative incidence of elimination versus other canine behavior problems have been reported elsewhere (Landsberg, 1991), making inappropriate elimination the second most commonly presented behavior complaint after aggression. Few situations generate more frustration than those associated with unsuccessful house training, either because the training efforts somehow go wrong or because a previously housetrained dog begins to eliminate indoors. A variety of elimination problems have been described and classified according to descriptive and functional features (Table 9.1).

Household Urine-marking Problems

Urine marking in the home can be a persistent and damaging habit. Dogs presenting with household-marking problems are often highly excitable and reactive to novelty. Marking behavior is frequently directed toward packages brought into the home (e.g., groceries laid on the floor) or new furniture—the Christmas tree is a prime target for urinary marking. Other dogs may be stimulated to mark in the presence of visiting guests or by the presence of strange dogs coming into the home. Some dogs may mark after observing other dogs or passersby (e.g., the mail carrier) through a window. Occasionally, a particularly dominant dog might exhibit the obnoxious habit of marking people rather than objects. The behavior modifier should attempt to identify the various situations in which marking occurs and then alter the environment or introduce appropriate counterconditioning procedures.

Olfactory cues appear to play a significant environmental role in the maintenance of

TABLE 9.1.   Description and etiology of elimination problems

Urine marking: Exhibited most commonly by adult, intact male dogs. Urine-marking dogs usually direct small squirts of urine against vertical objects, especially absorbent couches, chairs, and curtains. Smaller toy breeds most commonly present the problem, but large dogs also exhibit the habit.

Elimination (urination and defecation) in the owner's presence: Inadequate or inappropriate house training may cause dogs to develop a habit of eliminating indoors. A common cause of such problems is excessive crate training and failure to generalize the habit to other parts of the house.

Elimination (urination and defecation) in the owner's absence: Some dogs may abstain from eliminating indoors as long as the owner is present but will eliminate when the owner is away from the home. These cases require careful evaluation, since the unwanted elimination habit may be more directly related to separation anxiety than to inadequate house training.

Refusal to eliminate outdoors: A surprising number of dogs, especially those that have been poorly trained or not trained at all, refuse to eliminate outdoors. Such dogs often hold urine and feces while outdoors or during long walks and then race to their preferred spot upon entering the house.

Excitement elimination: Some highly excitable dogs may lose bladder control during periods of increased arousal or social stimulation. Excitement urination is distinct from submissive urination, although punishment of excitement urination may lead to submissive urination. Excitable dogs may urinate during play or at other times involving intense arousal.

Submissive urination: Young dogs and some adult dogs may eliminate when the owner returns home or enters a room where the dog is located. A submissive dog may also eliminate when guests enter or reach for it. The habit seems to be particularly prominent in females and certain breeds (e.g., the cocker spaniel, golden retriever, and German shepherd).

Fear-related elimination: Some highly fearful and reactive dogs may eliminate in response to strong fearful stimulation. Intense fear is sometimes associated with anal gland evacuation and defecation. Additionally, highly nervous dogs may develop elimination problems associated with diarrhea resulting from increased peristaltic activity.

Dietary etiology: Elimination problems can be traced to dietary causes. These include overfeeding, poor-quality food, the presence of ingredients that cause an excessive intake of water (e.g., excessive salt protein), sudden changes of food, and foods containing large amounts of fat.

Physical causes: Some elimination problems result from structural pathologies of the urinary tract or disease (e.g., renal failure, diabetes insipidus, cystitis, and obstructions). The most common sign of a urinary-tract problem is frequent urination and unusual difficulty to housetrain. Functional incompetence of the urethral sphincter is commonly treated with phenylpropanolamine (Voith and Borchelt, 1996). Urinary incontinence is sometimes observed in spayed dogs. Typically, incontinent dogs leak urine while lying down or dribble it while walking. This problem is caused by an endocrine imbalance which is often treated with hormonal supplementation (e.g., diethylstilboestrol). Older dogs often exhibit a loss of eliminatory control as part of a general aging process and deterioration of central control over the function. Some ongoing research indicates promising benefits resulting from L-deprenyl. Ruehl and colleagues (1994) have reported improvement with L-deprenyl therapy in 16 of 19 dogs with geriatric incontinence.

Genetic predisposition: Some breeds (e.g., beagles, Yorkshire terriers, and bassett hounds) appear to be more difficult to house train or more prone to lose the habit than others.

marking behavior. Dogs are attracted to areas that they have urine marked in the past, perhaps remarking those areas in an effort to keep the odor fresh. It makes sense, therefore, to carefully identify and clean such areas. In addition to scrubbing the area, the owner should also obtain cleaning agents that enzy-matically break down residual deposits of urine and kill the odor-producing bacteria associated with it. Melese-d'Hospital (1996) has emphasized the importance of thorough neutralization of urine odors in the treatment of urine-marking behavior problems. Several products are currently on the market for this purpose [e.g., KOE, Nature's Miracle, X-O and X-O plus, and ANTI-ICKY-POO (a genetically engineered combination of enzyme and bacteria designed to consume urine efficiently)].

Although olfactory cues are important controlling stimuli, they are not the only operative environmental stimuli maintaining the habit. The contextual stimuli associated with the area (e.g., substrate texture, visual cues, and location) may also control eliminatory behavior to some extent. It should be remembered that urination is an intrinsically reinforcing activity; that is, the dog obtains some degree of pleasure or relief as the result of eliminating. Environmental cues occurring contiguously with elimination may gradually become discriminative stimuli regulating the emission of the behavior. Consequently, the olfactory cues contained in urine may only represent a part of an overall stimulus situation controlling urinary-marking behavior.

To counteract these environmental influences, new associations must be formed with the soiled area. This task of forming new, noneliminative associations is accomplished in a variety of ways. The simplest method is to feed and water the dog near the marked area (Voith and Borchelt, 1985). Between feedings, the owner can periodically place treats around the previously soiled area as well, so that whenever the dog approaches the location it is likely to find some food. Chew toys can be permanently anchored to the area with a short length of twine. Another useful procedure is to tie the dog off near the area for short periods lasting between 10 and 20 minutes at a time. The area can also be associated with play, massage, and general obedience training. The central purpose of these recommendations is the formation of a new set of associations connected with the area that are incompatible with elimination. As a result of such training, the previously soiled area may come to be identified as a place promising the acquisition food, toys, affection, training, or restraint. Subsequently, the urge to eliminate will be gradually overshadowed by incompatible expectations associated with the area, making the dog less likely to urinate in the area than before. When the owner is away from home, the dog should be confined so

that marking is prevented until the problem is under control.

An intact dog presenting with a persistent urine-marking problem is usually referred to a veterinary surgeon for castration. In cases unresponsive to castration and behavior modification efforts, various psychotropic drugs or hormonal therapy may be prescribed by the veterinarian. A common medical intervention involves treatment with synthetic progesterone (Hart and Hart, 1985). Unfortunately, the beneficial effects of progestin therapy often decay once the medication is discontinued. Since the chronic use of progestins may produce a variety of adverse side effects (e.g., mammary hyperplasia, tumors, and diabetes mellitus), its long-term use is not recommended for the control of refractory urine marking.

Elimination in the Owner's Absence

Some otherwise well-house-trained dogs may eliminate in the house only when their owners are away, while they are in another room, or when asleep. Separation anxiety is frequently associated with such elimination problems, especially when "accidents" only occur shortly after the owner leaves the house (McCrave, 1991; Yeon et al., 1999). Dogs whose house soiling is diagnostically linked with separation anxiety must receive appropriate behavior modification to reduce the underlying emotional tensions associated with the loss of bowel and bladder control. Some separation-anxious dogs appear to respond positively to a change of place when left alone. Elimination problems are particularly prevalent in separation-anxious dogs that are confined to an unsocialized part of the home (e.g., the garage or basement). In general, most dogs appear to find confinement in such areas (especially the basement) aversive and prefer to be confined in more socially active parts of the home. In cases where elimination might be attributable to the place of confinement, the dog should be moved to a more socially congenial area, for example, the kitchen or, perhaps, even crated in a bedroom, especially if the dog is accustomed to sleeping there at night.

Although many dogs eliminate (urinate or defecate) in the owner's absence as the result of separation anxiety, some incompletely house-trained dogs may also selectively eliminate only in the owner's absence or do so secretly to avoid punishment while the owner is at home but out of sight. Incompletely house-trained dogs are given remedial training to help improve their habits. Various other causes of elimination problems have been identified and should be considered when performing behavioral assessments of eliminatory complaints (Table 9.2). Such training usually involves a combination of increased vigilance, confinement, and more opportunities to eliminate outdoors. Dogs that are unable to avoid house-soiling behavior during the day may benefit from the assistance of a dog walker who comes in at midday and then gradually delays the visit by an hour or so each day until the dog can accommodate the longer schedule.

The first step in working through elimination problems is to determine the incidence of the unwanted behavior and other pertinent information. Of particular importance in this regard is the schedule of feeding, type of food fed, opportunities to eliminate outdoors (and outcome), and the time/place of accidents occurring in the house. Consequently, careful feeding and elimination records are necessary in order to determine the explicit character of such patterns and how they might be altered to make training efforts more successful (Figure 9.2). Keeping daily records and logging outdoor opportunities often provide unexpected information that may not be obvious through casual observation alone. Such records provide the owner with orderly feedback concerning the dog's elimination behavior and an objective means for assessing its daily progress. Remedial house training can be an extremely frustrating process, and such records objectively show patterns of improvement (or lack thereof) and help to diffuse some of the emotional tensions associated with the process.

Occasionally, in the case of multidog households, it may be difficult to ascertain which dog is responsible for urinating in the owner's absence. Separating the dogs is an expeditious way to identify the dog responsi-

ble. However, when separation is not possible or practical, another method may be used to discover the culprit (Karofsy, 1987). The determination can be made by giving the suspected dog a tablet of aspirin before a meal. Within a short period, urination will contain traces of salicylate. When a urine spot is found, it is extracted with a paper towel and ferric chloride is applied to it. If the urine contains the salicylate contaminant, it will turn a burgundy color.

Crate confinement is often recommended to facilitate good eliminatory habits. Although close confinement usually inhibits elimination in most dogs, some dogs may continue to urinate or defecate even when confined to crates. Excluding separation anxiety and health problems [see Reisner (1991)], the most common causes are related to the size of the crate or the amount of time the puppy or dog is required to spend crated between outings. Crates that are too big may not promote fastidiousness, but even if the crate is sufficiently small, some dogs may still eliminate when confined. A contributing cause for this failure is a history of excessively lengthy periods of crate confinement, which exceed the dog's ability to hold. In essence, such confinement presents an uncontrollable situation in which elimination is physiologically unavoidable, perhaps promoting a progressive state of learned helplessness with respect to eliminatory functions. Repetition of such treatment may lead a puppy to simply give up trying to hold urine or feces. Since the effort to hold is useless and progressively uncomfortable, the puppy may respond to the earliest internal signals of need and eliminate withoug trying to hold for long.

Another common difficulty involves dogs that refuse to eliminate on walks or malinger when let outside. This problem is exasperating for the owner, who may walk the dog for long periods, only to return home and discover that the dog quickly runs off to a favorite location in the house to eliminate. Such dogs appear desperate to eliminate but are unable to do so outdoors. Some dogs may have developed overly exclusive substrate or location preferences, whereas others may fail to eliminate outdoors (especially if the owner is nearby) as of the result of a history of excessive punishment,

TABLE 9.2. Common causes of elimination in the owner's absence

TABLE 9.2. Common causes of elimination in the owner's absence

Inadequate or inappropriate training

Separation distress

Elimination inhibitions (e.g., fears associated with the outdoors, weather aversions, overly exclusive substrate preferences, and fear of eliminating in the owner's presence)

Irregular scheduling of feedings and outings

Insufficient opportunities to eliminate outdoors and too much freedom to eliminate indoors

Quality or amount of food fed to the dog

Urinary-tract disease (e.g., cystitis)

HOUSE-TRAINING DAILY LOG		
WEEK	**AM**	**PM**
Monday		
Tuesday		
Wednesday		
Thursday		
Friday		
Saturday		
Sunday		

Notes

Note the time of opportunity and outcome. Also, indicate the time and place of all incidents of house soiling. (D) Defecation (U) Urination (D/U) Defecation and Urination (A) Accident

FIG. 9.2. House-training daily log.

causing them to generalize the threat of punishment across both indoor and outdoor contexts. These dogs may simply be afraid to eliminate in close proximity with the owner. Giving them more room to move about in a fenced area or exercising them on a long line may help to encourage outdoor elimination, especially if they are prompted with a gentle voice and rewarded with treats for performing. Other dogs may have simply been improperly trained in the first place. To modify these types of problems, the puppy should be taken out at times of greatest need (e.g., in the morning) for brief periods lasting about 1 to 3 minutes (adult dogs, 3 to 5 minutes). A puppy that fails to eliminate is taken back inside and crated or tethered for 10 or 15 minutes and taken outside again. This pattern is repeated until the dog performs outside, whereupon it is reassured with praise and affection. Urination and defecation in such cases can often be facilitated with brief periods of ball play or other vigorous activities that help to promote motility and disinhibition.

Submissive Urination

Submissive urination is most commonly exhibited by young dogs and appears to be more prevalent in female dogs. In most cases, dogs gradually grow out of the problem as urethral sphincter control improves; however, some highly sensitive and excitable dogs may continue to urinate submissively into adulthood, especially if the initial presentation of the problem is mismanaged. Submissive urination is evoked by a variety of social situations: (1) when the puppy or dog is reached for or (2) leaned over (in what might be perceived as a threatening gesture or posture), or (3) during episodes of excited social interaction (e.g., greetings). Submissive urination appears to represent an appeasement display and is often exhibited by a puppy or dog that has been exposed to inappropriate punishment or excessive control efforts; that is, the behavior may be expressed to allay a perceived threat posed by the presence of an overbearing owner, person, or other dog. The behavior may be maintained by negative reinforcement, since it causes the owner to withdraw as urination occurs. Even

worse, though, sometimes submissive puppies are punished for urinating, causing them to urinate even more—an action that is also frequently associated with the termination of the owner's punitive efforts. Unfortunately, in such cases, the habit of submissive urination may be strongly reinforced, thus becoming progressively more exaggerated and difficult to resolve. Some cases of submissive urination appear to be linked to punitive interaction early in a puppy's development—for example, during house-training efforts when the puppy is physically punished while eliminating. During such interaction, the puppy may make a rapid transition from functional urination to submissive urination in response to the owner's inappropriate punishment. Consequently, as the owner leans over, reaches for, or touches the puppy, it may respond by urinating.

Although submissive urination is frequently driven by appeasement motivations, it is not always and exclusively due to excessive punitive interaction between the puppy and its owner. Some puppies appear to be predisposed to exhibit this habit spontaneously as the result of excitement and urethral incompetence but usually grow out of it—provided that they are not punished for it.

Submissive urination occurs most commonly during social transitions, that is, during homecomings or while greeting guests. In some cases, the mere sight of a particular family member entering a room may elicit a copious release of urine. The most common posture displayed is an incomplete squat with small amounts of urine being expressed, but some dogs may perform a full squat or actually roll on their side (lateral recumbency) and expose their belly before eliminating. Other signs of submission may also be present (a submissive grin, licking, ears back, or a crouched-down look), but these submissive elements are not always strongly presented.

Submissive urination probably stems from the mother's practice of stimulating reflexive urination in puppies. Fox (1974) has described the relationship between reflexive urination and submissive behavior:

> When two adult dogs or wolves make social contact with each other, one invariably orients

toward the groin of the other. Groin presentation is usually manifested by the subordinate individual. As a social gesture, it is perhaps analogous to a handshake in man. The next time you see a friendly dog approaching you, notice how he wiggles his head and swings one hip around, presenting the groin. If you touch him in the groin, he will remain completely passive and may even roll over onto one side in complete submission. He may then urinate submissively. Submissive urination is the final clue to the ontogenetic history of this behavior. When wolves, coyotes, and dogs are very young, they are unable to urinate, and the mother reflexively stimulates urination by licking the genitalia. During stimulation the pups remain passive while the mother nuzzles the groin region. Later, of course, the animals are able to control urination voluntarily, but the behavior trait of remaining passive when the groin is touched persists as part of their social repertoire. (42)

In fact, many infantile behaviors involved in nursing, food getting, and elimination appear to be elaborated into mature active and passive submission displays.

Many adult submissive urination problems appear to stem from an emotional etiology. Puppies and dogs with highly excitable temperaments, which exhibit approach-avoidance conflict during greetings, appear to be most prone to exhibit the problem. The treatment of submissive urination begins by carefully identifying eliciting stimuli. Sometimes the reaction to people is specific to one sex, with some dogs urinating only in the presence of males and not females or vice versa. Some dogs have such a low threshold for submissive urination that they respond as soon as the owner or visitor enters their personal space, whereas others may urinate only when being reached for, leaned over, or touched. As just noted, in the case of young puppies (under 16 weeks of age), this is a common and normal habit that usually disappears with maturity. In older puppies and adult dogs, the habit may become more persistent and compulsive, requiring carefully structured behavior-modification efforts to resolve it fully.

Gradual exposure and counterconditioning prove extremely effective in reducing submissive urination. In the typical scenario, the owner is instructed to give the dog a treat on every approach, at first tossing the food on the floor and then gradually requiring the puppy to sit and stay a moment before delivering the reward. Besides eating, the dog can be engaged in other activities such as fetching a toy or, perhaps, taken directly outdoors. This process is facilitated by repeated exposure involving mass trials; that is, by staging repeated contact rituals involving as many as ten approach and withdrawal trials per session, the exposure-counterconditioning process is made more effective. In the beginning, the owner should avoid leaning over or reaching for the puppy or dog. As progress occurs, more obtrusive actions like reaching and leaning over the dog can be attempted, first while the puppy is eating, later while holding a sit-stay, and, finally, under progressively more natural circumstances occurring during actual greetings with family members and guests. In refractory cases of submissive urination, a pharmacological intervention might be considered. Some success has been reported using the alpha-adrenergic agonist phenylpropanolamine—for further information, see Marder (1991) or Voith and Borchelt (1996). The muscles of the urethra are adrenergic, and the drug enhances general tone and control so that, when the dog becomes overly excited or squats, it is less likely to lose control. The drug has potential side effects, such as increased excitability and restlessness. Marder (1991) reported good results using imipramine (Tofranil), a tricyclic antidepressant that also possesses alpha-adrenergic agonist properties.

DEFECATION PROBLEMS

When defecation problems present separately, the usual causes include inadequate or inappropriate house training, separation-related distress, change of diet, or disease conditions affecting the bowel (Reisner, 1991). As already noted in the case of urine-marking behavior, defecation may occur in the house in response to environmental cues that have been associated with defecation in the past. Although dogs do not appear to use feces to mark in the same manner and frequency as they mark with urine, some do show a tendency to deposit fecal material on vertical objects, suggesting that fecal marking or advertising may occur in some dogs. Few dogs show as much interest in the fecal deposits of other dogs as they exhibit toward urine-marked areas. Anal fluids are secreted into fecal materials as defecation occurs. The exact function of anal secretions is unknown, but they may contain some pheromonal information that is communicated in the feces. In wolves, alphas secrete more anal fluids during defecation than other pack members and tend to concentrate their feces to one area (Asa et al., 1985). One authority has suggested that the dog scratches after defecating in order to spread the scent of feces. This possibility is unlikely, however, since dogs rarely disturb feces with their feet while performing the scratching ritual. Wolves appear to step away from fecal deposits deliberately before scratching (see *Biological and Social Functions of Smell* in Volume 1, Chapter 4).

FLATULENCE

Flatulence is a common complaint. Dogs fed a new diet may develop flatulence, at least until the gut adapts to the change. Some breeds appear to be more prone to the problem than others. For example, brachycephalic breeds frequently have the problem, perhaps because such breeds ingest excessive amounts of air (*aerophagia*) while eating. Aerophagia appears to be a significant cause of flatulence in both dogs and people (Hubbard, 1989). Since dogs ingest more air while eating a liquid diet, changing to a dry kibble may be beneficial in such cases. Another significant cause of flatulence is bacteria fermentation in the lower gut. Undigested food undergoes bacteria fermentation in the colon—a process that increases gas production. Older dogs may be more prone to exhibit flatulence due to an age-related decrease in colonic motility (constipation) and increased fermentation time. Foods that may contribute to flatulence are those containing a high percentage of indigestible fiber (e.g., soybeans). Also, milk may cause flatulence in adult dogs bereft of lactase as the result of the putrefaction of lactose in the gut. In addition

to dietary changes, exercise is a useful way to reduce flatulence, because it increases colonic motility and stimulates more bowel movements. Finally, excessive flatulence may indicate the presence of gastrointestinal disease (e.g., malabsorption and exocrine pancreatic insufficiency) and should be brought to the attention of a veterinarian.

GRASS BURN AND URINE

A common complaint of dog owners is the presence of burned spots or dead areas of grass caused by urination. Various putative causes have been suggested, especially the belief that dogs urine is either excessively acidic or alkaline. In fact, the relative acidity or alkalinity of the dog's urine has no effect on its propensity to burn grass. Consequently, it is of little value to feed dogs substances with the intention of reducing the acidity or alkalinity of their urine output. Similarly, putting such materials as gypsum or lime on the grass probably does not help either, at least with respect to neutralizing urine and making it less hazardous to grass. According to Allard (1981), the most likely cause of grass burn is the nitrogenous content of urine. Urine burns grass just as excessive fertilizer would damage it. Since the nitrate content of urine is related to the metabolism of proteins and associated waste products, one potential way to reduce the extent of grass burn is to reduce the intake of dietary protein. In fact, many dogs ingest protein in excess of their activity and physiological needs. A high-quality, reduced-protein food may not only be an effective preventive for lawn burn (especially in the case of resistant grass varieties), but it may also be a healthier diet for inactive house dogs. Also, providing dogs with ample drinking water may produce a beneficial effect by diluting the urinary output. A simple way to prevent grass burn is to walk the dog away from the home property. The dog can learn to treat the yard and garden as extension of the home and keep it clean. If such training is impractical, then daily watering of urine-soaked areas may be helpful. Allard reported that, when urine spots were watered up to 8 hours after elimination, burning was prevented (fescue), whereas urine left undiluted for 12 hours caused a slight burn, and, after 24 hours, a lack of watering resulted in moderate burning. Some grass varieties are more resistant to urine burn than others. For example, fescue and rye grass were found to be the most resistant to urine burn, whereas Kentucky bluegrass and Fairway crested wheat grass were both very sensitive and burned, even in the presence of highly dilute urine samples.

REFERENCES

Allard AW (1981). Lawn burn and dog urine. *Canine Pract,* 8:26–34.

Allen DL (1979). *Wolves of Minong: Their Vital Role in a Wild Community.* Boston: Houghton Mifflin.

Asa C, Mech LD, and Seal US (1985). The use of urine, faeces, and anal-gland secretions in scent-marking by a captive wolf (*Canis lupus*) pack. *Anim Behav,* 33:1034–1036.

Beach FA (1974). Effects of gonadal hormones on urinary behavior in dogs. *Physiol Behav,* 12:1005–1013.

Beaver BV (1981). Grass eating by carnivores. *Vet Med Small Anim Clin,* 76:968–969.

Beerda B, Schilder MBH, Van Hooff JARAM, et al. (1999). Chronic stress in dogs subjected to social and spatial restriction: I. Behavioral responses. *Physiol Behav,* 66:233–242.

Bekoff M (1979). Scent-marking by free-ranging domestic dogs: Olfactory and visual components. *Biol Behav,* 4:123–139.

Berg IA (1944). Development of behavior: The micturition pattern in the dog. *J Exp Psychol,* 34:363–368.

Berne RM and Levy MN (1996). *Principles of Physiology,* 2nd Ed. St Louis: CV Mosby.

Bjorbaek C, Elmquist JK, Frantz JD, et al. (1998). Identification of SOCS-3 as a potential mediator of central leptin resistance. *Mol Cell,* 1:619–625.

Bradshaw J and Thorne C (1992). Feeding behaviour. In C Thorne (Ed), *The Waltham Book of Dog and Cat Behaviour.* Oxford: Butterworth-Heinemann.

Brownell KD, Greenwood MRC, Stellar E, and Shrager EE (1986). The effects of repeated cycles of weight loss and regain in rats. *Physiol Behav,* 38:459–464.

Campbell WE (1975). The stool-eating dog. *Mod Vet Pract,* Aug:574–575.

Carlson NR (1994). *Physiology of Behavior.* Boston: Allyn and Bacon.

Chaucer, G (1929). *The Canterbury Tales.* WW Skeat (Trans). New York: Modern Libray.

Cloche D (1991). Coprophagia. *Tijdschr Diergeneeskd,* 116:1257–1258.

Crowell-Davis SL and Caudle AB (1989). Coprophagy by foals: Recognition of maternal feces. *Appl Anim Behav Sci,* 24:267–272.

Crowell-Davis SL and Houpt KA (1985). Coprophagy by foals: Effect of age and possible function. *Equine Vet J,* 17:17–19.

Crowell-Davis SL, Barry K, Ballam J, and LaFlamme DP (1995). The effect of caloric restriction on the behavior of pen-housed dogs: Transition from unrestricted to restricted diet. *Appl Anim Behav Sci,* 43:27–41.

Dunbar I, Buehler M, and Beach FA (1980). Development and activational effects of sex hormones on the attractiveness of dog urine. *Physiol Behav,* 24:201–204.

Dunbar I and Carmichael M (1981). The response of male dogs to urine from other males. *Behav Neural Biol,* 31:465–470.

Durrer JL and Hannon JP (1962). Seasonal variations in caloric intake of dogs living in an Arctic environment. *Am J Physiol,* 202:375–378.

Edney ATB and Smith PM (1986). Study of obesity in dogs visiting veterinary practices in the United Kingdom. *Vet Rec,* 118:391–396.

Feldman MD (1986). Pica: Current perspectives. *Psychosomatics,* 27:519–523.

Fox MW (1962). Psychogenic polyphagia (compulsive eating) in a dog. *Vet Rec,* 74:1023–1024.

Fox MW (1963). *Canine Behavior.* Springfield: Charles C Thomas.

Fox MW (1974). *Concepts of Ethology: Animal and Human Behavior.* Minneapolis: University of Minnesota Press.

Friedman JM (2000). Obesity in the new millennium. *Nature,* 404:632–634.

Friedman JM and Halaas JL (1998). Leptin and the regulation of body weight in mammals. *Nature,* 395:763–770.

Friedman JM, Maffei M, Halaas JL, et al. (1995) Leptin helps body regulate fat, links to diet (research summary). http://www.rockefeller.edu/pubinfo/leptin-level.nr.html.

Gustavson CR, Garcia J, Hankins WG, and Rusiniak KW (1974). Coyote predation control by aversive conditioning. *Science,* 184:581–583.

Hankin L, Heichel GH, and Botsford RA (1974). Newspapers and magazines as potential sources of dietary lead for dogs. *JAVMA,* 164:490.

Hansen I, Bakken M, and Braastad BO (1997). Failure of LiCl-conditioned taste aversion to prevent dogs from attacking sheep. *Appl Anim Behav Sci,* 54:251–256.

Hart BL (1974). Gonadal androgen and sociosexual behavior of male mammals: A comparative analysis. *Psychol Bull,* 81:383–400.

Hart BL (1985). *The Behavior of Domestic Animals.* New York: Freeman.

Hart BL and Hart LA (1985). *Canine and Feline Behavioral Therapy.* Philadelphia: Lea and Febiger.

Hopkins SG, Schubert TA, and Hart BL (1976). Castration of adult male dogs: Effects on roaming, aggression, urine marking, and mounting. *JAVMA,* 168:1108–1110.

Houpt K (1982). Ingestive behavior problems of dogs and cats. *Vet Clin North Am Symp Anim Behav,* 12:683–692.

Houpt KA (1991). *Domestic Animal Behavior.* Ames: Iowa State University Press.

Hubbard B (1989). Flatulence and coprophagia. *Vet Focus,* 1:51–53.

Impellizeri JA, Tetrick MA, and Muir P (2000). Effect of weight reduction on clinical signs of lameness in dogs with hip osteoarthritis. *JAVMA,* 216:1089–1091.

James WT and Gilbert TF (1955). The effect of social facilitation on food intake of puppies fed separately and together for the first 90 days of life. *Br J Anim Behav,* 3:131–133.

Johnson JI, Goy RW, and Michels KM (1962). Physiological mechanisms and behaviour patterns. In ESE Hafez (Ed), *The Behaviour of Domestic Animals.* Baltimore: Williams and Wilkins.

Kafka F (1976). *Complete Stories,* NN Glatzer (Ed). New York: Schocken.

Karofsky PS (1987). Identifying source of urine on rugs. *JAVMA,* 191:917.

Kealy RD, Lawler DF, and Ballam JM (1997). Five-year longitudinal study on limited food consumption and development of osteoarthritis in coxofemoral joints of dogs. *JAVMA,* 210:222–225.

Kienzle E, Bergler R, and Mandernach A (1998). A comparison of the feeding behavior and the human-animal relationship in owners of normal and obese dogs. *J Nutr,* 128:2779S–2782S.

Kluver H and Bucy P (1937). "Psychic blindness" and other symptoms following bilateral temporal lobotomy in rhesus monkeys. *Am J Physiol,* 119:352–353.

Landsberg GM (1991). The distribution of canine behavior cases at three behavior referral practices. *Vet Med,* Oct:1011–1018.

Landsberg G, Hunthausen W, and Ackerman (1997). *Handbook of Behaviour Problems of the Dog and Cat.* Oxford: Butterworth Heinemann.

Levine M, Rumsey SC, Daruwala R, et al. (1999). Criteria and recommendations for vitamin C intake. *JAMA,* 281:1415–1423.

Lindell EM (1997). Diagnosis and treatment of Destructive Behavior in Dogs. *Vet Clin North Am Prog Companion Anim Behav,* 27:533–547.

Lopez BH (1978). *Of Wolves and Men.* New York: Charles Scribner's Sons.

Marder AR (1991). Psychotropic drugs and behavioral therapy. *Vet Clin North Am Adv Companion Anim Behav,* 21:329–342.

Markwell PJ, Erk W, and Parkin GD (1990). Obesity in the dog. *J Small Anim Pract,* 31:533–537.

McCrave EA (1991). Diagnostic criteria for separation anxiety in the dog. *Vet Clin North Am Adv Companion Anim Behav,* 21:247–255.

McCuistion WR (1966). The search for digestive enzymes. *Vet Med Small Anim Clin,* May:445–447.

McKeown D (1996). Eating and drinking behavior in the dog. In L Ackerman (Ed), *Dog Behavior and Training: Veterinary Advice of Owners.* Neptune City, NJ: TFH.

McKeown D, Luesher A, and Machum M (1988). Coprophagia: Food for thought. *Can Vet J,* 29:849–850.

Melese-d'Hospital P (1996). Eliminating odors in the home. In VL Voith and PL Borchelt (Eds), *Readings in Companion Animal Behavior.* Philadelphia: Veterinary Learning Systems.

Mugford RA (1977). External influences on the feeding of carnivores. In MK Kare and O Maller (Eds), *The Chemical Senses and Nutrition,* 25–50. New York: Academic.

Nickel RF and Venker-van Haggen AJ (1999). Functional anatomy and neural regulation of the lower urinary tract in female dogs: A review. *Vet Q,* 21:83–85.

Nishizawa O and Sugaya K (1994). Cat and dog: Higher center of micturition. *Neurourol Urodyn,* 13:169–179.

Norris MP and Beaver BV (1993). Application of behavior therapy techniques to the treatment of obesity in companion animals. *JAVMA,* 202:728–730.

O'Farrell V (1986). *Manual of Canine Behavior.* Cheltenham, UK: British Small Animal Veterinary Association.

Panksepp J (1998). *Affective Neuroscience: The Foundations of Human and Animal Emotions.* New York: Oxford University Press.

Rashotte ME, Smith JC, Austin T, et al. (1984). Twenty-four-hour free-feeding patterns of dogs eating dry food. *Neurosci Biobehav Rev,* 8:205–210.

Rathore AK (1984). Evaluation of lithium chloride taste aversion in penned domestic dogs. *J Wildl Manage,* 48:1424.

Reed DH and Harrington DD (1981). Experimentally induced thiamine deficiency in beagle dogs: Clinical observations. *Am J Vet Res,* 42:984–991.

Reid JB, Chantrey DF, and Davie C (1984). Eliminatory behaviour of domestic dogs in an urban environment. *Appl Anim Behav Sci,* 12:279–287.

Reisner IR (1991). The pathophysiologic basis of behavior problems. *Vet Clin North Am Adv Companion Anim Behav,* 21:207–224.

Ross S (1950). Some observations on the lair dwelling behavior of dogs. *Behaviour,* 2:144–162.

Rothwell NJ, Saville ME, and Stock MJ (1982). Effects of feeding a "cafeteria" diet on energy balance and diet-induced thermogenesis in four strains of rat. *J Nutr,* 112:1515–1524.

Ruehl WW, DePaoli A, and Bruyette DS (1994). Treatment of geriatric onset inappropriate elimination in elderly dogs [Abstract]. *J Vet Internal Med,* 8:178.

Scott JP and Fuller JL (1965). *Genetics and the Social Behavior of the Dog.* Chicago: University of Chicago Press.

Serpell J and Jagoe JA (1995). Early experience and the development of behaviour. In J Serpell (Ed), *The Domestic Dog: Its Evolution, Behaviour, and Interaction with People.* New York: Cambridge University Press.

Shafik A (1994). Olfactory micturition reflex: Experimental study in dogs. *Biol Signals,* 3:307–311.

Sibley KW (1984). Diagnosis and management of the overweight dog. *Br Vet J,* 140:124–131.

Singh NN, Ellis CR, Crews WD, and Singh YN (1994). Does diminished dopaminergic neurotransmission increase pica? *J Child Adolesc Psychopharmacol,* 4:93–99.

Soave O and Brand CD (1991). Coprophagy in animals: A review. *Cornell Vet,* 81:357–364.

Sprague RH and Anisko JJ (1973). Elimination patterns in the laboratory beagle. *Behaviour,* 47:257–267.

Turner DC (1997). Treating canine and feline behaviour problems and advising clients. *Appl Anim Behav Sci,* 52:199–204.

Unwin D (1994). Stone swallowing. *Vet Rec,* 135:511.

Voith VL (1980). Destructive behavior in the owner's absence. In BL Hart (Ed), *Canine Behavior.* Santa Barbara, CA: Veterinary Practice.

Voith VL and Borchelt PL (1985). Elimination behavior and related problems in dogs. *Compend Continuing Educ Pract Vet,* 7:537–544.

Voith VL and Borchelt PL (1996). Elimination behavior and related problems in dogs: Update. In VL Voith and PL Borchelt (Eds), *Readings in Companion Animal Behavior.* Trenton, NJ: Veterinary Learning Systems.

Wolf AV (1950). Osmometric analysis of thirst in man and dog. *Am J Physiol,* 161:75–86.

Yeon SC, Erb HN, and Houpt KA (1999). A retrospective study of canine house soiling: Diagnosis and treatment. *J Am Anim Hosp Assoc,* 35:101–106.

Zook BC, Carpenter JL, and Leeds EB (1969). Lead poisoning in dogs. *JAVMA,* 155:1329–1342.

10

Cynopraxis

Ultimately, the dog, with its ambiguous roles and cultural values, its constant presence in human experience coupled with its nearness to the feral world, is the alter ego of man himself, a reflection of both human culture and human savagery. Symbolically, the dog is the animal pivot of the human universe, lurking at the threshold between wildness and domestication and all of the valences that these two ideal poles of experience hold. There is much of man in his dogs, much of the dog in us, and behind this much of the wolf in both the dog and man.

DAVID G. WHITE, *Myths of the Dog-Man* (1991)

CYNOPRAXIC COUNSELING

Although descriptive and functional information is useful, its effective and humane implementation depends on properly focusing intervention efforts. For behavioral intervention to

work, the *whole picture* must be embraced and kept in focus throughout the assessment and training process. This method is referred to as *cynopraxis.* The ultimate goals of cynopraxic assessment and training are determined by two imperatives: improving the human-dog relationship while raising the dog's quality of life (see *Cynopraxis: Training and the Human-Dog Relationship* in Volume 1, Chapter 10). Analyzing the behavioral complaint into specific functional components (establishing operations, discriminative stimuli, elicited and emitted behavior, and controlling consequences) and the numerous molar relations existing between them is not enough. In addition, cynopraxic counselors must be sensitive to subjective and intuitive considerations associated with the human-dog bond—ultimately the focus of all training and counseling efforts. Behavioral approaches that neglect a dog's physical and psychological needs or fail to appreciate the ultimate value of the human-dog relationship are incomplete, inadequate, and inhumane. Whether adaptive or maladaptive, a dog's behavior is acquired or extinguished by way of interactive exchanges and transactions interfacing or colliding with human needs and expectations. Within the context of a shared home, these combined human-canine needs and expectations are either mutually satisfied or result in conflict, with an inevitable elevation of interactive tension (anxiety and frustration) ensuing. Excessive anxiety or frustration underlies the development of many behavior problems (see *Learning and Behavioral Disturbances* in Volume 1, Chapter 9). Interactive harmony depends on the identification of a dog's basic needs and developing acceptable and cooperative ways to satisfy them. Dog behavior problems are human-dog problems. Sensitivity in this area makes the difference between mastery and mediocrity in the practice of companion-dog training and behavioral counseling.

Attaching, Bonding, and Relating

A cultural and ethical ambivalence informs the way animals are viewed and treated in our society. Animals are slaughtered for food by some people or honored as symbols of piety and mystical transcendence by others, and at times serving both purposes at once, as in the case of animal sacrifice. Our relationship with dogs is also guided by many conflicted cultural purposes and agendas (see *Theories of Pet Keeping* in Volume 1, Chapter 10). Adding to the confusion is the lack of a consistent terminology for describing the human-dog relationship. Scott (1991) notes that the terms *attachment* and *bond*, for example, are loaded with surplus connotations and often inappropriately used to describe the same phenomenon. However, attachments and bonds are qualitatively different and distinguished on a number of levels. Unlike bonds, attachments can be equally felt toward animate objects (social) and inanimate objects (places and things). Attaching to some object or place does not require mutual exchange between individuals. A bond, however, implies the existence of mutual *ties* between individuals, based on various modes of reciprocal interaction and relating to one another (e.g., transactions and exchanges). Further, bonds are not based entirely on friendly or affiliative transactions and exchanges. In fact, bonds may be strongly influenced by the exchange of aversive transactions and subsequent reconciliations. Bonding may also be enhanced by the exchange of threat and appeasement displays.

Finally, exchanges between bonded individuals involve a strong interpretive component based on past experience, mutual expectations, and their changing motivational disposition to interact. These collective attitudes and expectations define the relationship, and the range of possible exchanges and transactions that can take place, between a dog and others with whom it is bonded and interacts.

Cynopraxis and the Human-Dog Bond

The most fundamental unit of cynopraxic analysis is the *human-dog dyad*. A central cynopraxic assumption is that behavioral and emotional problems develop within a system of relations between a family and its dog. People and dogs relate to each other through the exchange of attractive and aversive emotional transactions. These interspecies emotional transactions, the basis of human-dog communication, result in an alteration of both human and canine feeling states, experienced simultaneously inwardly (within the self or organism) and empathically (toward the other). The formation and perpetuation of the human-dog relationship places tremendous demands on a dog's adaptive resources. Under conditions in which these demands exceed a dog's ability to adjust (e.g., under the influence of unpredictable or uncontrollable transactions), the dog may revert to rigid emotional or instinctual systems with which to guide its behavior. Relational conflicts result in varying degrees of anxiety or frustration, with resultant disturbance of behavioral adaptations. Under interactive conditions in which anxiety and frustration levels surpass a dog's ability to cope, it may progressively rely on rigid emotional or species-typical defensive repertoires, thereby side stepping cognitive appraisal of the situation and responding instinctively or dysfunctionally. Consequently, the dog's behavior may become progressively maladaptive, fearful, compulsive, hyperactive, or aggressive.

These functional disturbances of the human-dog relationship take place within the context of a home. Ultimately, the functional significance of a behavior problem is determined by the extent to which it interferes with a dog's ability to form satisfying relationships with humans and other animals with whom it shares a home. Cynopraxic therapy objectifies the human-dog relationship as the functional unit of behavioral adaptation or maladaptation, set within a context of numerous contributory environmental influences (e.g., nutrition, exercise, and sensory stimulation). These environmental influences composing a dog's *home* collectively define its quality of life. Cynopraxic training aims to enhance the human-dog relationship while simultaneously improving the dog's quality of life. The cynopraxic process is an end in itself, insofar as there are no objectives beyond the attainment of human-dog harmony, mutual appreciation, and well-being.

BEHAVIOR PROBLEMS AND THE FAMILY

For purposes of the following discussion, the term *family* refers to any cooperative social group of individuals that lives together and provides for one another's physical, psychological, and emotional needs by forming bonds based on reciprocal transactions and exchanges within the context of a home. The family is not defined or limited in terms of biological relatedness but in terms of emotional and ecological relations sustained within a home. The family may be as simple as a single owner and dog dyad or include complex social relations, as, for example, found in the traditional nuclear family. Whether traditional or nontraditional, many family dynamics and activities are patterned around the dog as an emotional center of gravity.

The mélange of social roles that the dog plays in the family underscores its behavioral adaptability to domestic life. According to Levinson (1969/1997), a dog's role will depend "upon the family's structure, its emotional undercurrents, the emotional and physical strengths and weaknesses of each of its members, and the family's social climate" (122). In most families, the dog is an important object of affection, care, and entertainment—often taken for granted but nonetheless accepted as a beloved member. A dog's

presence in the family is harmonious and welcome to the extent that its behavior is well adjusted to the family's needs and expectations. With the advent of a serious behavior problem, however, intense conflicts may compete with or overshadow the more positive aspects of dog ownership. For the family, a problem dog becomes a highly *objectified* presence often precipitating a sense of disequilibrium and familial crisis. As a result, the dog moves out of the fluid background of harmony into a sharp focus of attention, becoming the object of conflict and disruption for family members.

Much of what follows has been adapted from the contextual therapy techniques developed by Ivan Boszormenyi-Nagy (Boszormenyi-Nagy et al., 1991) but remains an eclectic composite containing many influences, especially prominent is the work of Salvador Minuchin (Minuchin and Fishman, 1981) and Murray Bowen (Papero, 1990). The primary emphasis of cynopraxic training is to focus training efforts on the relationship, rather than on simply altering the dog's behavior.

The response of the family to a problem dog varies, depending on several factors. In some dysfunctional family situations, a problem dog may have a disruptive and polarizing influence, with the dog becoming a scapegoat for displaced anger. Rather than searching for legitimate causes and solutions, the dog's unwanted behavior may be used by family members to shame one another. In some cases, a serious behavior problem might actually provide some degree of stability and cooperation within an otherwise conflicted and tenuous family situation. In such cases, the problem dog may give the family a common crisis point, drawing members together in a more or less common cause. Although dysfunctional situations exist (see below), one is much more likely to encounter functional families seeking advice and training for problem dogs. Generally, such families tend to adopt a rational perspective when faced with adversity. In contrast to the arguing and scapegoating that characterize a dysfunctional family, a functional or parenting family is more apt to join together in a cooperative effort, with each acknowledging their responsibility to contribute to the ultimate solution. Rather than assigning blame, the parenting family is galvanized by a supportive sense of unity and mutual appreciation and respect for one another.

Joining the Family

Although the causes underlying a dog's adjustment problem may implicate the client or another family member, it is important to provide such information without assigning blame. Direct attributions of fault and blame are always polarizing and destructive. Most dog owners seeking help seem to expect some criticism, but framing a behavior problem in terms of fault finding is not the same as exploring potential causes or fact finding. Any potentially critical evaluations should be presented in a manner that is nonaccusatory and followed immediately by positive alternatives. First and foremost, one should avoid direct critical commentary on the family's failings with respect to the dog. Instead of shaming the family, positive resources should be highlighted through merit ascription, recognition of needed abilities, and encouragement. To achieve this end, it is vital that the trainer-counselor *joins* with the family. Minuchin and Fishman (1981) describe the process of joining the family in terms that are highly relevant to the cynopraxic counseling process:

> Joining a family is more an attitude than a technique, and it is the umbrella under which all therapeutic transactions occur. Joining is letting the family know that the therapist understands them and is working with them and for them. . .. How does a therapist join a family? Like the family members, the therapist is "more human than otherwise," in Harry Stack Sullivan's phrase. Somewhere inside, he has resonating chords that can respond to any human [or animal] frequency. In forming the therapeutic system, aspects of himself that facilitate the building of common ground with the family members will be elicited. And the therapist will deliberately activate self-segments that are congruent with the family. But he will join in a way that leaves him free to jar the family members. He will accommodate to the family, but he will also require the family to accommodate to him. (31–32)

A trainer-counselor who joins the family while blaming and shaming it (regardless of how expert and correct) for the dog's behavior problem may be reflexively held at a distance or expelled psychologically—if not physically! Direct criticism may cause the family members to withdraw into defensiveness and potentially strengthen their own scapegoating tendencies toward one another. The goal is to find and acknowledge as many constructive aspects of the family's interaction with the dog as possible and to build on that foundation. Validation of the family by acknowledging its affirmative value and contribution to the dog's good qualities is beneficial on many levels. The process draws heavily on a spirit of family cooperation and provides an opportunity for members to sacrifice and compromise to attain some greater good for the sake of the group and the dog. It is a process of building on the dog's good behavior rather than a fruitless labor of accusation and penance. Nonjudgmental and fair counselors are better able to establish a working rapport with families and gain their willing and happy collaboration. Furthermore, family members will more likely extend their trust and disclose vital information necessary for an accurate evaluation. By emphasizing the positive aspects of the family dog, an opportunity to strengthen the family's commitment and loyalty to the dog may be garnered, perhaps helping to restore a healthy bond and attachment rather than risking further marginalization of the dog.

In some cases involving severe behavior problems, the relationship between the family and dog may be seriously jeopardized by anxiety, frustration, anger, and resentment. In such cases, it is particularly important to review all of the dog's merits and strong points in order to forge a constructive perspective on the problem situation. For some clients, it may be necessary to underscore the dog's strong points repeatedly and to stress the successes that they have achieved in rearing and training it. Emphasizing what makes the dog special and complimenting these strengths can be very useful. Also, it is of value to acknowledge the client's entitlement to feel angry and resentful but at the same time pointing out to them that rumination on such feelings is unproductive and may interfere with the dog's progress.

The cynopraxic trainer-counselor's role is first and foremost one of model and leadership. The counselor should exemplify in a direct and personal way how to behave constructively toward the dog, while stressing fairness by not becoming overly partial toward the dog or the family. Although many technical issues are involved in rehabilitating a problem dog, the overall manner or attitude of the counselor is often more influential than any specific recommendation. The trainer models the spirit of the thing in attitude and interaction with both the family and the dog. Essentially, the *work* of trainer-counselors is to resolve *conflict* in the family-dog relationship and restore interactive harmony through training and counseling. From the cynopraxic point of view, the ultimate goal of intervention is not training a dog to sit on command or to stop some unwanted habit but rather to mediate interspecies understanding, behavioral compromise, and interactive harmony— a process that may or may not involve obedience training or behavior-modification efforts.

Fairness and Empathic Appreciation

A central variable informing interactive harmony is a relational ethics based on fairness and empathic appreciation. Boszormenyi-Nagy and colleagues (1991) emphasized the role of fairness in the process of counseling the family: "The balance of fairness among people [and animals] is the most profound and inclusive 'cluster' of relationship phenomena. This is the context to which the term 'contextual therapy' applies" (204). To be effective mediators, cynopraxic trainer-counselors must embody, above all, the virtue of fairness. But, in addition to fairness, trainer-counselors should also express clear and frank opinions, display a friendly attitude toward family members, express and show fondness toward the dog, and impress both family and dog with a clarity of purpose. These are key elements of successful cynopraxic counseling.

Cynopraxic counseling and training aim to guide the client and dog into a more satisfying relationship through enhanced affection, cooperation, and trust. This process often

emphasizes the need to establish appropriate boundaries and realistic expectations. These boundaries are established and tempered by empathy, mutual understanding, and leadership. A counselor's role as a mediator often entails helping the client to establish appropriate boundaries and to set limits for the dog. Such structuring of interaction results in the dog developing attentional abilities, impulse control, and better organized and effective goal-directed behavior, while it helps the client to form a clearer set of expectations about the dog's behavior and to feel more in control of things. Although training is objectified in terms of controlled behavior and the formation of definite boundaries and limits, the real focus of training is a higher synthesis and resolution, eventually freeing both human and dog to behave spontaneously and freely with each other. The picture is one of mutual harmony, affection, unity, tranquility, and profound respect—what Fox (1979) has called transpersonal relatedness or an appreciation of the dog without contingency or reference to something else beyond the dog. Transpersonal appreciation involves a direct apprehension of the thing itself or what the poet Rilke has called *inseeing* (see Volume 1, Chapter 10: *Mysticism and the Dog*). Framed as such, the adjustment problem, rather than representing a threat to the family's equilibrium, becomes an opportunity for enhanced cooperation and growth for both the family and the dog.

Multidirected Partiality

As mediators, cynopraxic trainer-counselors should show equal concern for family members and the dog. Such so-called *multidirected partiality* (borrowing Nagy's terminology) embodies the all-important ethical principle of fairness. Effective cynopraxic intervention requires that the trainer-counselor acknowledge the client's expectations without losing sight of the dog's needs and limitations. For example, a client's feelings of anger, betrayal, and distrust are valid emotions to have after being bitten by a beloved dog. But an equally valid set of circumstances may have been responsible for the dog's decision to attack, including past learning experiences, adverse or inadequate socialization, or abusive behavior by the owner toward the dog in the past. The bite incident was not simply a factual event but a socially and psychologically significant transaction between the owner and dog. To assess the situation properly, the counselor must evaluate the incident both as a factual or behavioral event as well as stress its meaning as a transaction between close social affiliates. This process is facilitated by adopting an attitude of fairness toward both the client and the dog, thereby justly acknowledging their respective contributions to the transaction and assigning mutual responsibility for the consequences stemming from it. This attitude of fairness is not intended to justify the dog's behavior or the client's emotional reaction but to recognize that they exist and require *contextualization* (that is, need to be placed into a perspective based on fairness to both parties). The goal of contextualization is to organize the transaction into a more formal and objective problem picture, rendering it more receptive to intervention and change—not engaging in unproductive judgments, criticisms, and behavioral cul-de-sacs.

Coupled with the mediational importance of exercising fairness is analyzing the problem in terms of bidirectional causality. The purpose of counseling is not to assign blame but to develop a program of positive change in the direction of interactive harmony. *Bidirectional causality* means that both the client and the dog are assigned a fair degree of responsibility for the behavior problem. Neither the client nor the dog is blamed for the development of conflict, but both are held accountable for contributing to its resolution; that is, both the client and the dog must change in order to overcome the problem and to attain a more satisfying relationship. As such, the behavioral complaint is interpreted as a symptom and manifestation of an underlying interspecies conflict and failure to achieve interactive harmony, that is, a satisfying relationship.

PSYCHOLOGICAL FACTORS

The majority of dog owners view the dog as an integral extension of the family unit (Levinson, 1969/1997), exerting many subtle and pronounced influences on the family system. These various effects are bidirectional, with the family also exerting powerful influences on the dog's behavior. In addition to accepting the dog as a family member, most people appear to believe that dogs have minds and the ability to think—a perception that has direct bearing on their beliefs regarding how dogs should be treated (Davis and Cheeke, 1998). With the attribution of awareness, thoughts, and feelings, people are more likely to treat dogs humanely and to appreciate their experience empathically. These various attitudes and perceptions about dogs exert a significant influence on the human-dog relationship.

Influence of Owner Attitudes and Attachment

Precisely identifying, describing, and measuring the influence of owner attitudes on dog behavior has been of interest to researchers. For example, Serpell (1996) has reported suggestive evidence indicating that the owner's degree of attachment for a dog has a direct bearing on how satisfied or dissatisfied the person will be with the dog's behavior. A family feeling a strong attachment and affection for a dog tends to be more accepting and tolerant of its behavior. The power of attachment can be quite extraordinary in regards to how behavior is judged. Voith (1984), for instance, recounts an interview with a woman whose baby had been tragically killed by her dog. Surprisingly, she spoke lovingly of the dog and attributed "accidental" causes to the child's death, refusing to blame the dog and hold it accountable for its actions. The grieving woman greatly lamented the loss of the dog and had great difficulty reconciling her affectionate feelings toward the dog with the fact that it had, after all, killed her baby.

Owner Mental States and Behavior Problems

Although the supporting evidence is sparse and contradictory, owner and family attitudes and mental health appear to exercise a significant influence on a dog's behavior. How this occurs remains subject to considerable debate and controversy. Certainly, the manner in which the owner applies behavior-controlling events (e.g., rewards and punishments) will directly affect a dog's behavior through learning and training. Owners, as the result of mental illness or other causes (e.g., alcoholism), who are unable to interact with a dog in a consistent manner, would naturally exert a disorganizing influence on its behavior. Further, just as attachment levels appear to affect an owner's perception of a dog's behavior, his or her attitude and mental state may also have a direct bearing on the dog's emotional state. Speck (1965), a psychiatrist, reported observing a direct relationship between severe mental illness and a contagion effect on animals living in the same household. In one case report, he described how the agoraphobic symptoms of a mother, father, and schizophrenic daughter were mirrored in a dog and cat that also refused to leave the house. In another report, Speck (1964) noted that, when performing in-home psychiatric counseling with families in which dogs or other companion animals were present, the animals were apt to reflect the family's general attitude toward him. He claims to have learned to predict a friendly, angry, or indifferent session by the way that he was greeted by resident cats and dogs. Further, he reports making a "repeated observation" (152) that in disturbed families the dog may become ill as a result and, if harmony is not restored, may actually die.

These sorts of presumably strong social influences exerted by an owner or family on a dog have not been widely confirmed by practitioners working with problem dogs. Although most counselors and trainers would agree that an owner's attitude or mental state should exert some influence, what the influence might be has not been fully worked out. Some evidence has appeared in the literature in support of such effects, however. For example, O'Farrell (1995) notes that owners suffering from mental disturbances tend to project undesirable qualities and traits onto their dogs more frequently than do owners without such mental problems. Neurotic individuals also tend to report more problematic behavior in their companion dogs. In a relevant study, O'Farrell (1997) was not able to detect a causal relationship between the owners' anxiety levels and the

etiology or maintenance of common phobias in dogs (e.g., fear of thunder)—a contagion previously believed to exert a powerful influence on the development of fears (Beaver, 1982). Although not a causal factor, owner anxiety levels do appear to affect how troubling or disturbing the dog's fearful behavior is for the owner. Finally, Dodman and colleagues (1996) performed a small study (N = 10) to assess, among other things, the effects of owner personality traits on the expression and treatment of dominance-related aggression. They did not detect any significant personality-type differences between owners of dominant-aggressive dogs and a control group composed of 10 owners of nonaggressive dogs. The researchers did find, however, that *thinking-type* owners were more likely than *feeling-type* owners to achieve 50% or better improvement in their dogs as the result of implementing a nonconfrontational treatment program.

Triangular Relations

Nearly all families regard their dogs as full members (Cain, 1983; Voith et al., 1992), with some dogs enjoying a privileged status and receiving extraordinary care and affection, whereas others are marginalized and pushed outside of the family's inner circle. Feelings of attachment for the dog often widely differ between family members, with disagreements about the significance or acceptability of the dog's behavior being fairly common. The quality of attachment between family members and the dog may also undergo degradation or disturbance as the result of a behavior problem. Another common source of disturbance involves various patterns of triangulation. Triangles and triangular relations develop in situations where a third party is incorporated into a dyad relationship to deflect intense emotional states (e.g., anxiety and anger) and to secure stability (Papero, 1990). The family dog may be triangulated as an alternative object for feelings of affection, anxiety, or anger arising between family members. As a consequence of such triangular relations, Schurr-Stawasz (1997) suggests that the dog may be variously viewed by family members as a "peacemaker, tension-breaker, or scapegoat" (354). She describes an interesting triangle involving a dog that became aggressive whenever a teenage boy was yelled at by his mother. Interestingly, however, the dog refrained from barking when the boy initiated the yelling. The boy interpreted the dog's selective aggressive behavior as evidence of its having taken sides with him against the mother.

Triangulated relations may simultaneously enhance attachment and affection levels toward the dog by some family members while reducing these measures of affiliation felt by other members of the family for the dog. In the aforementioned case, the boy might feel closer to the dog when arguing with his mother, while she may feel increasingly irritable and angry at the dog at such times. Fogle (1983) describes an interesting triangle involving a husband, wife, and pet parakeet. Upon returning home from work, the husband would habitually say hello to the parakeet before acknowledging his wife. As a result, the wife gradually developed a "death wish" for the bird:

> Their relationship and attitude to the bird was as clear an indication as any that the marriage was going through a rocky stage (which, incidentally, they were acute enough to observe, strong enough to accept, and willing enough to overcome). The parakeet was a focus for their problems and for a time even made the situation worse. (146)

Given the general effects of attachment levels on a family's perception of the dog's behavior, the disruptive implications of adverse triangles should be apparent and addressed as part of the counseling process. As the result of these and various other considerations, it is of utmost importance that behavioral interventions include the family as a group whenever possible. This is particularly important in the case of interventions involving serious behavior problems, where numerous lifestyle changes and commitments of time might be required of family members. This process can be highly disruptive and frustrating for everyone closely involved with the dog. Consequently, for effective intervention to occur, trainer-counselors must appreciate the influence of family dynamics on a dog's behavior and be sensitive to a family's needs.

ATTRIBUTIONAL STYLES

A potentially valuable approach for understanding the influence of owner attitudes on dog behavior and adjustment problems is provided by analyzing the various ways or *styles* with which the owner interprets his or her influence over significant events [see Davison and Neale (1994)]. As discussed in Volume 1 (see Chapter 9: *Locus of control and Self-efficacy*), attitudes and biases exert a significant influence on learning and personal efficacy beliefs. Believing that control over events is within one's personal ability (*internal* locus) produces significantly different expectancies regarding one's efforts. For example, if one believed that the significant causes of some event were located outside of one's reach and influence (*external* locus), one probably would quickly lose hope and despair of influencing those particular events through personal effort. Attributional styles are not only influenced by locus of control tendencies but are also affected by general attributional characteristics associated with the identified causes, especially their relative generality (*global-specific* continuum) and persistence (*stable-unstable* continuum). Negative global and stable attributions in conjunction with a history of failure in coping with a dog's behavior may cause its owner to experience a high degree of anxiety and helplessness, thereby disrupting his or her ability to address the problem in a constructive or solution-oriented manner.

The extent and duration of a client's frustration or sense of *helplessness* appear to be strongly correlated with the character of internal and external attributions expressed by the client. For example, owners expressing the belief that they lack the necessary emotional qualities (*internal global* attributions) or physical abilities (*internal stable* attributions) needed to control their dog effectively may be expected to harbor a long-term sense of helplessness with regard to their ability to resolve a behavior problem that requires the *internal* attributes that they believe they lack. In addition to promoting a sense of helplessness, negative global or stable internal attributions may also adversely affect an owner's self-esteem, especially if the lacking quality or ability is perceived as a personal shortcoming. On the other hand, owners who express (or hear) global and stable external attributions, such as biological predispositions (external global attributions) or lasting behavioral deficits resulting from adverse epigenetic events (external stable attributions), may come to believe that their dog's behavior is not likely to change in response to personal efforts, since it is influenced by external causes beyond their control.

To be maximally effective, trainer-counselors must, first of all, help owners to identify faulty or destructive internal or external attributions that block effective intervention. Secondly, counselors should provide owners with more constructive ways with which to interpret and understand the dog's behavior, such as isolating and describing objective causes that can then be addressed through appropriate training and behavior modification. This is especially pertinent in cases involving global and stable internal attributions that compromise an owner's self-esteem.

Enabling and Facilitating

Negative or pessimistic attributional styles appear to express themselves in a variety of dysfunctional ways. Paradoxically, for example, unwanted behavior is often inadvertently perpetuated by owners. Such owners can be divided into two types: *enablers* and *facilitators*. Enablers are distinguished from facilitators by the degree of awareness the enablers possess regarding their contribution to the problem situation. Facilitators are usually much more consciously aware of their active role in the development and perpetuation of the dog's unwanted behavior than are enablers. Further, facilitators are more willing to view the dog's behavior problem in terms of externally objective and controllable factors. Enablers, on the other hand, are often unconscious or unaware of the active role they play in the maintenance of the dog's problem.

Enabling owners are among the most difficult to counsel. They are usually congenial, ostensibly open-minded, and sensitive, but they are often very inhibited with regard to discipline and often lack healthy assertive skills—characteristics that may reflect compromised self-esteem. In matters of professional careers, however, they are frequently very competent in controlling the people with whom they interact in supervisory capacities. I recall a psychologist who worked on a daily basis with violent offenders with great effectiveness as a prison psychotherapist, but who was entirely victimized by her Lhasa apso. It is very difficult to make enabling owners fully aware of their *actual* contribution or to explain how their behavior is impacting on the dog's behavior. They are typically defensive and inclined to place the locus of the dog's problem on the level of some personal shortcoming or failing, underscoring the role of personal self-esteem in such cases. Unfortunately, such internalization may serve to place the problem outside of objective control and change. The distinctive marks of enablers are denial, victimization, and helplessness.

Denial

Denial plays a very important role in such cases; in fact, denial is a distinctive feature of enablers. Habitual denial gives a dog's problem autonomy, placing it outside the reach of rational control. Instead of approaching the problem systematically, an unhealthy atmosphere of shame, resentment, anger, defeat, and hopelessness may begin to hang gloomily over the relationship. These emotions effectively disable an owner and preclude effective action. Denial takes many forms from simply refusing to recognize the existence of the problem to articulating complex pseudoexplanations and rationalizations to account for the dog's behavior. When the misbehavior happens to occur in public, the owner's positive self-image may be threatened or damaged, causing him or her to engage in various "excusing tactics" aimed at making amends for the dog's behavior while at the same time striving to restore their good public image (Sanders, 1999). When discussing their dog's behavior, such clients tend to disclose large amounts of irrelevant information, including detailed explanations, prefaces, justifying accounts, mitigating interpretations, spurious anthropomorphic causes, and tangential external attributes based on physical ailments or maturity issues. The entire interview may be seeped in a normative language, serving to justify the dog's behavior and making excuses for it, rather than attempting to identify and assess functional causes objectively. Under the influence of denial, the problem is further cultivated and simultaneously pushed out of the reach of effective intervention.

Sabotage

Cynopraxic counselors are not only faced with the very delicate job of objectifying a dog's behavior but also with overcoming a client's active and, more often than not, passive resistance and sense of helplessness. This resistance is not always conscious. In fact, most clients appear very frustrated with themselves for not being able to come to grips with their dog's behavior. Besides lacking the necessary assertive skills needed for effective training and the draining influence of passive resistance, training efforts are often sabotaged. Sabotage takes place on two levels. The dog's behavior problem may serve some dysfunctional purpose within the overall family system; for example, the dog may be triangulated within a family suffering general conflict and disturbance. In some unfortunate situations, the dog may represent the most stable and unifying point of interaction in the family. Occasionally, mental illness or alcoholism exists, and the dog's behavior problems are used by family members as a vehicle to act out or as a weapon directed against each other. Under such conditions, the dog is very likely to fall victim to abuse stemming from unpredictable and alternating mood swings involving affectionate and violent displays.

More often than not, sabotage is the result of enabling and denial. As already noted, enablers are not always aware of their behavior and how it can affect a dog. This is an outcome of the sometimes fanciful and unrealistic picture that clients can paint of dogs. Such owners may maintain and protect this mental escape by behaving in a manner consistent with its underlying presumptions. This state of affairs generally involves substantial emotional and psychological armoring against criticism—armor as amorphous and fluid as shifting sands, yet as hard and impenetrable as stone. In some cases where serious problems develop, instead of giving up the fantasy and emotional satisfaction derived from the myth, such owners simply give up the dog. This situation is reminiscent of Lorenz's (1955) observations with regard to many dog owners whose insensitivity and selfishness are grossly apparent:

> If I question a man who has just been boasting of the prowess and other wonderful properties of one of his dogs, I always ask him whether he has still got the animal. The answer, then, is all too often. . . "No, I had to get rid of him—I moved to another town—or into a smaller house—I got another job and it was awkward for me to keep a dog." (148)

Besides pervasive helplessness, one of the most striking features of enmeshed owners is a pronounced selfishness that weaves itself through the fabric of their relationship with the dog. Selfishness stands out like Pinocchio's nose on a facade of childlike devotion and love toward the dog. It is very interesting to note how much enabling owners complain of the sacrifices they make for their ungrateful canine companions.

Whenever it occurs, denial reflexively results in sabotage. If owners believe that the dog's elimination problem is calculated to make them feel upset or to keep them from going out or to prevent them from inviting a friend to visit, they are not likely to put sufficient effort into proper house-training measures to correct the problem, since they do not really believe that the dog has a house-training problem based on those sorts of causes. If they believe that the dog is compelled by a history of previous abuse to act out aggressively toward guests, they are unlikely to carry out the necessary corrective measures to modify the unwanted behavior. The failure of many training efforts is a direct result of denial and sabotage.

Futurizing

Finally, most people have a strong tendency to procrastinate—to put things off that make them feel uncomfortable. Some people, though, engage in an *unconscious* form of putting-off behavior that operates in combination with denial and sabotage. This form of denial is referred to as *futurizing*. A common form of futurizing occurs when puppy owners put off training, hoping that the dog will grow out of its misbehavior without their support and guidance. More problematic forms of futurizing occur when owners delay seeking help for a behavior problem and instead allow it to develop into a more unmanageable form, ostensibly believing that it will magically disappear. Futurizing as a form of denial is strongly influenced by collateral anxiety or a fear of failure associated with the process of coming to grips with the problem. Sometimes the issues surrounding the problem may simply be too painful for clients to face, and consequently seeking help is indefinitely put off.

PSYCHODYNAMIC FACTORS

The vast majority of clients with problem dogs possess constructive attitudes toward their dog's behavior problem. Occasionally, however, clients will have special needs that require additional understanding and patience. This is a complicated area of counseling that is highly speculative and influenced by psychodynamic concepts that are controversial among behaviorist practitioners. In those relatively rare cases where a dog behavior problem occurs in conjunction with a human psychiatric disorder or substance-abuse problem, counselors are strongly advised to consult with appropriate professionals familiar with such matters.

Dogs are sometimes conceptualized by owners as idealized children or *transitional objects*. Unfortunately, necessary boundaries and reasonable expectations are often suspended when dogs are thought of in such ways. As a result, an owner may lose sight of the dog as a dog, concealed as it is under a projected mask composed of an awkward and ill-balanced concatenation of fantasy and reality. This process of projective idealization incorporates dogs as transitional objects, similar in psychological function to stuffed bears for children. A child treats a stuffed animal as though it were an animated object with feelings and cognitions but realizing all the while that the toy is neither alive nor sentient. In many ways, dogs are sometimes treated as such toys, with the very different and problematic difference that they are both very much alive and sentient:

> That dogs serve as "transitional objects," in a fashion similar to teddy bears, security blankets, and any one of a number of the soft talismen that youngsters carry around to provide comfort when they have been disappointed or are feeling lonely, has been observed by some psychologists and psychiatrists. They do not reconcile that, however, with their equal certainty that dogs represent surrogate children. Although they do not say so, perhaps what they mean is that babying encompasses being babied in that people are giving what they want to get, or that in the minds of infants they and their mother are felt to be one. But there is an important difference between teddy bears and dogs. Dogs are not inanimate but living creatures with whom we have distinctive relationships as much shaped by their species characteristics and individual makeup as by ours. The teddy bear's responses are as we imagine them to be, but Rover's are really those of a dog. (Perin, 1981:81–82)

The result is that many psychological defenses like projection, transference, and splitting may be actively incorporated into the human-dog relationship, which may consequently become progressively fantastical and dysfunctional (Heiman, 1956). The resulting sense of closeness and affiliation may be intensely satisfying for owners, but fraught with many dangers for their dogs. Ensuing magical thought patterns may blur or entirely overshadow an owner's ability to assess and evaluate their dog's behavior objectively (see *Psychoanalysis and the Human-Dog Bond* in Volume 1, Chapter 10).

Such owners may appeal to strange anthropomorphic explanations and justifications for their dog's shortcomings. When problems arise, which they frequently do, the owners often resort to enabling denial and sabotage. They are also inclined to describe their dog's misbehavior in terms of self-centered concerns, especially the emotional pain it causes them. When a dog's behavior falls short of expectations (which are usually very idealized and unrealistic), such owners may feel personally affronted, deeply let down, often lamenting their attachment and love for the unappreciative dog, and, finally, express painful feelings of victimization and helplessness—the ultimate risks of dysfunctional emotional and psychological exploitation of dogs as attachment objects [see Rynearson (1978)].

SOCIAL PLACEBOS

Some authorities have speculated that a significant factor contributing to the effectiveness of holistic therapy procedures (e.g., homeopathy, acupuncture, and therapeutic massage) results from a special placebo effect or *effect of person* on receptive patients (Rosenthal, 1981). Such therapies share a number of characteristic features. Typically, holistic treatments are rather time intensive, requiring sustained doctor-patient interaction. During treatment sessions, patients are subjected to repeated positive suggestions about the effectiveness of treatment, frequent verbal and nonverbal expressions of care and interest, gentle and reassuring touch during examination, and positive predictions about recovery. The result of such positive interaction and prognostication is an *interpersonal expectancy effect* (IEE) or social placebo. Placebo effects appear to exert a significant impact on the efficacy of medications used to control dog behavior problems (White et al., 1999), perhaps as the result of owner perceptions of the dog's problem, as a result of changes in the interaction between the owner and the dog or both. Some recent research suggests that placebo effects may represent as much as 75% of the beneficial effects of many common antidepressants used to control human depression (Enserink, 1999). Unfortunately, most of the putative benefits of psychotropic drugs used to control dog behavior problems have been obtained as the result of clinical impressions and unblinded studies. Recently, efforts have been made to correct this shortcoming with the appearance of appropriately controlled and blinded studies to assess the *real* effects of these various medications objectively.

Rosenthal (1981) notes that opinions and nonverbally expressed attitudes (self-fulfilling prophecies) have a profound negative or positive effect on health, learning, and therapy.

For instance, patients told by an optimistic physician that they are going to recover from a disease as the result of taking some particular medication seem to do better than those told not to expect very much from the medicine. The tendency for such self-fulfilling prophecies to occur have been scientifically evaluated under a variety of controlled conditions. Placebo effects strongly influence experimental results in cases where the study design does not control against experimenter bias. For example, researchers biased by false information about their subjects tend to confirm the expectations in their data, leading to the necessity and use of experimental safeguards like double-blind procedures. Other influences of IEE have also been identified. Teachers misled to believe that certain students possess gifted learning abilities (even though they do not) unconsciously conspire to make the child's scholastic achievement measure up appropriately to those expectations. IEEs are mediated by many interpersonal devices, including indirect ones like tone of voice and body language. For example, children who have been falsely assigned special abilities are often given more opportunities for success and receive more affectionate support for their successes—they are treated as special people and begin to respond as such.

Skillful cynopraxic counselors utilize social placebos and engender positive expectancies in the client-family toward the problem dog. Emphasizing the dog's strong points, placing focus on positive resources, and forming an optimistic perspective on the behavior problem can exercise a very powerful and beneficial influence over the outcome of behavioral training. At the very least, establishing a positive relationship with the client and family will make it more likely that they will accept instructions and carry out training recommendations. On the other hand, a trainer who fails to *join* (borrowing Minuchin's term) the family, or is actively rejected by it as the result of negative interaction or unwelcome criticism, will not likely engender confidence or willing cooperation. Placing the training process on a positive, optimistic level, while applying effective behavioral strategies and maintaining an objective assessment of progress, is an art that cynopraxic counselors must master to be effective.

THE CYNOPRAXIC TRAINER'S ATTITUDE

In addition to embracing scientific knowledge, cynopraxic trainer-counselors acknowledge the value of play, esthetic appreciation, emotional empathy, compassion, and ethical constraint. The cynopraxic trainer's attitude is distinguished by four overlapping characteristics and qualities that mediate connectedness, facilitate the bonding process, and support behavioral healing: composure, sincerity of purpose, presence, and playfulness. *Attitude* refers to a trainer-counselor's mental, emotional, and physical orientation toward the client-owner and the dog. Skilled and effective trainers appear elegant and efficient, cheerful, and gentle, even when setting the most definitive boundaries and limits on a dog's behavior. A cynopraxic trainer's movements are coordinated to *connect* optimally with a dog's behavior in a spirit of harmonious cooperation. Mental and physical composure and consistency make such connectedness possible. Composed trainers show a keen awareness and sensitivity to detail and the ability to focus attention in such a way that training activities possess a quiet presence and precision, without evidence of stifling hesitation, indecision, or doubt. Composure of the *mind and heart* is facilitated by formal and disciplined training activities and humane education in the arts and philosophy. Perhaps the most distinguishing quality of a cynopraxic trainer's character is spontaneity—the cumulative outcome of self-discipline and acquired skills, combined with a beginner's spirit of humility, wonder, and love for dogs.

Sincerity of purpose is closely related and dependent on composure and is the hallmark of a good trainer. *Sincerity* refers to a state of transparent honesty and an ability to express precisely and immediately what is appropriate and fair in response to a dog's behavior. All training interaction with the dog is carried out in a manner that is ever consistent with what the trainer believes necessary to actualize the dog's potential. Josephine Rine (1936) nicely described the value of sincerity of purpose in dog training:

> Look right at the dog as you talk to him, and endeavor to make your tone of voice carry out your meaning no less than your words. The dog is very sensitive to his master's facial expression so be consistent and look pleased or severe as the occasion demands and the spoken words imply. In other words, be sincere with your dog if you would have him retain his confidence in you. Don't expect too much, but on the other hand, don't demand one thing and accept another. (199)

Through sincerity, a direct and reflexive connection is established between what a trainer believes to be in a dog's best interest and what the trainer does. As a result, the trainer becomes a source of consistent, predictable, and controllable interaction, providing a vital foundation for the nurturance of affection, communication, and trust.

Presence is a necessary corollary of composure and sincerity, insofar as a trainer is able to maintain a constructive working relation and *connection* with a dog over time. Dogs live in the moment and, if trainers wish to live and work in close harmony with dogs, they must learn to relate to dogs in terms of a moment-to-moment connection. On a most fundamental level, orientating and concentrating on the present moment is a necessary stance for observing a dog's behavior and properly timing the delivery of training events. All training activities take place in the present tense, and a vital connection between a human and a dog is formed by collecting and focusing on the present. People and dogs connect and bond in the moment, with every simple joy and transformation taking place within the opening and closing of a perpetual threshold between the past and the future. Within the moment, a shared "now" is revealed around which we choose to stay together, cooperate, and live. A dog's experience is in the present moment, with the past and future having little significance, except insofar as they possess meaning for the present.

This present-tense orientation is most effectively organized and mediated through cynopraxic training and play. Training gradually attunes human and dog awareness to the same moment of shared exchange and cooperation or interactive harmony. Remaining true to the moment is most harmoniously achieved through the agency of play. The German philosopher Friedrich Schiller (1795/1981) observes that play is an essential aspect of our humanity, boldly stating that "Man plays only when he is in a full sense of the word a man, and *he is only wholly a Man when he is playing*" (80). According to Schiller, an artist's ability to make art and our ability to appreciate it as a thing of *beauty* are fully dependent on our play impulse. Similarly, the ability to train dogs is an art that depends on a trainer's ability to play and a dog's ability to play in turn. Where there is no play, there is no relationship or meaning. Play opens the portals of affection and trust between humans and dogs. *Humane* dog training is playing with a purpose, or as Heine Hediger (1955/1968) correctly surmised: "Good training is disciplined play" (139). Cynopraxic trainers embody a playful spirit and value above all else the dog's gift of play.

References

Beaver BV (1982). Learning—part one: Classical conditioning. *Vet Med*, 77:1348–1349.

Boszormenyi-Nagy I, Grunebaum J, and Ulrich D (1991). Contextual therapy. In AS Gurman and DS Kniskern (Eds), *Handbook of Family Therapy*, Vol 2. New York: Brunner/Masel.

Cain AC (1983). A study of pets in the family system. In AH Katcher and AM Beck (Eds), *New Perspectives on Our Lives with Companion Animals*. Philadelphia, PA: Univ of Pennsylvania Press.

Davis SL and Cheeke PR (1998). Do domestic animals have minds and the ability to think? A provisional sample of opinions on the question. *J Anim Sci*, 76:2072–2079.

Davison GC and Neale JM (1994). *Abnormal Psychology*, 6th Ed. New York: John Wiley and Sons.

Dodman NH, Moon R, and Zelin M (1996). Influence of owner personality type on expression and treatment outcome of dominance aggression in dogs. *JAVMA*, 209:1107–1109.

Enserink M (1999). Can the placebo be the cure? *Science*, 284:238–240.

Fogle B (1983). *Pets and Their People*. New York: Viking Penguin.

Fox MW (1979). The values and uses of pets. In RD Allen and WH Westbrook, *The Handbook of Animal Welfare: Biomedical, Psychological, and Ecological Aspects of Pet Problems and Control*. New York: Garland STPM.

Hediger H (1955/1968). *The Psychology and Behavior of Animals in Zoos and Circuses*, G Sircom (Trans). New York: Dover (reprint).

Heiman, M (1956). The relationship between man and dog. *Psychoanal Q*, 25:568–585.

Levinson BM (1969/1997). *Pet-oriented Child Psychotherapy*. Springfield: Charles C Thomas (reprint).

Lorenz K (1955). *Man Meets Dog*. Boston: Houghton Mifflin.

Minuchin S and Fishman HC (1981). *Family Therapy Techniques*. Cambridge: Harvard University Press.

O'Farrell V (1995). The effect of owner attitudes on behaviour. In J Serpell (Ed), *The Domestic Dog*. New York: Cambridge University Press.

O'Farrell V (1997). Owner attitudes and dog behaviour problems. *Appl Anim Behav Sci*, 52:205–213.

Papero DV (1990). *Bowen Family System Theory*. Boston: Allyn and Bacon.

Perin C (1981). Dogs as symbols in human development. In B Fogle (Ed), *Interrelations Between People and Pets*. Springfield, IL: Charles C Thomas.

Rine JZ (1936). *The Dog Owner's Manual*. New York: Tudor.

Rynearson EK (1978). Humans and pets and attachment. *Br J Psychiatry*, 133:550–555.

Rosenthal R (1981). Pavlov's mice, Pfungst's horse, and Pygmalion's PONS: Some models for the study of interpersonal expectancy effects. *Ann NY Acad Sci*, 364:182–198.

Sanders CR (1999). *Understanding Dogs: Living and Working with Canine Companions*. Philadelphia: Temple University Press.

Schurr-Stawasz RL (1997). Social work and behavioral problems: Implications for treating the problem pet and for the family. In K Overall (Ed), *Clinical Behavioral Medicine for Small Animals*. St Louis: CV Mosby.

Scott JP (1991). The phenomenon of attachment in human—nonhuman relationships. In H Davis and D Balfour (Eds), *The Inevitable Bond: Examining Scientist-Animal Interactions*. Cambridge: Cambridge University Press.

Serpell JA (1996). Evidence for an association between pet behaviour and owner attachment levels. *Appl Anim Behav Sci*, 47:49–60.

Schiller F (1795/1981). *On the Aesthetic Education of Man*, R Snell (Trans). New York: Frederick Ungar (reprint).

Speck RV (1964). Mental health problems involving the family, the pet, and the veterinarian. *JAVMA*, 145:150–154.

Speck RV (1965). The transfer of illness phenomenon in schizophrenic families. In AS Friedmann et al. (Eds), *Psychotherapy for the Whole Family.* New York: Springer-Verlag.

Voith VL (1984). Human/animal relationships. In RS Anderson (Ed), *Nutrition and Behavior in Dogs and Cats.* New York: Pergamon.

Voith VL, Wright JC, Danneman PJ, et al. (1992). Is there a relationship between canine behavior problems and spoiling activities, anthropomorphism, and obedience training? *Appl Anim Behav Sci,* 34:263–272.

White DG (1991). *Myths of the Dog_Man.* Chicago, Il: Univ of Chicago Press.

White MM, Neilson JC, Hart BL, and Cliff KD (1999). Effects of clomipramine hydrochloride on dominance-related aggression in dogs. *JAVMA,* 215:1288–129.

Index